T0139857

Current Cancer Research

Series Editor
Wafik El-Deiry

More information about this series at http://www.springer.com/series/7892

Kumaravel Somasundaram
Editor

Advances in Biology and Treatment of Glioblastoma

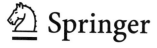 Springer

Editor
Kumaravel Somasundaram
Department of Microbiology and Cell Biology
Indian Institute of Science
Bangalore, Karnataka, India

ISSN 2199-2584   ISSN 2199-2592   (electronic)
Current Cancer Research
ISBN 978-3-319-86010-7   ISBN 978-3-319-56820-1   (eBook)
DOI 10.1007/978-3-319-56820-1

This Springer imprint is published by Springer Nature
The registered company is Springer International Publishing AG
The registered company address is: Gewerbestrasse 11, 6330 Cham, Switzerland

Preface

Glioblastoma (GBM), the grade IV astrocytoma, is the most common primary adult brain tumor. GBM is a fast-growing and most aggressive type of central nervous system tumor. During the last decade, the scientific community is witnessing an incredible amount of progress and successes in cancer research including glioblastoma biology, especially with the use of various high-throughput studies like genomics, proteomics, and next-generation sequencing. While the median survival remains low despite advances on many aspects, we have begun to understand this extremely complex disease primarily because of the coordinated effort between surgeons, pathologists, oncologists, radiologists, and basic research scientists. Many gene signatures for risk stratification and targets for developing novel therapies have been identified. In this aspect, the efforts made by The Cancer Genome Atlas, USA, are highly commendable.

Unlike many books, this book focuses on various aspects of GBM biology. The chapters are written by experts in their field. The first chapter by Dr. Sujit S Prabhu and his colleagues describes the various adjuncts in the maximal safe surgical resection, which remains the first and most important line of therapy for GBM. The second chapter by Dr. Vani Santosh and her colleagues discusses the recent WHO 2016 classification of glioblastoma, which uses molecular parameters in addition to histology. The next five chapters deal with advances and current understanding of GBM therapy. Drs. Puduvalli and Giglio and their colleagues provide an outline of current treatments and also examine many promising newer approaches. While Chap. 4 by Dr. Kesari and his colleagues describes the current status of various targeted therapies in GBM, Dr. Sanchez-Gomez and her colleagues discuss in their chapter the biology and the current understanding of EGFR targeting in GBM. Dr. Arvind Rao and his colleagues in Chap. 6 present a case for a complementing role for radiogenomics and histomics (computational histology) in the practice of GBM personalized medicine. In the next two chapters contributed from my laboratory, there is an emphasis on the importance of next-generation sequencing in GBM-targeted therapy and a summary of the origin and biology glioma stem-like cells as tumor-initiating cells, their role in therapy resistance and potential methods to target them. Dr. M. Squatrito and his colleagues examine in Chapter 9 the various animal models to study the biology of GBM and for developing therapeutic strategies. In the last chapter (Chap. 10), Dr. Chitra Sarkar and her colleagues give an update about the pediatric glioma, which is the most common solid tumors of childhood.

The chapters presented in this book deals with various aspects of GBM including biology, pathology, improved surgical resection, and various therapeutic options. There is also an emphasis on the translational potential of various aspects. I sincerely hope this book would be highly useful to clinicians, basic scientists, and more to the students. Further, I would like to acknowledge the contribution of all authors and the team of production group of Springer.

Kumaravel Somasundaram
Department of Microbiology and Cell Biology
Indian Institute of Science
Bangalore, Karnataka, India

Contents

1 **Maximal Safe Resection in Glioblastoma: Use of Adjuncts** 1
Daria Krivosheya, Marcos Vinicius Calfatt Maldaun,
and Sujit S. Prabhu

2 **Molecular Pathology of Glioblastoma- An Update** 19
Vani Santosh, Palavalasa Sravya, and Arimappamagan Arivazhagan

3 **Current Therapies and Future Directions
in Treatment of Glioblastoma** 57
Joshua L. Wang, Luke Mugge, Pierre Giglio, and Vinay K. Puduvalli

4 **Recent Advances for Targeted Therapies in Glioblastoma** 91
Michael Youssef, Jacob Mandel, Sajeel Chowdhary,
and Santosh Kesari

5 **Targeting EGFR in Glioblastoma: Molecular Biology
and Current Understanding** 117
Juan Manuel Sepúlveda, Cristina Zahonero, and Pilar Sánchez Gómez

6 **Radiogenomics and Histomics in Glioblastoma: The Promise
of Linking Image-Derived Phenotype with Genomic Information** 143
Michael Lehrer, Reid T. Powell, Souptik Barua, Donnie Kim,
Shivali Narang, and Arvind Rao

7 **Next-Generation Sequencing in Glioblastoma Personalized
Therapy** 161
Jagriti Pal, Vikas Patil, and Kumaravel Somasundaram

8 **Glioma Stem-Like Cells in Tumor Growth
and Therapy Resistance of Glioblastoma** 191
Abhirami Visvanathan and Kumaravel Somasundaram

**9   Animal Models in Glioblastoma: Use in Biology
     and Developing Therapeutic Strategies** 219
     A.J. Schuhmacher and M. Squatrito

10 Pediatric High Grade Glioma 241
     Chitra Sarkar, Suvendu Purkait, Pankaj Pathak, and Prerana Jha

Index 267

Author Biography

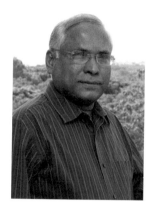 Kumaravel Somasundaram is a Professor in the Department of Microbiology and Cell Biology, Indian Institute of Science, Bangalore, India. He obtained his Veterinary Medicine degree (1985) from Madras Veterinary College, Masters in Biotechnology (1987) and Ph.D. in Bacterial Genetics (1993) from Madurai Kamaraj University, Madurai, India. Subsequently, he did his post-doctoral training at Northwestern University and University of Pennsylvania in Cancer Biology before moving to Indian Institute of Science (1999) as a faculty. The major focus of his laboratory is genetics of glioma, the most common primary adult brain tumor.

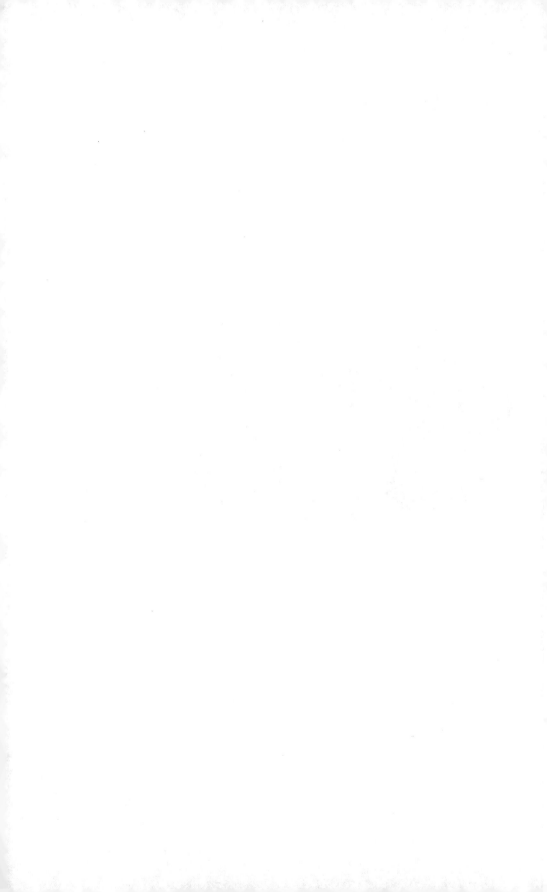

Chapter 1
Maximal Safe Resection in Glioblastoma: Use of Adjuncts

Daria Krivosheya, Marcos Vinicius Calfatt Maldaun, and Sujit S. Prabhu

Abstract Glioblastoma is a malignant primary brain neoplasm for which no cure exists due to the infiltrative nature of this tumor. Maximal safe resection is the cornerstone of treatment that was shown to prolong patient survival. To maximize the extent of resection while preserving neurological status of the patient, good understanding of tumor anatomy as well as location of eloquent cortex and subcortical pathways is required. A number of imaging and functional adjuncts can be used before and during surgery to achieve both of these goals. This chapter first describes the use of preoperative adjuncts such as functional MRI, diffusion tensor imaging, navigated transcranial magnetic stimulation, and others, to help with preoperative planning. Furthermore, it describes the principles of intraoperative techniques such as fluorescence, direct electrical stimulation, and awake craniotomy, that allow intraoperative visualization of tumor tissue as well as mapping of functional cortical and subcortical areas to safely accomplish maximal tumor resection.

Keywords Glioma • Glioblastoma • Cortical mapping • Awake craniotomy • Functional MRI • Diffusion tensor imaging • Navigated transcranial magnetic stimulation

1.1 Introduction

Gliomas are primary brain neoplasms that diffusely infiltrate the brain thus making it difficult to achieve a cure. Over the last decades much effort was extended to determine factors that affect patient survival. While radiation and chemotherapy are important to control tumor progression, surgery has the advantage of reducing tumor burden acutely. Furthermore, the extent of tumor resection has been shown to

D. Krivosheya • S.S. Prabhu, MD (✉)
Department of Neurosurgery, University of Texas M. D. Anderson Cancer Center, 1400 Holcombe Boulevard, Room FC7.2000, Unit 442, 77030 Houston, TX, USA
e-mail: sprabhu@mdanderson.org

M.V.C. Maldaun
Division of Neurosurgery of Sírio Libanês Hospital, São Paulo, Brazil

K. Somasundaram (ed.), *Advances in Biology and Treatment of Glioblastoma*,
Current Cancer Research, DOI 10.1007/978-3-319-56820-1_1

correlate with overall and progression-free survival in low- and high-grade gliomas (Coburger et al. 2016; Jakola et al. 2012; Lacroix et al. 2001; Li et al. 2016; Sanai et al. 2011). On the other hand, a new postoperative neurological deficit negatively affects patient outcome resulting in decreased overall survival (McGirt et al. 2009). Therefore, glioma surgery is a balance of maximal resection and avoidance of post-operative neurological deficits, i.e. maximal safe resection. To achieve this goal, there are a number of imaging modalities available that help delineate tumor anatomy and functional areas of brain in the vicinity of the tumor, but all modalities have limitations that will be discussed in this chapter. This information is used for a careful preoperative planning added to advanced intraoperative technique to ensure maximal amount of tumor is resected in a safe manner. This chapter focuses on first describing some of the preoperative adjuncts that can be used to better characterize the tumor and the surrounding functional cortical areas. The second part of this chapter focuses on describing techniques that can be used intraoperatively to maximize safe tumor resection.

1.2 Preoperative Investigations

1.2.1 Magnetic Resonance Imaging

Understanding tumor anatomy and its relationship to the surrounding eloquent cortical areas and subcortical structures is paramount for surgical planning. High quality magnetic resonance study is the foundation of understating of tumor anatomy in relation to the surrounding structures. In the case of high-grade gliomas, contrast enhanced T1-weighted images are key in delineating the extent of the aggressive part of the tumor. These tumors derive their blood supply from abnormally formed blood vessels that lack blood-brain barrier and therefore allow for contrast to accumulate in tumor tissue. The surrounding high FLAIR (fluid-attenuated inversion recovery) signal is thought to represent surrounding vasogenic edema (Fouke et al. 2015). Recent evidence shows, however, that it may also represent the infiltrative part of the tumor, as resecting greater than 50% of the surrounding T2 signal was shown to improve patient survival (Li et al. 2016). Revised Assessment in Neuro-Oncology (RANO) criteria also use T1- and T2-weighted MRI images to describe the extent of high-grade glioma resection, as well as response to treatment. In contrast, lower grade neoplasms have an intact blood brain barrier and do not enhance. The area of infiltration is thought to correlate with high T2 or FLAIR signal. Several additional advanced MRI sequences can also be used to further characterize tumor ultrastructure and help identify hypermetabolic areas that could be targeted for biopsy or to be included in resection. These include MR spectroscopy, diffusion and perfusion weighted imaging techniques (DWI and PWI), the latter including dynamic contrast enhanced and susceptibility contrast MRI studies (DCE and DSC). PWI seems to be a great complementary MRI sequence that allows better understanding of biological behavior to differentiate between early progression, pseudoprogression, and radionecrosis during follow up.

1.2.2 Functional MRI

Functional MRI (fMRI) has evolved as an important adjunct to preoperative surgical planning for the purpose of mapping of eloquent language and motor areas. This technique relies on the phenomenon of neurovascular coupling that detects increased blood flow, i.e. oxygenation of areas of cortical activation as the patient is performing a particular task. It is widely used for mapping of motor cortex. Functional motor cortical areas identified with fMRI were shown to correlate well with the results of intraoperative direct cortical stimulation with greater than 95% specificity and sensitivity (Kuchcinski et al. 2015; Trinh et al. 2014). This is in contrast to mapping of language areas using fMRI that has sensitivities in the 37–91% range and specificity of 64–83% when compared to results of intraoperative language mapping (Kuchcinski et al. 2015; Trinh et al. 2014). Therefore, fMRI is mainly used for determination of hemispheric language dominance (Krings et al. 2002; Trinh et al. 2014). It can also be used to highlight areas involved in different aspects of speech production and comprehension (Fig. 1.1). Awake intraoperative mapping of language areas using direct electrical stimulation, however, remains the gold standard for language mapping due to poor spatial resolution of fMRI data.

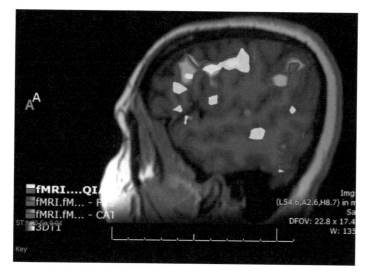

Fig. 1.1 Functional MRI mapping of speech areas. Sagittal view showing overlap of speech paradigms used for identifying speech areas using fMRI. The sentence completion task highlights both Wernicke's and Broca's areas of speech (*fMRI functional MRI, CAT category naming task, FAS word generation task, QIAC sentence completion task*)

The widespread use of fMRI in preoperative planning is in part due to minimal additional equipment requirements for performing the test, as no additional equipment is required. There are a couple of caveats with the use of fMRI in preoperative planning, however. First, fMRI highlights all areas that are activated during task execution, and cannot make the conclusion as of whether a particular cortical area is required for that function. Furthermore, vascularity of the tumor may result in neurovascular uncoupling phenomenon at the margins of the lesion, resulting in false-negative mapping (Schreiber et al. 2000; Ulmer et al. 2004). Similarly perilesional edema may induce false-positive activations. Overall, despite poor spatial resolution of this study modality, it is accurate at localizing motor areas, thus helping with preoperative planning and minimizing the time of intraoperative mapping.

1.2.3 Magnetoencephalography

As cortical areas are activated during task performance, magnetic fields are produced as a result of neuronal electrical activity. Magnetoencephalography (MEG) is a technique that allows detection of these magnetic fields and thus identification of the corresponding areas of cortical activation through cross-referencing with patient's MRI. Currently, MEG can be used for mapping of motor, visual, and auditory cortex, and assist in determination of language dominance. The studies correlating MEG results with intraoperative DCS mapping show high degree of correlation (Korvenoja et al. 2006; Tarapore et al. 2012). The cost of equipment however is the main limitation of widespread use of this technology. Cortical magnetic fields are of very low values requiring a magnetically shielded room for testing and superconductors for detection, which contributes to high equipment cost resulting in its limited availability.

1.2.4 Navigated Transcranial Magnetic Stimulation

The main limitation of fMRI and MEG functional mapping is that they provide a "passive" or observational information with respect to cortical eloquent areas. In addition, patient cooperation is required for accurate functional mapping. While direct cortical stimulation (DCS) remains the gold standard for motor and language mapping, transcranial magnetic stimulation is the equivalent of DCS that can be performed outside of the operating room environment (Fig. 1.2a). The TMS coil sets up magnetic field that induces electrical current in the underlying cortical area during transcranial stimulation. Motor evoked potentials (MEPs) are recorded during the stimulation and do not require patient cooperation for testing. During language testing, a short train of impulses is administered to create a temporary cortical lesion with subsequent speech arrest that is observed while the patient is naming objects. Recent advances in imaging technology allow cross-referencing the TMS

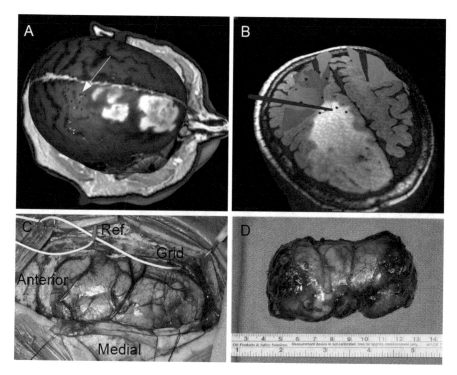

Fig. 1.2 Using nTMS, DAT, and intraoperative DES for mapping of eloquent motor cortical areas in a patient with a left-frontal high-grade glioma. (**a**) Navigated-TMS demonstrating areas of leg (*red pegs*) and arm (*yellow pegs*) activation just posterior to enhancing areas of left frontal glioma. (**b**) Deformable anatomic template image displaying projection of descending corticospinal tracts that corresponded with good accuracy to the results of pre-operative nTMS and intraoperative direct electrical stimulation. (**c**) Intraoperative photograph displaying the stimulation set-up for continuous monitoring of leg function. A 4 × 2 silicone grid is placed over the motor area and sutured to dura for the duration of the case. Continuous monitoring of motor evoked potentials during tumor resections provides information on corticospinal pathway integrity. (**d**) En-bloc resection of left frontal glioblastoma specimen (*nTMS navigated transcranial magnetic stimulation, DAT deformable anatomic template, DES direct electrical stimulation, Ref reference electrode*)

coil with the patient head position and the preoperative high-definition MRI image thus resulting in high precision stimulation. The accuracy of this testing is about 5 mm, and correlation with DCS has demonstrated good agreement between the two modalities in the range of 5–15 mm (Krieg et al. 2012a; Lefaucheur and Picht 2016; Tarapore et al. 2012).

Preoperative use of nTMS has been shown to improve outcomes and result in longer patient progression-free survival (Frey et al. 2014; Krieg et al. 2014; Picht et al. 2016). More importantly, the results of the nTMS stimulation can affect surgical strategy, help estimate the extent of possible resection, and can be used to improve accuracy of subcortical fiber mapping using diffusion tensor imaging (DTI) protocols when used as a seed point for subcortical fiber tracking to improve their accuracy. In addition, nTMS can be used to follow patients longitudinally to identify

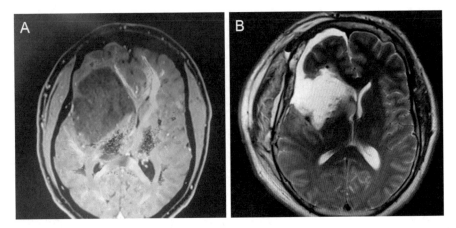

Fig. 1.3 Right frontal low-grade glioma resection. (**a**) Preoperative DTI tractography results are overlaid onto T1-weighted MRI image with contrast enhancement. This demonstrated that descending corticospinal tracts (*in blue and pink*) are displaced rather than infiltrated by tumor. (**b**) A complete surgical resection was achieved preserving patient's neurological function (*DTI diffusion tensor imaging*)

patients in whom eloquent cortical areas may have shifted due to previous surgery or tumor involvement as a result of neural plasticity. The ease of use and relatively low cost of the equipment contribute to the increased use of this modality in preoperative planning across different neurosurgical centers.

1.2.5   Diffusion Tensor Imaging

Mapping of eloquent cortical areas is important to avoid damage to these areas and subsequent neurological deficit. However, it is important to appreciate that damaging the subcortical fibers can result in a neurological deficit that may be just as severe, and therefore they must be respected. Diffusion tensor imaging (DTI) is the only preoperative imaging modality that allows mapping the location of subcortical white matter tracts. DTI is a T2-weighted MRI protocol that detects the preferential movement of water, or anisotropy, along the axon (Fig. 1.3). Further computational processing involving fiber tracking algorithms estimate the location of the corticospinal tracts and major tracts involved in language processing, such as arcuate fasciculus and inferior orbitofrontal fasciculus. The reliability of DTI fiber tracking mapping of corticospinal tracts were confirmed using intraoperative direct electrical stimulation (DES) (Zhu 2012). Using DTI for surgical planning and during the resection reduces the risk of postoperative deficit and results in longer median patient survival (Wu et al. 2007).

It is important to be aware of some of the limitations of using DTI for operative planning. Diffusion tensor imaging is a computational process and subject to variability depending on the protocol used. Proximity of neoplastic tissue and peritumoral edema can further affect the results of DTI rendering (Pujol et al. 2015). In infiltrative tumors it is at times difficult to establish the real relationship between lesion and tracts that could be infiltrated, dislocated or disrupted. While technological advances and use of higher definition technologies such as diffusion spectrum imaging (DSI) (Wedeen et al. 2005) and high angular resolution diffusion imaging (HARDI) (Tuch et al. 2002) may overcome some of these limitations at the expense of longer imaging acquisition times and more complex computational processing, intraoperative DES of subcortical white matter tracts should be used intraoperatively to delineate their exact location relative to tumor.

1.2.6   Deformable Anatomic Templates

Many functional areas in the brain are consistently localized to specific gyri and thus could be determined by identifying specific anatomical landmarks. Deformable anatomic templates (DAT) are derived from a set of generic MRI images that contain information on cortical functional areas and subcortical tracts. These templates can be co-registered with the patient's MRI scan and subjected to three-dimensional deformation to closely match patient's MRI. The resulting scan provides functional and structural information about the areas surrounding the tumor and can be used in preoperative planning as well as intraoperatively (Figs. 1.2b and 1.4a) (Kumar et al. 2013; Vabulas et al. 2014). Special training and software are required, however, to apply this technology as imaging matching is performed manually. Furthermore, at present application of this technology is only limited to cases of small tumors with minimal or no mass effect that minimally disrupt their environment (Vabulas et al. 2014).

1.3   Intraoperative Adjuncts

1.3.1   Intraoperative Image Guidance Techniques

Several techniques using imaging technology are available to help guide surgical tumor resection in the operating room. Frameless stereotaxy was introduced over two decades ago and since has become the tool that is used almost ubiquitously in neurosurgery, and especially during neurooncology cases. Most commercially available systems use infrared technology where a combined infrared emitter and camera detects the location of reflective markers in space. Typical setup includes a reference array that is rigidly connected to the patient's head fixation device. Image guidance probe containing several reflector markers is then registered relative to the frame and tracked in real time. The patient's head position is registered relative to the frame, and a high definition CT or MRI set is used to create a 3D rendering of intracranial contents. The imaging probe subsequently can be used to identify

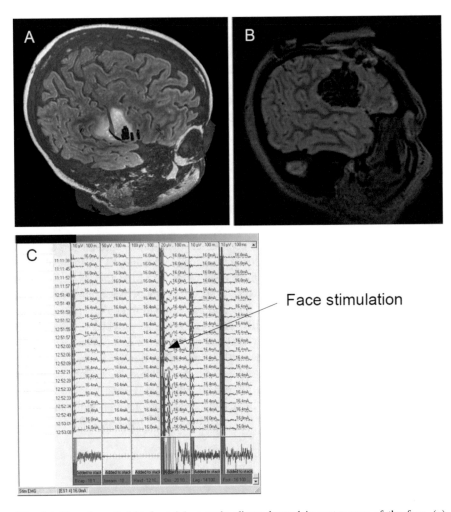

Fig. 1.4 Resection of right frontal low-grade glioma located in motor area of the face. (**a**) Deformable anatomic template MRI of patient with low-grade glioma (high signal on FLAIR MRI) in face motor area. The red areas in the tumor are areas of fMRI activation for tongue. The lower end of the DAT overlay (*blue, gray and purple areas*) overlying the face and tongue area are within the tumor (**b**) Intraoperative MRI FLAIR sequence demonstrating complete resection of the lesion. (**c**) Intraoperative direct cortical stimulation record demonstrating motor evoked potentials in face when stimulating in the area of the tumor (*fMRI functional* MRI, *DAT deformable anatomic templates*)

different structures intracranially. Frameless stereotaxy helps optimize the location of surgical incision and location of craniotomy to ensure adequate exposure for surgical resection (Willems et al. 2006).

Frameless stereotaxy is excellent at identifying surface landmarks and structures that are fixed in space. In brain surgery however, with the CSF egress and with tumor removal, so call "brain shift" occurs which makes intraoperative navigation inaccurate. To obtain updated information on the progress of resection one can use intraoperative ultrasound. Over 80% of low-grade gliomas and nearly all high-grade gliomas can easily be identified with ultrasound (Gerganov et al. 2011; Le Roux et al. 1992; Serra et al. 2012). Given that the information obtained with ultrasound is more difficult to interpret and is user dependent, additional features such as cross-referencing ultrasound probe with preoperative MRI scan, or using contrast enhanced ultrasound techniques can facilitate ultrasound image interpretation (Prada et al. 2014; Rivaz et al. 2015).

To obtain updated high resolution imaging, intraoperative MRI can be used. It is excellent at identifying remaining tumor, provides an updated high-resolution scan that can be used for subsequent neuronavigation (Fig. 1.4b). The use of iMRI results in improved extent of resection and was correlated with improved neurological outcomes of tumor patients with longer survival times (Knauth et al. 1999; Senft et al. 2011). The main disadvantage of using iMRI is very high cost of the scanner and increased length of procedure due to additional scans acquisition.

1.3.2   5-Aminolevulinic Acid

Another way of visualizing the remaining tumor intraoperatively is to use fluorescent compounds, such as 5-aminolevulinic acid (5-ALA). It is administered in liquid form that the patient drinks aporoximately one hour before the procedure. The compound is absorbed, traverses the blood brain barrier, and further metabolized inside the tumor cells to photoporphyrin IX. The latter is a fluorescent compound that can be detected as pink fluorescence under blue light when using intraoperative microscope. At present, it can only be used effectively for high-grade glioma resection, as it does not accumulate in low-grade gliomas in concentration that would sufficient for its detection under the microscope. The use of 5-ALA has been shown to increase the rate of complete tumor resection by 50% (Nabavi et al. 2009; Stummer et al. 2006). During the resection however the surgeon needs to be aware that tissue overhangs or blood may obscure some areas of fluorescence. Furthermore, this technique provides purely anatomical information, and while eloquent areas may be involved and thus fluoresce, clinical judgment is required of whether those areas should be excised or spared. Overall, the ease of use of this technology has a potential to be of benefit in glioma surgery to improve the rates of complete resection.

1.3.3   Functional Cortical and Subcortical Mapping

For gliomas involving eloquent brain, functional mapping of cortical and subcortical eloquent areas help guide surgical resection and minimize the risk of new postoperative deficit. Direct electrical stimulation (DES) remains the gold standard for functional characterization of eloquent areas (Fig. 1.4c). The original protocol was established by Penfield and Bodrey in 1930s and involves current delivery to cortical area in question to obtain a behavioral response thus allowing to map cortical eloquent regions (Penfield and Boldrey 1937). At present, DES is used to identify eloquent motor and language areas. There are several fundamental differences in how motor and language areas are mapped out. The fundamentals of stimulation are common to both mapping protocols. Therefore, we will first review the basic principles of electrical stimulation followed by focused discussion of details relating to motor and language mapping.

1.3.4   Principles of Direct Electrical Stimulation

There are three components to electrical stimulation: the generator, the electrical stimulus administered during mapping, and the probe that is used to deliver the stimulus. There are two types of generators that are available commercially: constant current and constant voltage. Constant current generators are used more commonly since it is more reliable as it is not affected by tissue impedance resulting in known amount of charge delivered during stimulation.

Stimulation parameters describe the characteristics of the electrical pulse delivered to the brain tissue. There are two different protocols that are commonly used: low- and high-frequency stimulation. In the low-frequency protocol used for cortical mapping, the typical peak current used in brain stimulation ranges from 2.5 to 8 mA with biphasic or monophasic pulses lasting 0.2 to 0.5 ms delivered at frequency of 50 or 60 Hz. The high-frequency stimulation is used for monopolar cortical and subcortical stimulation and uses train of five pulses of 0.5 ms duration that are delivered at a frequency of 250–500 Hz (Taniguchi et al. 1993). Peak current values used with this technique ranges from 1 to 20 mA. It is essential to have a good understanding of the technique and the timing of stimulation during surgery between the surgeon and the neurophysiologist. This interaction plays an important role to obtain a better functional result.

Two types of probes that are used for DES of the brain are monopolar and bipolar. In stimulation with a monopolar probe the current is delivered in a radial pattern thus allowing for stimulation of larger area of tissue and of targets that are further away from the probe. Anodal current is used in cortical stimulation, whereas cathodal current is employed in stimulation of subcortical white matter. The bipolar probe consists of two electrodes one representing an anode and the other cathode separated by 5 mm. This configuration allows for focused current delivery between the electrodes, and thus higher precision mapping. This is, however, at the expense of higher likelihood of triggering seizures due to higher density of charge delivered over a smaller cortical area.

1.3.5   Motor Mapping and Monitoring

1.3.5.1   Somatosensory Evoked Potentials

There are a number of surface landmarks that help predict the location of the primary motor cortex. Presence of the tumor however frequently distorts normal brain anatomy making it difficult to reliably identify precentral gyrus. In such situations, measuring somatosensory evoked potentials (SSEPs) may help reliably identify the central sulcus thus helping with the intraoperative identification of primary motor cortical area. A platinum grid electrode consisting of 4×2 or 8×1 electrodes is placed over the cortical area. The contralateral median nerve is then stimulated and SSEPs are recorded. There is a change in dipole direction as the current traverses over central sulcus resulting in "phase reversal" observed in SSEP recordings. This technique of motor cortex identification is successful in over 90% of patients, and can be conducted in patients under general anesthesia (Cedzich et al. 1996). The cortical grid can subsequently be used to monitor for after-discharges or seizure activity during cortical stimulation, or used throughout the case for continuous motor evoked potentials (cMEPs) monitoring of integrity of motor system (Fig. 1.2c).

1.3.5.2   Motor Evoked Potentials

Following identification of the primary motor cortex, motor function can be monitored thought the case by recording MEPs. To accomplish this, a small strip of electrodes is placed on the motor cortex and one of the contacts is used as a monopolar probe to stimulate motor pathways at regular intervals while the tumor is resected (Fig. 1.2c). The latency to MEPs and the amplitude is recorded, while the amount of current that is administered to the cortex remaining the same. Potential compromise to the motor system is assumed if the amplitude is reduced by 50% or there is a need to go up on the current more than 4 mA to obtain MEP response with the same amplitude (Kombos et al. 2001; Krieg et al. 2012b; Seidel et al. 2013). In situations were these parameters improve later in the surgery, the patient will most likely sustain a reversible neurological deficit. If the MEP are permanently decreased or lost during surgery, the patient will wake up with a new neurological deficit (Krieg et al. 2012b). In 4.5% of cases, the patient will have a new neurological deficit postoperatively despite unchanged cMEP recordings during surgery (Krieg et al. 2012b). In those cases, the new deficit was secondary to postoperative stroke, hematoma, resection of supplementary motor area, or lack of monitoring in that limb. Therefore, cMEPs are quite accurate in predicting postoperative neurological outcome from surgical resection alone with a false negative rate that is essentially zero. It has a limited role, however, in alerting the surgeon to the impending neurological damage as only 60% of intraoperative changes are reversible (Seidel et al. 2013).

1.3.5.3   Cortical Stimulation

For higher precision mapping of motor cortex, direct cortical stimulation may be employed. Low-frequency parameters using bipolar stimulation are typically used in an awake patient, whereas high-frequency train of five technique using monopolar probe can be used in a patient that is awake or asleep, and requires smaller amount of charge delivered to neural tissue thus minimizing the risk for seizures. Cortical stimulation of motor cortex allows differentiation of primary motor cortex from premotor areas by observing resulting movement: clonic and at lower stimulation threshold in stimulation of primary motor areas, and tonic contractions at higher thresholds in stimulation of premotor areas. Furthermore, inhibition of movement can occur with stimulation of supplementary motor areas, and should be distinguished from patient fatigue.

1.3.5.4   Subcortical Stimulation

Recently much more emphasis has been placed on stimulation not only cortical areas, but also the descending white matter tracts. Transection of descending corticospinal tracts results in a significant neurological deficit and an accompanying loss of cMEPs in the corresponding limb. Preoperative studies that include DTI and tractography can predict the location of corticospinal fibers relative to tumor. During tumor resection, as brain shift occurs, the fibers can shift 4–15 mm (Nimsky et al. 2007). The direction of the shift is unpredictable, however, thus making intraoperative subcortical stimulation an important adjunct to prevent new neurological deficit. Low-frequency bipolar stimulation can be used, and the assumption is that stimulation of the white matter tracts occurs at a distance of 2–5 mm from the stimulating electrode. High-frequency monopolar stimulation is used more commonly now for mapping of descending corticospinal tracts. Furthermore, the distance to the descending tracts is proportional to the amount of current that is delivered to elicit MEPs. A linear relationship was shown with 1 mA equivalent to 1 mm of distance to the descending fibers (Nossek et al. 2011; Ohue et al. 2012; Prabhu et al. 2011). Tumor resection up to 5 mA of stimulation threshold was shown safe in avoiding a new postoperative deficit (Prabhu et al. 2011). Yet other studies demonstrated that resection of the tumor to the threshold up to 1 mA may be safe with only 3% of rate of new permanent neurological deficit at 3 months (Raabe et al. 2014). Overall, a combination of cortical and subcortical stimulation is encouraged to minimize risk of postoperative neurological deficit.

1.3.6   Language Mapping

While motor mapping can be performed in a patient that is awake or asleep, not requiring patient cooperation, language mapping can only performed in an awake and cooperative patient. Awake craniotomy is performed in many centers as it was shown to result in greater extent of resection while minimizing postoperative deficits. Awake craniotomy is well tolerated by patients with very low failure rates of 0.5–6.4% (Hervey-Jumper et al. 2015; Nossek et al. 2013). Since the patient is woken up in the middle of surgery, preoperative preparation of the patient for the awake craniotomy should include a detailed explanation of the procedure, of the tests performed intraoperatively, as well as introduction of the members of surgical and medical teams to ensure successful procedure.

The craniotomy is planned to expose at least 2–4 cm of cortical tissue around the tumor to allow for mapping. Low-frequency stimulation protocol using a bipolar probe is used most commonly. The stimulation current starting at 1 mA and going up on the current in 0.5 mA increments to a maximum of 6–8 mA. The cortex is systematically stimulated at 5–10 mm intervals with the duration of stimulation of 2–4 s. Stimulation for longer periods of time as well as repetitive stimulation of the same areas of cortex should be avoided as it predisposes to higher incidence of seizures. Stimulation is performed while the patient is performing language tests that may include naming, counting, dual task (simultaneous object-naming and movement task), repetition, or semantic tasks. Areas of mistakes or speech arrest are noted and a sterile marker placed to denote observed abnormality. An intraoperative photograph may be taken at the end of stimulation for documentation of eloquent areas and future reference in cases of repeat resection.

Intraoperative seizure activity is one of the most common complications of awake craniotomy occurring in about 3% of cases (Hervey-Jumper et al. 2015). It is therefore important that patients who are on antiepileptic medication take their medication on the day of surgery. Electrocorticography is commonly used during the stimulation to detect after-discharges and non-convulsive seizure activity. Most seizures are extinguished by applying ice-cold Ringer's saline to cortical surface. In resistant cases a small bolus of propofol can be administered to end seizures.

Recently, the appreciation of importance of white matter pathways for speech production has evolved (Chang et al. 2015). As a consequence, many groups perform subcortical mapping of speech pathways in addition to identifying speech cortical areas. Subcortical stimulation is for the most part performed in a manner similar to cortical stimulation protocols. The monopolar stimulation with train-of-five protocol has also been attempted with good success (Axelson et al. 2009).

1.3.7 Resection Principles

Once functional areas around the tumor have been established, the consideration is given to the mode of resection. In general, tumors infiltrating eloquent areas are resected in piecemeal fashion. En-block resection is the preferred method of tumor resection, however, whenever possible. The latter makes use of naturally present planes, such as cortical sulci to define the extent of resection. Each sulcus is followed to its depth until white matter is encountered at which point the interface between the tumor and white matter is established and followed circumferentially (Fig. 1.2d). Subcortical eloquent areas are identified early in such cases using DES and are avoided.

1.4   Conclusion

In summary, a variety of techniques are available to functionally characterize cortical and subcortical areas of brain in the vicinity of tumor. Preoperative investigations provide great anatomic detail of the area in question and preliminary functional
information that may guide the choice of intraoperative adjuncts to be used during
the resection. Combining adjuncts that enable better tumor visualization with direct
cortical and subcortical stimulation for functional mapping allows us to maximize
glioma resection while minimizing the risk of postoperative neurological deficit.

References

Axelson, H.W., G. Hesselager, and R. Flink. 2009. Successful localization of the Broca area with
short-train pulses instead of "Penfield" stimulation. *Seizure* 18: 374–375.
Cedzich, C., M. Taniguchi, S. Schäfer, and J. Schramm. 1996. Somatosensory evoked potential
phase reversal and direct motor cortex stimulation during surgery in and around the central
region. *Neurosurgery* 38: 962–970.
Chang, E.F., K.P. Raygor, and M.S. Berger. 2015. Contemporary model of language organization:
An overview for neurosurgeons. *Journal of Neurosurgery* 122: 250–261.
Coburger, J., A. Merkel, M. Scherer, F. Schwartz, F. Gessler, C. Roder, et al. 2016. Low-grade
glioma surgery in intraoperative magnetic resonance imaging: Results of a multicenter retro-
spective assessment of the German study group for intraoperative magnetic resonance imaging.
Neurosurgery 78: 775–786.
Fouke, S.J., T. Benzinger, D. Gibson, T.C. Ryken, S.N. Kalkanis, and J.J. Olson. 2015. The role of
imaging in the management of adults with diffuse low grade glioma. *Journal of Neuro-
Oncology* 125: 457–479.
Frey, D., S. Schilt, V. Strack, A. Zdunczyk, J. Rösler, B. Niraula, et al. 2014. Navigated transcranial
magnetic stimulation improves the treatment outcome in patients with brain tumors in motor
eloquent locations. *Neuro-Oncology* 16: 1365–1372.
Gerganov, V.M., A. Samii, M. Giordano, M. Samii, and R. Fahlbusch. 2011. Two-dimensional
high-end ultrasound imaging compared to intraoperative MRI during resection of low-grade
gliomas. *Journal of Clinical Neuroscience* 18: 669–673.
Hervey-Jumper, S.L., J. Li, D. Lau, A.M. Molinaro, D.W. Perry, L. Meng, et al. 2015. Awake craniotomy to maximize glioma resection: Methods and technical nuances over a 27-year period.
Journal of Neurosurgery 123: 325–339.
Jakola, A.S., K.S. Myrmel, R. Kloster, S.H. Torp, S. Lindal, G. Unsgård, et al. 2012. Comparison
of a strategy favoring early surgical resection vs a strategy favoring watchful waiting in low-
grade gliomas. *JAMA* 308: 1881–1888.
Knauth, M., C.R. Wirtz, V.M. Tronnier, N. Aras, S. Kunze, and K. Sartor. 1999. Intraoperative MR
imaging increases the extent of tumor resection in patients with high-grade gliomas.
AJNR. American Journal of Neuroradiology 20: 1642–1646.
Kombos, T., O. Suess, O. Ciklatekerlio, and M. Brock. 2001. Monitoring of intraoperative motor
evoked potentials to increase the safety of surgery in and around the motor cortex. *Journal of
Neurosurgery* 95: 608–614.
Korvenoja, A., E. Kirveskari, H.J. Aronen, S. Avikainen, A. Brander, J. Huttunen, et al. 2006.
Sensorimotor cortex localization: comparison of magnetoencephalography, functional MR
imaging, and intraoperative cortical mapping. *Radiology* 241: 213–222.

Krieg, S.M., J. Sabih, L. Bulubasova, T. Obermueller, C. Negwer, I. Janssen, et al. 2014. Preoperative motor mapping by navigated transcranial magnetic brain stimulation improves outcome for motor eloquent lesions. *Neuro-Oncology* 16: 1274–1282.

Krieg, S.M., E. Shiban, N. Buchmann, J. Gempt, A. Foerschler, B. Meyer, et al. 2012a. Utility of presurgical navigated transcranial magnetic brain stimulation for the resection of tumors in eloquent motor areas. *Journal of Neurosurgery* 116: 994–1001.

Krieg, S.M., E. Shiban, D. Droese, J. Gempt, N. Buchmann, H. Pape, et al. 2012b. Predictive value and safety of intraoperative neurophysiological monitoring with motor evoked potentials in Glioma surgery. *Neurosurgery* 70: 1060–1071.

Krings, T., M. Schreckenberger, V. Rohde, U. Spetzger, O. Sabri, M.H.T. Reinges, et al. 2002. Functional MRI and 18F FDG-positron emission tomography for presurgical planning: Comparison with electrical cortical stimulation. *Acta Neurochir (Wien)* 144:889–99– discussion 899.

Kuchcinski, G., C. Mellerio, J. Pallud, E. Dezamis, G. Turc, O. Rigaux-Viodé, et al. 2015. Three-tesla functional MR language mapping: Comparison with direct cortical stimulation in gliomas. *Neurology* 84: 560–568.

Kumar, V.A., J. Hamilton, L.A. Hayman, A.J. Kumar, G. Rao, J.S. Weinberg, et al. 2013. Deformable anatomic templates improve analysis of gliomas with minimal mass effect in eloquent areas. *Neurosurgery* 73: 534–542.

Lacroix, M., D. Abi-Said, D.R. Fourney, Z.L. Gokaslan, W. Shi, F. DeMonte, et al. 2001. A multivariate analysis of 416 patients with glioblastoma multiforme: prognosis, extent of resection, and survival. *Journal of Neurosurgery* 95: 190–198.

Le Roux, P.D., M.S. Berger, K. Wang, L.A. Mack, and G.A. Ojemann. 1992. Low grade gliomas: comparison of intraoperative ultrasound characteristics with preoperative imaging studies. *Journal of Neuro-Oncology* 13: 189–198.

Lefaucheur, J.-P., and T. Picht. 2016. The value of preoperative functional cortical mapping using navigated TMS. *Neurophysiologie clinique = Clinical neurophysiology* 46: 125–133.

Li, Y.M., D. Suki, K. Hess, and R. Sawaya. 2016. The influence of maximum safe resection of glioblastoma on survival in 1229 patients: Can we do better than gross-total resection? *Journal of Neurosurgery* 124: 977–988.

McGirt, M.J., D. Mukherjee, K.L. Chaichana, K.D. Than, J.D. Weingart, A. Quinones-Hinojosa. 2009. Association of surgically acquired motor and language deficits on overall survival after resection of glioblastoma multiforme. *Neurosurgery* 65:463–9– discussion 469–70.

Nabavi, A., H. Thurm, B. Zountsas, T. Pietsch, H. Lanfermann, U. Pichlmeier, et al. 2009. Five-aminolevulinic acid for fluorescence-guided resection of recurrent malignant gliomas: A phase ii study. *Neurosurgery* 65:1070–6– discussion 1076–7.

Nimsky, C., O. Ganslandt, P. Hastreiter, R. Wang, T. Benner, A.G. Sorensen, et al. 2007. Preoperative and intraoperative diffusion tensor imaging-based fiber tracking in glioma surgery. *Neurosurgery* 61:178–85– discussion 186

Nossek, E., A. Korn, T. Shahar, A.A. Kanner, H. Yaffe, D. Marcovici, et al. 2011. Intraoperative mapping and monitoring of the corticospinal tracts with neurophysiological assessment and 3-dimensional ultrasonography-based navigation. Clinical article. *Journal of Neurosurgery* 114: 738–746.

Nossek, E., I. Matot, T. Shahar, O. Barzilai, Y. Rapoport, T. Gonen, et al. 2013. Failed awake craniotomy: a retrospective analysis in 424 patients undergoing craniotomy for brain tumor. *Journal of Neurosurgery* 118: 243–249.

Ohue, S., S. Kohno, A. Inoue, D. Yamashita, H. Harada, Y. Kumon, et al. 2012. Accuracy of diffusion tensor magnetic resonance imaging-based tractography for surgery of gliomas near the pyramidal tract: A significant correlation between subcortical electrical stimulation and postoperative tractography. *Neurosurgery* 70:283–93– discussion 294.

Penfield, W., E. Boldrey. 1937. Somatic motor and sensory representation in the cerebral cortex of man as studied by electrical stimulation. *Brain* 60: 389–443.

Picht, T., D. Frey, S. Thieme, S. Kliesch, and P. Vajkoczy. 2016. Presurgical navigated TMS motor cortex mapping improves outcome in glioblastoma surgery: a controlled observational study. *Journal of Neuro-Oncology* 126: 535–543.

Prabhu, S.S., J. Gasco, S. Tummala, J.S. Weinberg, and G. Rao. 2011. Intraoperative magnetic resonance imaging-guided tractography with integrated monopolar subcortical functional mapping for resection of brain tumors. Clinical article. *Journal of Neurosurgery* 114: 719–726.

Prada, F., l. Mattei, M. Del Bene, L. Aiani, M. Saini, C. Casali, A. Filippini, F.G. Legnani, A. Perin, A. Saladino, I.G. Vetrano, L. Solbiati, A. Martegani, and F. DiMeco, 2014. Clinical StudyIntraoperative Cerebral Glioma Characterization with Contrast Enhanced Ultrasound. BioMed Research International 2014, 1–9. doi:10.1155/2014/484261.

Pujol, S., W. Wells, C. Pierpaoli, C. Brun, J. Gee, G. Cheng, et al. 2015. The DTI challenge: Toward standardized evaluation of diffusion tensor imaging tractography for neurosurgery. *Journal of Neuroimaging* 25: 875–882.

Raabe, A., J. Beck, P. Schucht, and K. Seidel. 2014. Continuous dynamic mapping of the corticospinal tract during surgery of motor eloquent brain tumors: evaluation of a new method. *Journal of Neurosurgery* 120: 1015–1024.

Rivaz, H., S.J.-S. Chen, and D.L. Collins. 2015. Automatic deformable MR-ultrasound registration for image-guided neurosurgery. *IEEE Transactions on Medical Imaging* 34: 366–380.

Sanai, N., M.-Y. Polley, M.W. McDermott, A.T. Parsa, and M.S. berger. 2011. An extent of resection threshold for newly diagnosed glioblastoma. *Journal of Neurosurgery* 115: 3–8.

Schreiber, A., U. Hubbe, S. Ziyeh, and J. Hennig. 2000. The influence of gliomas and nonglial space-occupying lesions on blood-oxygen-level-dependent contrast enhancement. *AJNR. American Journal of Neuroradiology* 21: 1055–1063.

Seidel, K., J. Beck, L. Stieglitz, P. Schucht, and A. Raabe. 2013. The warning-sign hierarchy between quantitative subcortical motor mapping and continuous motor evoked potential monitoring during resection of supratentorial brain tumors. *Journal of Neurosurgery* 118: 287–296.

Senft, C., A. Bink, K. Franz, H. Vatter, T. Gasser, and V. Seifert. 2011. Intraoperative MRI guidance and extent of resection in glioma surgery: A randomised, controlled trial. *The Lancet Oncology* 12: 997–1003.

Serra, C., A. Stauffer, B. Actor, J.-K. Burkhardt, N.H.-B. Ulrich, R.-L. Bernays, et al. 2012. Intraoperative high frequency ultrasound in intracerebral high-grade tumors. *Ultraschall in der Medizin* 33: E306–E312.

Stummer, W., U. Pichlmeier, T. Meinel, O.D. Wiestler, F. Zanella, H.-J. Reulen, et al. 2006. Fluorescence-guided surgery with 5-aminolevulinic acid for resection of malignant glioma: A randomised controlled multicentre phase III trial. *Lancet Oncology* 7: 392–401.

Taniguchi, M., C. Cedzich, and J. Schramm. 1993. Modification of cortical stimulation for motor evoked potentials under general anesthesia: Technical description. *Neurosurgery* 32: 219–226.

Tarapore, P.E., M.C. Tate, A.M. Findlay, S.M. Honma, D. Mizuiri, M.S. berger, et al. 2012. Preoperative multimodal motor mapping: a comparison of magnetoencephalography imaging, navigated transcranial magnetic stimulation, and direct cortical stimulation. *Journal of Neurosurgery* 117: 354–362.

Trinh, V.T., D.K. Fahim, M.V.C. Maldaun, K. Shah, I.E. McCutcheon, G. Rao, et al. 2014. Impact of preoperative functional magnetic resonance imaging during awake craniotomy procedures for intraoperative guidance and complication avoidance. *Stereotactic and Functional Neurosurgery* 92: 315–322.

Tuch, D.S., T.G. Reese, M.R. Wiegell, N. Makris, J.W. Belliveau, and V.J. Wedeen. 2002. High angular resolution diffusion imaging reveals intravoxel white matter fiber heterogeneity. *Magnetic Resonance in Medicine* 48: 577–582.

Ulmer, J.L., L. Hacein-Bey, V.P. Mathews, W.M. Mueller, E.A. DeYoe, R.W. Prost, et al. 2004. Lesion-induced pseudo-dominance at functional magnetic resonance imaging: Implications for preoperative assessments. *Neurosurgery* 55:569–79– discussion 580–1.

Vabulas, M., V.A. Kumar, J.D. Hamilton, J.J. Martinez, G. Rao, R. Sawaya, et al. 2014. Real-time atlas-based stereotactic neuronavigation. *Neurosurgery* 74:128–34– discussion 134.

Wedeen, V.J., P. Hagmann, W.-Y.I. Tseng, T.G. Reese, and R.M. Weisskoff. 2005. Mapping complex tissue architecture with diffusion spectrum magnetic resonance imaging. *Magnetic Resonance in Medicine* 54: 1377–1386.

Willems, P.W.A., M.J.B. Taphoorn, H. Burger, Berkelbach van der Sprenkel JW, and C.A.F. Tulleken. 2006. Effectiveness of neuronavigation in resecting solitary intracerebral contrast-enhancing tumors: A randomized controlled trial. *Journal of Neurosurgery* 104: 360–368.

Wu, J-S., L.-F. Zhou, W.-J. Tang, Y. Mao, J. Hu, Y.-Y. Song, et al. 2007. Clinical evaluation and follow-up outcome of diffusion tensor imaging-based functional neuronavigation: A prospective, controlled study in patients with gliomas involving pyramidal tracts. Neurosurgery 61:935–48– discussion 948–9.

Zhu, F.-P., J.-S. Wu, Y.-Y. Song, C.-J. Yao, D.-X. Zhuang, G. Xu, et al. 2012. Clinical application of motor pathway mapping using diffusion tensor imaging tractography and intraoperative direct subcortical stimulation in cerebral glioma surgery: A prospective cohort study. *Neurosurgery* 71: 1170–1183.

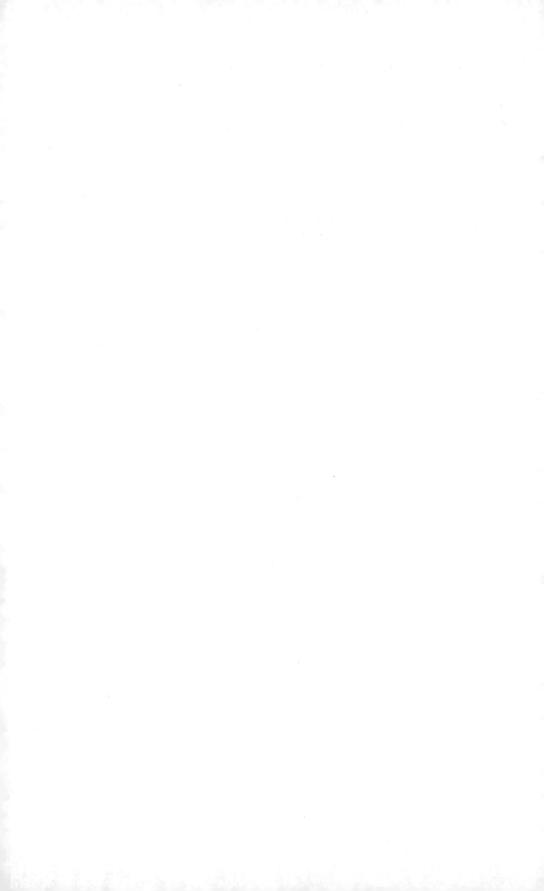

Chapter 2
Molecular Pathology of Glioblastoma- An Update

Vani Santosh, Palavalasa Sravya, and Arimappamagan Arivazhagan

Abstract Glioblastoma, the most common primary brain malignancy, has piqued the interest of researchers for decades. As a result, it is one of the most studied brain malignancies. Advancement in technology in recent years has had a tremendous impact on the understanding of this dreaded disease. Deepening insight into its molecular pathology has brought about a paradigm shift in the knowledge of this disease. The WHO has made significant changes in the classification of glioblastoma with emphasis on the molecular changes, thus advocating a histomolecular diagnosis, as opposed to the purely histological diagnosis which was the gold standard until recently. The molecular diagnostics aid the decision making in the management of the disease. This chapter discusses the histomorphology of glioblastoma, new WHO classification of glioblastoma, recent molecular contributions of various research groups leading to changing concepts and also the less explored avenues like intra-tumor heterogeneity and tumor recurrence in glioblastoma.

Keywords Glioblastoma • WHO 2016 • Molecular pathology • IDH1 • MGMT • Recurrence

2.1 Introduction to Adult Diffuse Gliomas and Glioblastoma with Emphasis on Changing Concepts

Gliomas are the most common primary brain tumors in adults and are the focus of research in neuro-oncology. Until recently, they have been grouped together according to what was believed to be their cell of origin. Hence, they were classified as astrocytic, oligodendroglial, oligoastrocytic and ependymal tumors. Initially, the cell

V. Santosh (✉)
Department of Neuropathology, NIMHANS, Bengaluru, India
e-mail: vani.santosh@gmail.com

P. Sravya
Department of Clinical Neurosciences, NIMHANS, Bengaluru, India

A. Arivazhagan
Department of Neurosurgery, NIMHANS, Bengaluru, India

© Springer International Publishing AG 2017
K. Somasundaram (ed.), *Advances in Biology and Treatment of Glioblastoma*,
Current Cancer Research, DOI 10.1007/978-3-319-56820-1_2

of origin was predicted solely based on the morphological similarities of the neo-plastic cells to the different glial cells. However, with advancing technology, the picture of molecular landscape of gliomas has become sharper and the family trees have been re-drawn. It is now understood that the various diffusely infiltrating glio-mas are more nosologically similar to each other than to the circumscribed gliomas sharing similar cellular morphology.

Thus, according to the latest WHO 2016 classification, adult diffuse gliomas, whether astrocytic or not, now fall under one category and comprise the WHO grade II and grade III astrocytoma, grade II and grade III oligodendroglioma, grade II and grade III oligoastrocytoma-'Not Otherwise Specified(NOS)' and grade IV glioblas-toma . Previously, pediatric gliomas were grouped along with their adult counter-parts, despite the known differences in their biological behavior. Increasing insights into the molecular aberrations in pediatric gliomas have enabled sharper demarca-tion in the subtypes. One such group defined in the new classification is the diffuse midline glioma, H3 K27 M mutant. Overall, the most notable change in the way gliomas are now viewed at is the integration of molecular markers in defining the entities.

Diffuse gliomas are potentially malignant or overtly malignant tumors, glioblas-toma being the most aggressive of all. Its inexorable progression and the inevitabil-ity of death it brings about within 14–16 months of diagnosis despite the best available treatment makes it the nightmare of patients, clinicians and researchers alike. Glioblastoma has plagued the minds of researchers ever since the entity came to be known. Diagnosis of this tumor is not so much of a challenge, but predicting its clinical behavior is. This tumor is so varied in its composition that heterogeneity, both inter and intra tumor, is one of the characteristic features of glioblastoma. Prior to the advent of technologies to decipher the molecular makeup of glioblastoma, histopathology was the only modality available to characterize the tumor and its variants.

In glioblastoma, the heterogeneity is such that if each pattern were to be consid-ered a variant, there would be many variants which are of doubtful prognostic sig-nificance and which would not, with the present knowledge, aid the prediction of clinical and biological behavior. Hence, the WHO has identified only those patterns as variants which would throw light on possible clinical course. WHO 2007 classi-fication had identified Glioblastoma as one codified tumor entity with two variants-Gliosarcoma and Giant cell glioblastoma.

With the advent of molecular profiling which picked up speed in the last decade, the understanding of the tumor has moved up by several notches and the latest WHO 2016 classification now identifies two entities of glioblastoma based on mutational status of IDH (Isocitrate dehydrogenase) gene-IDH wild type glioblastoma and IDH mutant glioblastoma. A new variant of IDH wild type glioblastoma also has been penned down, which is epithelioid glioblastoma. Glioblastoma with primitive neu-ronal component has been described as a pattern.

It is evident that there was an enormous inflow of molecular data which com-pelled the scientific community to reconsider the approach to gliomas. Discoveries of note are 1p and 19q codeletion (oligodendroglioma specific), IDH point mutations, ATRX mutations, TP 53 mutations, TERT mutations, EGFR amplifications, PTEN mutations and others. This flood of molecular findings has brought about a revolution in the diagnosis and prediction of clinical behavior of gliomas, including glioblastoma. The ISN Haarlem guidelines have played a central role in bringing about this change.

2.2 ISN Haarlem Guidelines and Evolution of WHO 2016

The inadequacy of the WHO 2007 guidelines in prognosticating the patient's response to treatment and the inter-observer variability which was prevalent when WHO 2007 classification failed to guide the pathologists in arriving at an unequivocal diagnosis, instigated the International Society for Neuropathology to convene at Haarlem, Netherlands in order to discuss the need for incorporation of pertinent molecular discoveries into the existing diagnostic criteria and classification. This crucial meeting, called the "WHO'S NEXT" has set the stage for the new WHO classification. However, the WHO authorized an 'update' of the WHO 2007 4th edition but not the release of a 5th edition. This update features predominantly a combination of morphology and genetics resulting in a major restructuring in the classification of several brain tumour entities, the gliomas in particular.

The ISN Haarlem guidelines suggested that a "layered diagnosis with histological classification, WHO grade and molecular information listed below to derive an integrated diagnosis" be made routinely (Louis et al. 2014) (Table 2.1).

With this, the picture became clearer and several unresolved issues have successfully attained a greater resolution.

2.3 WHO 2007 Classification Versus 2016 Classification w.r.t Glioblastoma (Table 2.2)

Following the suggestions made by ISN Haarlem consensus and taking into account the advancement in understanding of molecular pathogenesis, the WHO 2016 has made significant changes in the classification of gliomas. One major change is the regrouping of the gliomas as 'diffuse astrocytic and oligodendroglial tumors ',

Table 2.1 Multilayered reporting format as per ISN haarlem consensus (Louis et al. 2014)

Layer 1: Integrated diagnosis (incorporating all tissue-based information)
Layer 2: Histological classification
Layer 3: WHO grade (reflecting natural history)
Layer 4: Molecular information

Table 2.2 Differences between WHO 2007 (Louis et al. 2007) and WHO 2016 (Louis et al. 2016) classification w.r.t glioblastoma

WHO 2007	WHO 2016
Astrocytic tumors:	**Diffuse gliomas:**
Glioblastoma ICD code 9440/3	Glioblastoma IDH wild type*ICD code 9440/3*
Giant cell glioblastoma *ICD code 9441/3*	Giant cell glioblastoma *ICD code 9441/3*
Gliosarcoma*ICD code 9442/3*	Gliosarcoma*ICD code 9442/3*
	Epitheloid glioblastomaICD code 9440/3
	Glioblastoma IDH mutant*ICD code 9445/3*
	Glioblastoma NOS[a]*ICD code 9440/3*

[a]*NOS* Not otherwise specified

'other astrocytic tumors', 'ependymal tumors' and 'other gliomas' as opposed to the WHO 2007 that includes; 'astrocytic tumors', 'oligodendroglial tumors', 'oligoastrocytic tumors', 'ependymal tumors' and 'other neuroepithelial tumors'. Another significant change in WHO 2016 is the inclusion of entity defining molecular information in the classification. Now, various entities are defined by their molecular signatures.

Both these major changes apply to Glioblastoma, too. It is now grouped with diffuse gliomas which are now believed to arise from a common bipotential precursor cell/ a neural stem cell which undergoes sequential mutations that directs its evolution to the different types of diffuse glioma. A new entity namely "Glioblastoma-IDH mutant" is recognized. This change is guided by accumulating evidence that IDH mutant glioblastoma confers a significantly better prognosis than IDH wild type glioblastoma.

2.4   Glioblastoma: Gross Pathology, Histomorphology and the New Definitions

Even though histomolecular approach has now taken over pure histological approach for brain tumor diagnosis, it must, however, be re-iterated that histology is the key entry point, which is especially true for glioblastoma. The holistic understanding of glioblastoma is only complete when one is well versed with its histomorphology. Few human malignancies display the heterogeneity which glioblastoma exhibits. The cellular composition is varied and as a result, there are numerous histological patterns of glioblastoma which have been described in great detail.

Glioblastomas are disproportionately large for the duration of symptoms with which the patient presents. The tumor, in no time, completely infiltrates an entire lobe. In fact, one of the earliest descriptions (1928) of treatment for glioblastoma was that of hemispherectomy by neurosurgeon Walter Dandy, despite which the patients succumbed due to contralateral hemisphere involvement (Bahuleyan et al. 2013). This vignette clearly shows how aggressively the tumor grows.

While a vast majority of glioblastomas show such aggressive biological and clinical behaviour, a small group of glioblastomas present with long duration of symptoms and usually occur in younger adult patients. These tumors are believed to evolve from a lower grade astrocytoma to glioblastoma over a long duration. These are referred to as "clinico-pathologically defined secondary glioblastomas" whereas the aggressive glioblastomas, without evidence of a less malignant precursor lesion, are called "clinico-pathologically defined primary glioblastomas or de novo glioblastomas". The secondary glioblastoma is found to have a significantly longer survival than the primary glioblastoma. The discovery of IDH mutations provided the reason for this dramatic difference. It was later understood that the clinico-pathologically defined secondary glioblastoma corresponds very well to the IDH mutant glioblastoma.

The lesions, though usually unilateral, may present as supratentorial bilateral tumor mass due to extension along the myelinated structures, especially the corpus callosum and the commissures (Fig. 2.1a, b). Multifocal glioblastoma as visualized on radiological imaging is not unusual. Whether the seemingly independent multi-

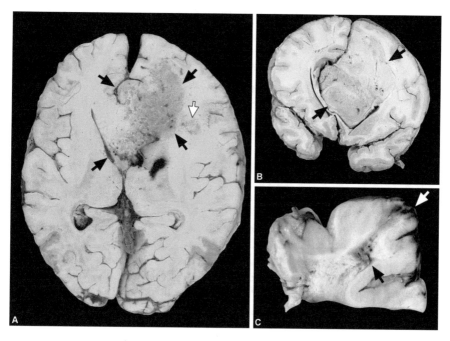

Fig. 2.1 Gross morphology of glioblastoma. (**a**) Depicts tumor in the right frontal region showing diffuse infiltration of the white matter, overlying grey matter, including cingulate gyrus and spreading across the corpus callosum (*black arrows*). Another small tumor nodule is noted beyond the discernible margin of the main tumor mass indicating spread (*white arrow*). Tumor shows a variegated appearance with discoloration indicating necrosis and hemorrhage. (**b**) Shows tumor in the right frontal region diffusely infiltrating the parenchyma resulting in compression of right lateral ventricle and shift of midline structures with compression of contralateral lateral ventricle (*black arrows*). (**c**) Depicts a coronal slice of a resected glioblastoma tumor showing tumor located superficially in the white matter (*black arrow*) with areas of hemorrhage and with spread into the overlying grey matter (*white arrow*)

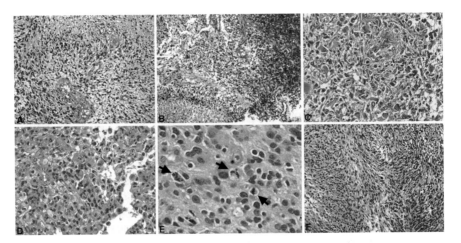

Fig. 2.2 Heterogeneous cellular composition of glioblastoma showing fibrillary (**a**), undifferentiated (**b**), pleomorphic (**c**) and gemistocytic (**d**) morphology. Brisk mitotic activity (*black arrows*) is seen (**e**). The tumor occasionally imparts a sarcomatous appearance on histology (**f**) (Microscopic images **a–c** and **f** – original magnification ×80; **d**- original magnification ×160 and **e**- original magnification ×320[All H&E])

ple lesions are truly multifocal is to be determined. Truly multifocal gliomas are usually seen in inherited neoplastic syndromes. But outside of this setting, true multifocal gliomas are relatively rare, with studies reporting about 2.4% glioblastomas to be truly multifocal with different foci showing different clonality (Batzdorf and Malamud 1963).

Most glioblastomas arise from the white matter of cerebral hemispheres but sometimes, they may be largely superficial (Fig. 2.1c). They are diffusely infiltrating, peripherally greyish with central areas of yellowish necrosis. There may also be extensive hemorrhages and macroscopic cysts containing liquefied necrotic tissue.

Microscopically, glioblastoma appears as a highly cellular tumor, composed of a wide variety of anaplastic astroglial cells. A heterogeneous cellular composition prevails with cell types such as fibrillary, undifferentiated, pleomorphic, gemistocytic, lipidized, multinucleated and granular astrocytic cells, with significant nuclear atypia and brisk mitosis (Fig. 2.2a–e). The cells are dispersed over a variably fibrillated stroma with occasional microcystic change. At times, the spindle shaped astrocytes can be arranged in interlacing fascicles imparting a sarcomatous appearance to the tumor (Fig. 2.2f). The cells may also be large with well delineated borders and at times resemble an epithelial malignancy or melanoma. This extent of cellular variety necessitates that the diagnosis of glioblastoma be based on the tissue pattern rather than on the individual cell type. Thus, the essential diagnostic features are the presence of pleomorphic anaplastic glial cells with nuclear atypia, brisk mitosis and prominent microvascular proliferation (MVP) and/or necrosis. Prominent MVP is a histopathological hallmark of glioblastoma. On light microscopy, it typically appears as glomeruloid tufts of multilayered endothelial cells which are mitotically active along with smooth muscle cells or pericytes (Fig. 2.3a). This is often found

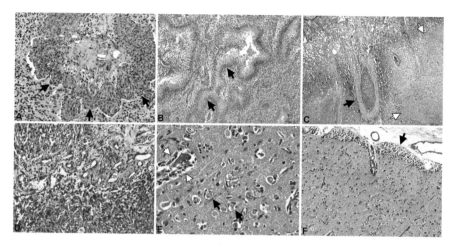

Fig. 2.3 Representative photomicrographs of glioblastoma depicting the vascular changes, necrotic pattern and the spreading front. Microvascular proliferation often has a glomeruloid appearance (**a**- *black arrows*). Necrosis can be palisading (**b**-*black arrows*) or confluent (**c**-*white arrows*), the latter accompanied by sclerosed thrombosed blood vessels (**c**- *black arrow*). Florid neovascularization is seen in most glioblastomas (**d**). The spreading front of glioblastoma shows characteristic peri-neuronal spread (**e**- *black arrows*), peri-vascular spread (**e**- *white arrows*) and subpial spread (**e**- *black arrow*) (Images **a**, **d** and **f** – original magnification ×80; **b** and **c** – original magnification ×32; **e**- original magnification ×160[All H&E])

around necrosis and is directionally oriented to it (Haddad et al. 1992). Tumor necrosis is a fundamental feature of glioblastoma and may be of geographic(confluent) or palisading (historically called pseudo palisading) type (Fig. 2.3b, c). Necrosis is one of the strongest predictors of aggressive behavior among the diffuse gliomas. Another striking feature of glioblastoma is the angiogenesis (neovascularization). Glioblastoma is a highly vascular tumor and sprouting capillaries from pre-existing vessels, vessel cooption by migrating tumor cells are commonplace in glioblastoma (Fig. 2.3d). The tumor may be studded with fresh and/or old bleeds. Other salient features of glioblastoma include sclerosed and thrombosed blood vessels (Fig. 2.3c), tumor infiltrating lymphocytes and secondary structures such as satellitosis, which is the phenomenon where tumor cells line up in the sub pial/subependymal region/ around neurons and blood vessels (Fig. 2.3e, f). The secondary structures, highly suggestive of infiltrating glioma, were earlier referred to as Scherer's structures, in appreciation of the scientist whose visionary description demonstrated the most common sites for glioma invasion (Scherer and Structural 1938).

Previously, glioblastoma was called "Glioblastoma multiforme". Though the terminology is now obsolete, it reflects on the extreme variability of the histopathology of the tumor. Some of the histological patterns observed in glioblastoma are:

1. Small cell glioblastoma (Fig. 2.4): This pattern consists of highly monomorphic small cells with round to elongated hyperchromatic nuclei with minimal cytoplasm. They tend to mimic lymphocytes and due to their uniformity, micro calcifications and chicken wire like blood vessels, they may be confused with

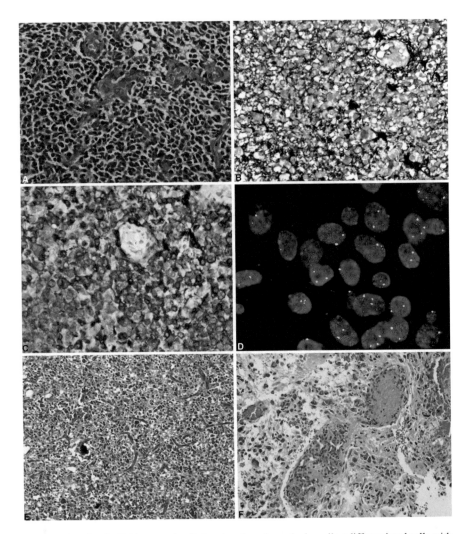

Fig. 2.4 Small cell glioblastoma (**a–d**) showing densely packed small undifferentiated cells with hyperchromatic nucleus dispersed over a vascularized stroma, mimicking an undifferentiated anaplastic oligodendroglioma (**a**). The tumor cells are minimally positive for GFAP, whilst the stromal fibrils are variably positive (**b**). Uniform and strong membrane/ cytoplasmic EGFR expression is seen (**c**). FISH image (**d**) showing EFGR amplification (orange signals) in the interphase nuclei. (**e**) and (**f**) show glioblastoma with oligodendroglial component. The oligodendroglial component is highlighted in (**e**) and astrocytic component with microvascular proliferation in (**f**) (Images **a–c** – original magnification ×160; Images **e** and **f**- original magnification ×80; Image **d** – original magnification ×800[Fig. A,E&F are H&E]

anaplastic oligodendroglioma (Fig. 2.4a). They may show minimal immunoreactivity to GFAP, which is a marker for astrocytes (Fig. 2.4b). However, the increased understanding of molecular signatures of gliomas has made this pattern easily discernible. The WHO 2016 has acknowledged that unlike the other tumors that come up as differential diagnosis, small cell glioblastomas frequently have EGFR amplifications/overexpression (Fig. 2.4c, d) and chromosomal arm 10q losses. Also, 1p and 19q co-deletion which is the defining feature for anaplastic oligodendroglioma, is absent in small cell glioblastoma.

2. Glioblastoma with Oligodendroglial component (Glioblastoma-O) (Fig. 2.4e, f): This pattern had caused quite a debate while laying down the WHO 2007 classification. It was identified by C.R. Miller et al. through studies involving large cohorts of patients with mixed glioma encompassing astrocytic and oligodendroglial components and with large areas of necrosis. They found that these patients had a worse prognosis than those without necrosis (Miller et al. 2006). They had suggested that this pattern be called anaplastic oligoastrocytoma grade IV. But the majority of pathologists who convened at the WHO 2007 consensus meeting opined that more clinico-pathological data should be available before this tumour is considered a new disease entity. Thus it was decided that this pattern be termed as 'glioblastoma with oligodendroglioma component'. Then came the histomolecular coup which has overthrown the diagnosis of oligoastrocytoma altogether in the WHO 2016 classification. With this, it is possible to classify such tumors as 'Glioblastoma, IDH wild type', 'Glioblastoma, IDH mutant' or 'Anaplastic oligodendroglioma, IDH mutant and 1p/19q codeleted'.

3. Granular cell Glioblastoma (Fig. 2.5a): Glioblastoma sometimes consists of large cells with a granular eosinophilic cytoplasm which stains with periodic acid Schiff (PAS), usually scattered and sometimes as foci within the tumor. When granular cells predominate, the histology closely resembles that of other granular cell tumors like those arising from the pituitary stalk or other tissues. Occasionally, these cells, though more granular and larger, may be mistaken for macrophages and the lesion may be misinterpreted as macrophage-rich condition such as a demyelinating lesion, especially in the context of perivascular chronic inflammation. Such cells may be immunoreactive for macrophage markers like CD68 but not for specific markers such as CD163. GFAP may show peripheral positivity in occasional cells. Glioblastoma with this pattern has an aggressive behavior. In other diffuse gliomas too, granular cell pattern has been reported to confer poorer prognosis (Rao et al. 2017).

4. Heavily lipidized glioblastoma (Fig. 2.5b, c): Occasional glioblastomas consist of cells with foamy cytoplasm. However, rarely such cells predominate but when they do, the pattern is called heavily lipidized glioblastoma. The lipidized cells may be grossly enlarged and juxtaposed lobules of fully lipidized cells may mimic adipose tissue.

5. Glioblastoma with primitive neuronal component (Fig. 2.5d–f): This newly recognized pattern in WHO 2016 classification, was earlier referred to as 'Glioblastoma with PNET component' (Song et al. 2011). An otherwise classical high grade diffuse glioma with one or more foci of sharply demarcated primitive nodules showing neuronal differentiation constitutes this pattern. These foci are markedly cellular, even more than the adjacent glioma, display a high nuclear-to-cytoplasmic ratio and mitosis- karyorrhexis index and may contain variable features like Homer-Wright rosettes, cell wrapping and other features that resemble

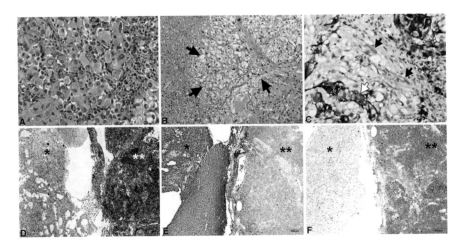

Fig. 2.5 Representative microphotographs of granular cell glioblastoma (**a**), heavily lipidized glioblastoma (**b**, **c**) and glioblastoma with primitive neuronal component (**d–f**). Granular cell glioblastoma shows several large cells with abundant granular, eosinophilic cytoplasm (**a**). Heavily lipidized glioblastoma shows tumor cells with abundant, foamy cytoplasm(**b**). GFAP staining (**c**) reveals that several lipidized tumor cells are negative for GFAP while few others show moderate patchy staining (*black arrows*) and small groups of cells are intensely staining (*white arrows*). Glioblastoma with primitive neuronal component (**d–f**) showing astrocytic (**d***) and primitive neuronal component (**d****). The astrocytic component stains positive for GFAP (**e***) and negative for synaptophysin (**f***). The primitive neuronal component is negative for GFAP (**e****) and positive for synaptophysin (**f****) (Images **a** and **c**- original magnification ×160. Image **b**- original magnification × 80. Images **d–f**- original magnification × 32[Fig.A,B&D are H&E])

CNS embryonal neoplasms. Similar to the primitive neuronal cells, these foci show immunoreactivity for synaptophysin, loss of GFAP expression and a high Ki-67 index. One notable feature is that though the genetic makeup is similar to glioblastoma in general, this subtype may be seen in either a de-novo glioblastoma or in a clinicopathologically defined secondary glioblastoma. However, it must be noted that be it primary or secondary, the glioblastomas with primitive neuronal component have similar survival times, with a few studies suggesting that this subset has a relatively more favourable outcome (Song et al. 2011; Joseph et al. 2013). The distinctive feature of this pattern is its high rate of cerebrospinal fluid dissemination and the frequency of MYCN or MYC gene amplification which is restricted to the primitive neuronal nodules.

Thus, there exists a great cellular pleomorphism in glioblastoma. But every histological pattern does not reflect on clinical and biological behavior of the tumor. While histopathology is quintessential for establishing diagnosis of glioblastoma, it has failed to predict the clinical behavior of the tumor based on phenotypic patterns. One classical example for this is the attempt at understanding the biological behavior of patients with glioblastoma with oligodendroglial component (He et al. 2001; Wang et al. 2012). It was previously understood that glioblastoma with oligodendroglial component had a better prognosis than classical glioblastoma (He et al.

2001). Nevertheless, later studies proved that this group was, in fact, a heterogeneous one with differing IDH mutational status and some of tumors previously categorized as glioblastoma-O may have in fact been aggressive anaplastic oligodendrogliomas with 1p and 19q codeletion, which is now known to be Oligodendroglioma specific (Wang et al. 2012; Homma et al. 2006).

Hence, as explained earlier, the molecular composition, which aids greatly in the prediction of the behavior of the tumor, has been included in mainstream diagnostics. Thus, the entities of glioblastoma, as defined by the WHO 2016 are; Glioblastoma, IDH-wild type; Glioblastoma, IDH-mutant and Glioblastoma, NOS(reserved for cases where complete IDH evaluation was not done).

2.4.1 Glioblastoma, IDH-Wild Type

This is defined as *a 'high grade glioma with predominantly astrocytic differentiation; featuring nuclear atypia, cellular pleomorphism (in most cases), mitotic activity, and typically a diffuse growth pattern, as well as microvascular proliferation and/or necrosis; and which lacks mutations in the IDH genes'*(D N Louis et al. 2016).

The microscopic picture is as described above with high cellular pleomorphism, MVP and/or necrosis. In addition, the WHO 2016 classification defines this entity by the absence of IDH mutations. The immunophenotype of this entity is diverse with different variants showing different immunoreactivity. GFAP expression is usually the norm in glioblastoma. However, the degree of reactivity is markedly different among variants. Other typically expressed markers in glioblastoma are S-100, Nestin and Vimentin. Nestin may be of diagnostic use when attempting to differentiate glioblastoma from other high grade gliomas. When faced with a poorly differentiated tumor, the expression of OLIG2 may help identifying astrocytomas and oligodendrogliomas as it is not so often expressed in ependymomas and non-glial tumors. Classical glioblastoma sometimes also express cytokeratin AE1/AE3 or EMA. Apart from these markers, certain subsets of glioblastoma express markers specific to their genetic makeup, ex. P53 immunoreactivity in tumors with TP53 mutation leading to p53 mutant protein expression, EGFR expression in those with EGFR gene amplification, EGFR vIII expression as a result of mutation in a relatively smaller subset, H3 K27 M mutant expression, and others. Glioblastoma, IDH wild type has three variants, two of which were described in the WHO 2007 classification with a new addition in the WHO 2016 classification. The three variants identified are observed to possess a genetic profile which is more or less characteristic of the variant.

The variants are as under:

(i) Giant cell glioblastoma (Fig. 2.6a–d): This is a rare histological variant characterized by large, bizarre multi nucleated giant cells with vesicular nuclei and prominent nucleoli and an occasionally abundant reticulin network. The giant cells may contain few to >20 nuclei and occasionally contain intra nuclear

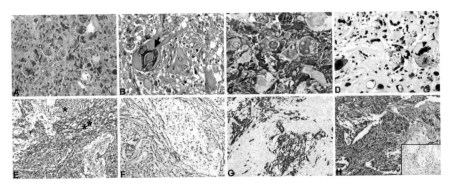

Fig. 2.6 Representative microphotographs of Giant cell glioblastoma (**a–d**) and gliosarcoma (**e–h**). Giant cell glioblastoma showing several bizarre multinucleated tumor giant cells (**a**), with some of the giant cells containing intra-nuclear cytoplasmic inclusions (**b**- *black arrow*). Most of the giant cells are positive for GFAP (**c**) and show strong immunopositivity for p53 (**d**). Gliosarcoma shows a biphasic pattern with intermingled glial (**e***) and sarcomatous component (**e****). The sarcomatous component shows dense pericellular reticulin which is not seen in the glial component (**f**). The glial but not the sarcomatous component shows strong GFAP expression (**g**) and both components stain for Vimentin (**h**). *Inset* in (**h**) shows high MIB-1 labeling in both the components (Images **a–d**- original magnification × 160 and **e–h**- original magnification × 80[Fig.A,B&E are H&E])

cytoplasmic inclusions. A commonly found feature of this variant is the formation of pseudo-rosette like pattern with tumor cells accumulating around the blood vessels. Unlike the classical glioblastoma, microvascular proliferation is not common in this variant. The immunophenotype of this variant is characterized by the consistent but varying level of expression of GFAP and frequent positivity for p53 mutant protein expression arising as a result of TP53 mutation (>80%). Genetically, this subset is conspicuous in its lack of EGFR amplification and homozygous CDKN2A deletion. They also frequently harbor TP53 mutations (80%) and PTEN mutations (33%).The clinical outcome of giant cell glioblastoma is somewhat better than that of classic glioblastoma.

(ii) Gliosarcoma (Fig. 2.6e–h): This variant is characterized by a biphasic tissue pattern with alternating areas displaying glial and sarcomatous components. The glial component shows typical features of glioblastoma whereas the sarcomatous component consists of bundles of spindle cells surrounded by reticulin fibres. Gliosarcoma, though usually occurs in classic glioblastomas, may also arise in ependymomas and oligodendrogliomas. A subset of gliosarcomas show additional features of mesenchymal differentiation like formation of bone, cartilage, muscle and lipomatous features. In some instances, a glioblastoma with fibroblastic proliferation due to meningeal invasion or extensive vascular sclerosis can be mistaken for a gliosarcoma. However, in gliosarcoma, significant nuclear atypia and mitosis are present in both components. GFAP stains the glial component only and not the sarcomatous component, though isolated spindle cells may be positive. The sarcomatous component variably expresses other markers like alpha-1 antitrypsin, actin and EMA. Vimentin, which is an immature glial cell marker, shows itself in both the glial as well as sarcomatous component. This variant is largely negative for IDH1 R132H-mutant protein. TP53 mutation is infrequent and hence p53 immunoreactivity is unusual. When positive for p53, it is identified in both glial and sarcomatous components. The occurrence of genetic alterations like TP53 mutations and IDH mutations, when present in gliosarcoma, in both glial and sarcomatous components suggest that the variant is monoclonal in origin as opposed to the earlier belief that it was polyclonal. Genetically, it differs from giant cell glioblastoma in that it contains CDKN2A deletions. EGFR amplification is infrequent in this variant, too. The clinical course of gliosarcoma differs slightly from classical glioblastoma in that it was reported in occasional cases to disseminate systemically and sometimes penetrate the skull. But the studies on the difference in outcome of gliosarcoma and glioblastoma have, so far, yielded conflicting and inconclusive results.

(iii) Epithelioid Glioblastoma: This is a newly recognized, relatively rare variant of glioblastoma (IDH wild type) is the latest addition to the glioblastoma group, added in the WHO 2016 classification. It consists of densely packed epithelioid-like cells with eosinophilic cytoplasm and paucity of cytoplasmic processes, absence of interspersed neuropil and an eccentric nucleus. Epithelioid glioblastoma is an aggressive tumor which occurs mainly in young adults and children and is associated with a particularly poor prognosis. Most commonly, it is located in the cerebrum or diencephalon (Ellison, Kleinschmidt-DeMasters, and Park 2016). BRAF V600E mutation is more common in epithelioid glioblastoma compared to other glioblastomas. VE1 antibody which recognizes V600E mutant BRAF show positivity in about 50% of these cases (Kleinschmidt-DeMasters et al. 2015). The tumor also displays retention of SMARCB1 and SMARCA4 while not expressing markers such as desmin, myoglobin, smooth muscle actin or melan A. Also, it shows immunopositivity for Vimentin and S100, expresses epithelial markers like EMA and cytokeratin and lacks IDH1 and IDH2 mutations. Copy number alterations in genes observed in adult IDH wild type glioblastomas, such as EGFR amplification and chromosome 10 losses are occasionally present (Ellison, Kleinschmidt-DeMasters, and Park 2016; Broniscer et al. 2014).

2.4.2   Glioblastoma, IDH Mutant (Fig. 2.7)

This entity is defined as a 'high grade glioma with predominantly astrocytic differentiation; featuring nuclear atypia, cellular pleomorphism (in most cases), mitotic activity, and typically a diffuse growth pattern, as well as microvascular proliferation and/or necrosis; with a mutation in either the IDH1 or IDH2 gene' (Ohgaki et al. 2016). Histologically, the IDH mutant glioblastomas are similar to the IDH-wild type glioblastoma, with only two significant differences. Large areas of ischemic and/or palisading necrosis are less frequent in IDH mutant glioblastoma than the IDH wild types glioblastoma (Nobusawa et al. 2009). Another difference is that focal oligodendroglioma component is more frequent in the IDH mutant glioblastoma (Lai et al. 2011).

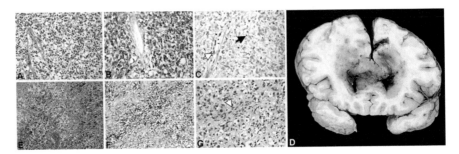

Fig. 2.7 Depicts a case of anaplastic astrocytoma (WHO grade III) (**a–c**) with malignant progression over 2 years. The patient succumbed to the illness and autopsy revealed a secondary glioblastoma(WHO grade IV) (**d–g**). Anaplastic astrocytoma showing a cellular astrocytic tumor (**a**), with tumor cells exhibiting diffuse and strong IDH1- R132H positivity (**b**) and loss of ATRX expression (**c**). Coronal slice of the cerebral hemisphere shows a bifrontal hemorrhagic necrotic tumor spreading across the corpus callosum and infiltrating the ventricular walls (**d**). Histology revealed features of glioblastoma with focal necrosis (**e**). The tumor cells are diffusely positive for IDH1- R132H (**f**) and show loss of ATRX expression (**g**). Note that in Fig C and G, the endothelial cells (*white arrows*) and a few over-run native glial cells (*black arrow*) show retained ATRX expression, serving as internal controls (Images **a–c** and **g**- original magnification × 160; **d**, **e**- original magnification × 80[Fig. A&E are H&E])

The characteristic immunophenotype of this entity is that of IDH1-R132H mutant positivity in over 90% of cases. The remaining tumors harbor rare IDH mutations. Mutations in ATRX gene (loss of expression) are the norm rather than exception in these tumors. Also, TP53 overexpression is frequent and EGFR amplification is rare in IDH mutant glioblastomas. Another typical feature of this entity is the hypermethylator phenotype it shows. All in all, the genetic makeup of this entity confers a significantly better prognosis than the wild type glioblastoma (Table 2.3).

2.5   Molecules That Define Glioblastoma in Detail

The earliest molecules which were studied in glioblastoma are TP53 and MGMT. These were identified when attempting to understand treatment resistance of glioblastoma. Epigenetic silencing of MGMT gene through its promoter methylation resulting in better response to Temozolomide was the most advocated prognostic marker in glioblastoma for nearly a decade (Hegi et al. 2005).The twenty first century has seen a tremendous advancement of technology which opened the flood gates for molecular research and inundated the scientific world with overwhelming information on the genetic and molecular make up of various malignancies. Glioblastoma was among the earliest to be targeted by large scale molecular profiling platforms like comparative genomic hybridization (CGH), single nucleotide polymorphism (SNP) arrays and others. The Cancer Genome Atlas (TCGA), an initiative by NIH, USA, applied multiplatform profiling to systematically and comprehensively define the genomic landscape of glioblastoma (Cancer Genome Atlas Research Network 2008).

Table 2.3 Key clinical and molecular characteristics of IDH-wildtype and IDH-mutant glioblastomas (Ohgaki et al. 2016)

	IDH wild type	IDH-mutant
Corresponds to	Clinico-pathologically defined primary Glioblastoma	Clinico-pathologically defined secondary Glioblastoma
Evolution	De novo	From lower grade astrocytoma
Proportion of glioblastomas	~90%	~10%
Age at diagnosis	Usually >60yrs	Younger adults
Clinical history	Brief	Long
Overall survival with Surgery+ radiotherapy+ chemotherapy	~15 months	~30 months
CpG methylator phenotype	Less frequent	More frequent
EGFR amplification	More frequent	Rare
TP53 overexpression	Less frequent	More frequent

The rich data has hauled several molecules into focus which hitherto evaded the notice of researchers. This has allowed the sub classification of glioblastoma into prognostically relevant molecular subgroups. In 2006, Phillips H.S et al. have classified high grade gliomas into three subgroups- Proneural, Proliferative and mesenchymal with the proneural group showing best prognosis. They used Olig2, DLL3, BCAN(Proneural), PCNA, TOP2A(proliferative), YKL-40, CD44 and VEGF (mesenchymal) as markers to histologically identify these subtypes (Phillips et al. 2006). In the seminal paper in 2008, Parson D. W.et al. have brought to centre stage, the star molecule IDH1 (Isocitrate dehydrogenase 1) whose recurrent mutations in a small subset of glioblastoma significantly correlated with better prognosis (Parsons et al. 2008). In later years, Verhaak R.G.W et al. have revamped the molecular classification and identified 4 subgroups namely Proneural, Neural, Classical and Mesenchymal. Their study focused on alterations in PDGFRA, IDH1, EGFR, and NF1 and further highlighted the importance of IDH1 mutation which was seen in the proneural group predominantly (Verhaak et al. 2010). Though both these groups of scientists used distinct methodologies and sample sets, the proneural and mesenchymal groups were robustly concordant in their molecular profiling (Table 2.4).

In the same year, H.Noushmehr's group identified the existence of CpG Island hypermethylator phenotype in a distinct subset of gliomas (G-CIMP). The highlights of this landmark paper are the findings that G-CIMP is tightly associated with IDH1 mutation, G-CIMP patients are younger at diagnosis and display improved survival, G-CIMP is more prevalent among low- and intermediate-grade gliomas and that G-CIMP tumors belong to the proneural subgroup.

All the high throughput studies on glioblastoma yielded an ocean of information on molecular alterations which may dictate the tumor progression. Many of these alterations were further studied and possible pathway involvement has been assessed. The subsequent sections detail each of these molecules that changed the face of glioblastoma research.

Table 2.4 Common findings between molecular classification of Glioblastoma proposed by Philips H.S et al (Phillips et al. 2006) and Verhaak R.G.W et al (Verhaak et al. 2010)

Philips	Proneural	Proliferative		Mesenchymal
Verhaak	Proneural	Neural	Classical	Mesenchymal
Signature	Olig2/DDL3/SOX2	MBP/MAL	EGFR/AKT2	YKL40/CD44
Mutated genes	TP53, PI3K, PDGFRA		Chr.7 gain, chr.10 loss, PDGFRA	NFkB, NF1

2.5.1 IDH Mutations

The discovery of IDH mutations is arguably the most significant contribution to the molecular pathobiology of glioblastoma. It has kick-started an era of genetic and molecular research and diagnosis. *IDH* enzyme is of three subtypes- *IDH1*, *IDH2*, *IDH3* (Yan et al. 2009). Five genes encode for these three subtypes. *IDH1* is predominantly cytosolic whereas *IDH2* and *IDH3* are predominantly found in the mitochondrial matrix. *IDH3* catalyses the conversion of isocitrate to α-ketoglutarate(α-KG) and NAD+ to NADH(Kreb's cycle).The other two isoforms catalyze the same reaction, but outside of the Kreb's cycle and reduce NADP + to nicotinamide adenine dinucleotide phosphate(NADPH).These products are essential for the generation of ATP required for the cell survival. Also, studies have shown that cells with low levels of *IDH* became more sensitive to oxidative damage. Thus, in addition to being a major enzyme in the citric acid cycle, *IDH* also plays an important role in cellular defense against oxidative stress (Marko and Weil 2013).

A multi-institutional study in 2008 by Parson et al., found point mutations in *IDH* 1 gene in a small subset of glioblastoma samples (Parsons et al. 2008). Further analysis showed that the IDH mutant glioblastomas corresponded pretty convincingly to the clinicopathologically defined secondary glioblastomas. This landmark finding set off further studies on grade II and grade III tumours which revealed that *IDH* 1 mutation is common in low grade diffuse gliomas and that *IDH2* mutation also was present occasionally. The patients with *IDH1/IDH2* mutated tumour had a better survival than those who did not harbour these mutations (Yan et al. 2009).

Later, when Verhaak R.G.W et al. molecularly classified glioblastoma based on gene expression, they have defined the proneural subtype as the group possessing mutations in the PDGFRA or in IDH1/2. The proneural GBM is further subdivided into G-CIMP positive and negative subgroups based on characteristic DNA methylation patterns that are directly linked to the IDH1/2 mutational status and better prognosis (Noushmehr et al. 2010) (Noushmehr H. et al., 2010).

IDH 1 mutations observed in gliomas are most often point mutations at position 132 (R132H) (Parsons et al. 2008), where wild type Arginine is replaced by Histidine. This mutation is also popularly referred to as canonical *IDH* 1 mutation. The nucleotide change causing this mutation is G395A, i.e., change of nucleotide from G to A at the position 395.Other rarer mutations at this position include R132C(Arginine to Cysteine), R132S (Serine), R132L (Leucine), R132G (Glycine), R132V (Valine). All these mutations are missense and heterozygous mutations (Table 2.5).

Table 2.5 Summary of *IDH* mutations and their respective nucleotide changes (Yan et al. 2009)

IDH 1:	
Arg132His(R132H)	395G>A
Arg132Cys (R132C)	394C > T
Arg132Ser (R132S)	394C > A
Arg132Gly (R132G)	394 C > G
Arg132Leu (R132L)	395G > T
Arg132Val (R132V)	394_395 CG > GT
IDH2:	
Arg172Lys (R172K)	515G > A
Arg172Met (R172M)	515G > T
Arg172Trp (R172W)	514A > T
Arg172Ser (R172S)	516G > T
Arg172Gly (R172G)	514A > G

The R132 residue is evolutionarily conserved being located in the active site of the enzyme and is essential for isocitrate binding (Xu et al. 2004). The mutation at R132 makes the protein incompatible with binding to isocitrate and abolishes its' normal catalytic activity. This results in reduced levels of α-KGand NADPH, which is an important cofactor, and essential for the maintenance of normal levels of reduced glutathione (GSH) to combat reactive oxygenspecies. R132 mutated *IDH1* has an altered binding site favouring α-KetoGlutarate (α-KG) over isocitrate which results in increased production of 2-hydroxyglutarate (2-HG), which is an oncometabolite, in the cells harbouring the mutation (Dang et al. 2010). 2-HG competitively inhibits the activity of many α-KG-dependent dioxygenases which are a diverse group of enzymes that have control over several important physiological processes like hypoxia sensing, chromatin remodeling through demethylation of histone, demethylation of hypermethylated DNA, fatty acid metabolism, and collagen modification, among others (Loenarz and Schofield 2008). Thus, *IDH1* mutations lead to a series of events like DNA hypermethylation of CpG Islands in the promoters of various genes (G-CIMP), histone hypermethylation, etc. Both DNA and histone hypermethylation are thought to arrest cellular differentiation by transcriptional silencing of a broad spectrum of target genes (Turcan et al. 2012).

IDH2 is the only human protein homolog of *IDH1* that uses NADP+ as a proton acceptor. What R132 is to *IDH1*, is what R172 is for *IDH2*. Five point mutations have been identified in *IDH2*, where arginine at 172(R172) is replaced with glycine (R172G), methionine (R172 M), lysine (R172 K), serine (R172S), and tyrosine (R172Y).

Studies focusing on temporal sequence of genetic alterations have found that *IDH1* mutations occur early in the development of IDH-mutant diffuse gliomas. This discovery saw the light of day when Watanabe et al. performed serial biopsies from single patient and *IDH* 1 mutation was found to occur before the development of 1p and 19q co-deletion which lead to oligodendroglioma development and *TP53* mutation which later became diffuse astrocytoma (Watanabe et al. 2009). Subsequently, *ATRX* mutation was found to be characteristic of diffuse astrocytomas. However, the IDH wild type gliomas, comprising predominantly the glioblastomas, are thought to develop through a separate sequence of molecular events (Fig. 2.8).

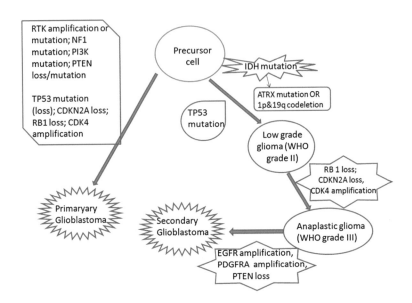

Fig. 2.8 Illustrates the sequence of genetic changes occurring in the evolution of primary and secondary glioblastoma

IDH mutations, due to the clinical relevance they carry, have found their way into routine diagnostics. *IDH* mutational analysis was previously done by sequencing the *IDH* gene. But eventually, Capper et al. have successfully raised the monoclonal antibody to mutant *IDH1* R132H protein in mouse (Capper et al. 2009). This antibody is now used routinely for immunohistochemistry on formalin fixed paraffin embedded tissue. Since R132H is the most common mutation (nearly 90%), this modality of testing has gained popularity. At present, IHC for *IDH1*(R132H) is performed routinely to characterize all adult diffuse gliomas (Thota et al. 2012).

Raising the antibody to IDH-1 R132H mutant protein spiked the interest of researchers across the world and immunotherapy enthusiasts went ahead and developed a vaccine against the mutant *IDH1* for immunotherapy for the patients harbouring the mutation (Schumacher et al. 2014). But despite the great advancement in technology, we are still a far way behind in identifying therapeutic strategies using IDH1 mutations. Other genetic alterations that are common in IDH wild type glioblastoma are TERT promoter mutation (~80%), homologous deletion of CDKN2A/CDKN2B (~60%), loss of chromosome 10 p (~50%) and 10q (~70%), EGFR alterations (mutations/ rearrangement, altered splicing and/or amplification, ~55%), PTEN mutation/deletion (~40%), TP53 mutations (25–30%), PI3K mutations (~25%) (WHO, 2016).

Glioma CpG Island Methylated Phenotype (G-CIMP), often associated with IDH mutations, frequent in the proneural group, confers better prognosis and, shows hypermethylation of CpG islands in the promoter regions of various genes. Hypermethylation is the most commonly observed epigenetic alteration resulting in silencing of the promoter regions of genes, thus altering (decreasing) gene expression. Promoters of several genes such as cyclin-dependent kinase inhibitor 2A

(CDKN2A), RB1, PTEN, TP53, MGMT, etc., have been described, of which *MGMT* gene promoter methylation is by far the most essential in predicting the prognosis of glioblastoma (Wick et al. 2014; Hegi et al. 2008).

2.5.2 O^6-Methyl Guanine DNA Methyl Transferase (MGMT) Gene Promoter Methylation

MGMT has been extensively studied in glioblastoma. Being a DNA repair enzyme, it has attracted the attention of scientists in oncology for a very long time. Towards the end of the 20th century, study of MGMT expression and its importance in gliomas began picking up speed. Starting with protein expression studies which showed inconclusive results, the research centered on this gene in gliomas has gone a long way due to its association with response to alkylating agents, especially Temozolomide in gliomas (Hegi et al. 2005).Epigenetic silencing of MGMT gene through promoter methylation has established itself as a significant event in a subset of glioblastomas.

MGMT is the gene encoding O^6-Methyl Guanine DNA Methyl Transferase which is a DNA repair enzyme which removes alkyl groups (such as methyl groups) from the O^6 position of guanine within the DNA. This phenomenon is of particular importance in glioblastoma as the chemotherapeutic agent, Temozolomide, which is the current standard treatment for Glioblastoma, acts by causing damage to the tumour cell DNA by adding methyl groups to the O^6 position of guanine. Such damage is usually repaired by MGMT. Thus, a tumour with high *MGMT* activity would be resistant to the chemotherapy. Methylation of the promoter region of this gene will silence the gene and prevent the repair of chemotherapy induced DNA damage, thus, possibly making the tumour more responsive to chemotherapy.

Due to its clinical significance, MGMT promoter methylation status has been considered in various clinical trials assessing treatment response in glioblastoma (Hegi et al. 2008; Malmström et al. 2012; Stupp et al. 2009; Stupp et al. 2014; Hart et al. 2011). The earliest clinical trials showed that a combined treatment approach (temozolomide with radiotherapy) seemed to have better outcomes with improved progression-free and overall survival compared to either treatment modality alone, raising the question of the utility of routinely testing for MGMT promoter methylation status (Hegi et al. 2005), (Stupp et al. 2009). The Nordic trial found that the patients aged over 60 years, treated with temozolomide who had tumour MGMT promoter methylation had significantly longer survival than those without MGMT promoter methylation. Standard-dose TMZ (5 out of 28 days) was found to be superior to standard radiotherapy in patients older than 70 years with methylated MGMT promoter (Malmström et al. 2012). Based on the findings of various clinical trials like NOA-8, Nordic trial, Stupp's study, and others, the EANO suggests that the patients who are not thought to be candidates for standard chemo-radiotherapy(based on performance status), may be provided either radiation or temozolomide monotherapy, depending on their MGMT methylation status (Taylor and Schiff 2015),

(Weller et al. 2014).Thus, testing for MGMT promoter methylation is recommended for elderly patients with glioblastoma as this could aid in the decision of the course of management. However, in younger patients, though a methylated MGMT promoter confers a good prognosis, it does not determine the choice of management, as a combined therapy is shown to be associated with better survival than monotherapy in these patients.

With increasing awareness of personalized medicine, testing for MGMT promoter methylation status is gaining impetus and is now being performed for all patients with the diagnosis of glioblastoma, if not for treatment decision, at least to understand the prognosis. *MGMT* gene promoter methylation testing becomes especially important in a subset of patients who develop pseudoprogression after the onset of treatment with Temozolomide. Pseudoprogression is defined by an increase in contrast-enhancement accompanied sometimes with clinical symptomatology, but there is subsequent improvement and stabilization. Its underlying mechanism could be induced by a local inflammatory reaction, with abnormal vessel permeability and edema (Hygino da Cruz et al. 2011). If an MGMT-methylated tumor under treatment with temozolomide develops pseudoprogression on imaging, chemotherapy should not therefore be stopped (Jansen et al. 2010). On the other hand, if clinical and radiological features suggestive of pseudoprogression are present in temozolomide-treated non MGMT-methylated glioblastoma, they likely represent bonafide tumor progression, and a change in therapy should be considered. More often than not, MGMT promoter methylation is seen in the patients presenting with pseudoprogression, according to a study by Stupp's group (Weller et al. 2010) .

Various methods of MGMT promoter methylation testing were assessed for accurate estimation. Immunohistochemistry was assessed for its efficiency at detecting MGMT protein expression which did not correlate significantly with promoter methylation and with survival (Christmann et al. 2010).Methylation specific PCR was made popular by Esteller M et al. which correlated significantly with survival (Esteller et al. 1999). Though various other methods like quantitative MSP (Vlassenbroeck et al. 2008), methylation specific multiplex ligation- dependent probe amplification (Kim et al. 2015) (Van den Bent et al.), combined bisulphate analysis (Mikeska et al. 2012), pyrosequencing (Christians et al. 2012) (Ronaghi et al., Christians et al.), HM27K and HM450k Bead chip (Bady et al. 2012), High Resolution melt analysis (Switzeny et al. 2016), etc. are being investigated for their efficacy, the methods being widely used clinically are semi quantitative methylation specific PCR (MS PCR) (Hegi et al. 2008), quantitative real time MS PCR(qRT-PCR) and pyrosequencing.

2.5.3   ATRX Mutation

The latest contribution to molecular diagnosis of gliomas is the discovery of Alpha Thalassemia/Mental Retardation Syndrome X-Linked (*ATRX*) gene (Wiestler et al. 2013). The gene is so named because germline mutations in *ATRX* are associated with alpha thalassemia mental retardation X-linked (ATR-X) syndrome (Gibbons et al. 1995).*ATRX* gene is located at Xq21.1 and is a DNA helicase and chromatin remodeling protein. *ATRX* mutations are loss-of-function mutations. A primary function of *ATRX* is incorporation of histone H3.3 monomers into chromatin in collaboration with the histone chaperone protein DAXX (Death-associated protein 6) (Goldberg et al. 2010; Lewis et al. 2010). This form of chromatin remodeling is essential for maintenance of inactive proportion of the genome in a compact organization which is refractory to regulatory activity (Brennan et al. 2013). Thus, a mutation in ATRX would result in loss of this compact chromatin organization and thereby exposure of the region of genome which should be inactive.

It was in 2012 that *ATRX* mutations were identified in adult and paediatric gliomas (Kannan et al. 2012; Liu et al. 2012; Schwartzentruber et al. 2012). Shortly after the discovery, it had quickly gained impetus and redefined the classification of adult gliomas, as suggested by a publication from Von Deimling's group (Wiestler et al. 2013). *ATRX* loss characterizes astrocytoma and is mutually exclusive with 1p and 19q codeletion which is seen in oligodendroglioma. Thus, a tumor which would have previously been thought of as a glioblastoma-O, can now be characterized using 1p and 19q codeletion status and ATRX mutational status. ATRX mutations are relatively rare in IDH wild type glioblastoma. Among the IDH mutant gliomas, about 60–70% of them show ATRX mutation (Foote et al. 2015).

ATRX loss (mutation) is strongly associated with *TP53* mutation which is again, a more common feature of IDH mutant gliomas. *ATRX* has also been found to play a role in the regulation of telomere length as shown by studies which found that the ALT phenotype (alternative lengthening of telomeres) was significantly correlated with *ATRX* loss (Wiestler et al. 2013). This regulation of telomere length is essential for tumor cell immortality.

Molecular testing for *ATRX* is now routinely done using Immunohistochemistry (IHC). Since the mutation predominantly results in a truncated protein or abrogated protein expression, the mutant phenotype is evidenced by the loss of expression of the protein. During IHC interpretation, it is important to note that retention of *ATRX* expression is seen in the normal endothelial cells, native and reactive glial cells and overrun neurons. This serves as an internal control. Therefore it is important to assess ATRX immunoreactivity in the tumor core rather than its' infiltrating front.

2.5.4 TP53 Mutation

TP53 is the most widely studied gene in cancer research. Popularly known as the guardian of the genome, its mutations have been implicated in numerous human cancers. TP53 mutation was initially thought to be the earliest mutation leading to glioma genesis, as with other cancers. It was only much later that the identification of IDH mutations being the earliest changes, even prior to TP53 mutation, surprised the world (Watanabe et al. 2009). TP53 mutations, along with IDH and ATRX mutations are now considered molecular hallmark features of diffuse and anaplastic astrocytomas (WHO grades II and III) as well as clinicopathologically defined secondary glioblastoma (Liu et al. 2012; Gillet et al. 2014). It is also of interest to note that giant cell glioblastomas usually possess TP53 mutations (Meyer-Puttlitz et al. 1997). The cascade of molecular events triggered by the mutation of TP53 gene involving the p53/MDM2/p14ARF pathway is one of the key events in gliomagenesis.

2.5.5   TERT Promoter Mutation

Maintenance of the telomeres in the tumour cells is an essential step towards cancer cell immortality. As mentioned earlier, alternate lengthening of telomere (ALT) phenotype is associated with ATRX mutation. Another mechanism by which the tumour cells maintain the telomeres is through the telomerase reverse transcriptase (TERT) (Horn et al. 2013). It is a catalytic subunit of the enzyme telomerase. Telomerase is an enzyme which essentially maintains the telomere length. This is repressed under physiological conditions leading to progressive shortening of telomeres. The mutations leading to aberrant expression would maintain telomere length, thus imparting immortality to the cell.

TERT gene promoter mutations are point mutations usually affecting positions −228 and −250 in the promoter region, substituting a cytosine for a thymine (228 C > T, 250C > T). This unmasks a binding site for GA-binding protein (GABP) transcription factor which binds to the mutant promoter, causing aberrant expression of TERT (Koelsche et al. 2013; Arita et al. 2013).

These mutations were first discovered in melanoma, and are thought to increase the expression of telomerase, thereby maintaining telomere length and enabling repeated cell division (Horn et al. 2013).These mutations have later been identified in many CNS tumours, including glioblastoma (Killela et al. 2013). TERT mutations are more common in IDH wild type glioblastomas than in the IDH mutant form. Within the IDH wild type glioblastoma, TERT promoter mutation is inversely related to the TP53 mutations (Brennan et al. 2013; Nonoguchi et al. 2013). The IDH mutant glioblastoma preferentially makes use of ATRX mutation induced alternate lengthening of telomere pathway. TERT promoter mutations and polymorphisms have been reported to be associated with shorter survival in several studies (Mosrati et al. 2015; Spiegl-Kreinecker et al. 2015; Yuan et al. 2016).

2.5.6   Cytogenetic Abnormalities

A wide variety of chromosomal alterations are found in glioblastoma, of which, the most common alterations are gain of chromosome 7 and loss of chromosomes 9,10 and 13. The combination of gain of 7p and loss of 10q (7p+/ 10q-) is most frequently encountered in glioblastoma (Homma et al. 2006). Chromosome 7 harbours

EGFR gene on its short arm and the key gene affected by loss of 10q is PTEN. Hence, EGFR amplification and PTEN deletion are associated with 7p+/10q-. However, mutations in these genes are less frequently encountered. Another combination of chromosomal alteration found, though less often, in glioblastoma is the combined gain of chromosomes 19 and 20.

2.5.7 EGFR Amplification and Mutation

As discussed above, 7p gain is associated with EGFR (Epithelial Growth Factor Receptor)gene amplification. It is more common in clinicopathologically defined primary glioblastoma and other IDH wild type gliomas and is often found in the classical glioblastomasubtype (Verhaak et al. 2010). EGFR, under normal physiological conditions, plays a central role in various normal cellular processes such as cell proliferation, differentiation and development.

EGFR is located on the short arm of the chromosome 7 (7p12) which encodes a cell surface receptor tyrosine kinase, a member of erb-1 family of receptors (Hatanpaa et al. 2010). Binding of growth factor ligand to extracellular domain and phosphorylation on the intracellular domain activates EGFR and this initiates signal transduction cascades (Ras/MAPK and PI3K /Akt) leading to increased DNA transcription, angiogenesis, anti-apoptosis and cellular proliferation.

In addition to amplification, mutations are also commonplace in glioblastoma. Several mutants may be present in one tumor itself, contributing to intra-tumor heterogeneity. EGFR mutant (EGFR vIII) is detected in about 50% of tumours with EGFR amplification. EGFR vIII is generated from a deletion in exon 2–7 of the EGFR gene which results in the frame shift deletion of 267 amino acids in the extracellular domain of EGFR (Hatanpaa et al. 2010).EGFR vIII does not bind to the growth factor ligand as the receptor is truncated with a short extracellular domain, but is constitutively phosphorylated. This structural abnormality mimics the effect of ligand binding and induces conformational change in the receptor, followed by increased intracellular signaling and cell proliferation (Nishikawa et al. 1994). Studies have shown that EGFR vIII expressing cells not only drive their own intrinsic growth but also increase the proliferation of adjacent wild type EGFR expressing cells by paracrine signaling through cytokine receptors (Inda et al. 2010).

Another mutant EGFR vII is also generated by deletion of exon 2–7 of the EGFR gene and is present in 9% of focally EGFR amplified cases. Constitutive expression of EGFR vII results in the downstream activation of Akt signaling similar to that of EGFR vIII.

In the light of molecular studies, it has become clear now that various genetic alterations involving EGFR in glioblastoma are distinct from those observed in other EGFR altered cancers. In glioma, focal EGFR amplification occurs at extremely high level. Vast majority of other mutations are EGFR vIII point and missense mutations which are found exclusively in the extracellular domain (Lee et al. 2006), while most mutations in other non-glioma cancer are found in the intracellular domain

(Jänne et al. 2005). EGFR phosphorylation of EGFRvIII leads to nuclear transport of EGFRvIII and enhanced formation of a complex between EGFRvIII and STAT3 in the nucleus suggesting that EGFR and EGFRvIII coordinate to drive enhanced and prolonged STAT3 activity in the nucleus (Fan et al. 2013).

Though EGFR is clearly an important genetic alteration found in glioblastoma, various groups studying its association with survival and its prognostic significance have produced disagreeing results. While some groups found that EGFR vIII over-expression along with EGFR amplification was associated with poor prognosis in younger patients (Shinojima et al. 2003), other studies showed that EGFR overexpression was associated with poor prognosis in older individuals (Srividya et al. 2010). Yet another study showed that EGFR over expression did not carry prognostic significance in the natural history of disease (Heimberger et al. 2005).

Thus identifying the EGFR gene status in glioblastoma may be useful only for identifying the subset of patients who may benefit from EGFR targeted therapy.

2.5.8   PTEN Mutation

The chromosomal arm 10q harbours the gene *PTEN* (phosphatase and tensin homolog deleted on chromosome 10), which was originally identified in 1997 as a tumour suppressor gene that was mutated in prostate, breast and brain tumours, including glioblastoma (Li et al. 1997). PTEN protein catalyses the dephosporylation of the 3` phosphate of the inositol ring in PIP3, resulting in the biphosphate product PIP2. This dephosphorylation is important because it results in inhibition of the AKT signaling pathway. PI3K/AKT pathway is usually dormant in differentiated and quiescent cells. When this pathway is activated, cell cycle regulation goes hay-wire and oncogenesis ensues. *PTEN* deletion primarily acts through AKT and PI3K pathway by functioning as a lipid phosphatase (Endersby and Baker 2008).Thus, *PTEN* deletion and loss of 10q (including *PTEN*) are associated with more aggressive phenotype (Srividya et al. 2011).

2.5.9   Platelet Derived Growth Factor Receptor Alpha(PDGFRA)

PDGFRA makes its appearance during normal CNS development and regulates normal glial cell proliferation and oligodendrocyte differentiation (Richardson et al. 1988). PDGFRA expression has been shown to be increased in various cancers including brain tumor (Shih and Holland 2006).

The gene encodes a transmembrane protein belonging to the class III family of receptor tyrosine kinases (RTKs). The binding of ligand to this receptor triggers downstream signaling pathways like, MAPK, PI3K/AKT and JAK/STAT and plays an important role in cell proliferation, cell migration and angiogenesis (Lu et al.

2001). Thus, an enhanced expression of PDGFRA would result in excessive proliferation, angiogenesis, etc. which are features of malignancy.

In glioblastoma, amplification of the PDGFRA gene is found in 15% of all
tumors,

mainly in the proneural subtype of GBM (Verhaak et al. 2010). PDGFRA may
be altered through various genetic mechanisms such as amplification, mutation and
truncation (Phillips et al. 2013).*PDGFRAΔ8, 9* is the frequent gene rearrangement
in PDGFRA-amplified GBM, formed by an in-frame deletion of 243 bp in exons 8
and 9 of the extracellular portion (Kumabe et al. 1992). In addition to this deletion,
in-frame gene fusion of the extracellular domain of KDR/VEGFR-2 and the intracellular domain of PDGFRA has also been found, and both of these mutant proteins
were shown to be constitutively active, display transforming ability and could be
inhibited using inhibitors of PDGFRA (Cancer Genome Atlas Research Network
2008).A recent study on PDGFRA amplification in a large set of pediatric and adult
high grade gliomas showed that, PDGFRA amplification had no prognostic significance in pediatric high grade glioma patients but is associated with worse overall
survival in adult IDH1 –R132H mutant, Glioblastoma (Phillips et al. 2013).

2.5.10 Neurofibromatosis Type 1 Gene (NF1)Inactivation

NF1 gene is a potent tumor suppressor gene which codes for neurofibromin, whose
negative regulation of Ras and mTOR signaling in astrocytes is responsible for antitumor effect. Hence, an inactivation of this gene can cause tumorigenicity. The
genetic alterations in NF1 gene in glioblastoma are deletions and inactivating mutations. Mutations of NF1 are predominantly seen in mesenchymal subgroup of glioblastoma (Verhaak et al. 2010). NF1 loss results in increased cell proliferation and
migration that is dependent on Ras mediated hyperactivation of mTOR. Evidence
from experiments using genetically engineered mouse models shows that NF1 loss
in glial cells, in combination with a germline p53 mutation, results in fully penetrant
malignant astrocytomas (Zhu et al. 2005), which progress to glioblastoma upon
deletion of PTEN (Kwon et al. 2008).

2.5.11 Signaling Pathways Altered in Glioblastoma:

– **Receptor tyrosine kinase/ PI3K/ PTEN/AKT/mTOR pathway** (**Altered in
  88% glioblastomas** (Cancer Genome Atlas Research Network 2008)) (Fig. 2.9):
– The PI3K/AKT/mTOR pathway is an intracellular signaling pathway which is
  important in regulating the cell cycle. Under normal physiological conditions,
  this pathway is essential to promote growth and proliferation over differentiation
  of adult stem cells and neural stem cells specifically (Peltier et al. 2007). The first
  intracellular component of this pathway is phosphatidylinositol 3-kinase (PI3K)

Fig. 2.9 Illustrates the P53 and the RB pathways. $\triangle$ Indicates gene activating alterations like amplification and $\triangledown$ indicates gene inactivating alterations like deletion. The more commonly altered genes are highlighted in purple. Inhibition is indicated by – and activation is indicated by +

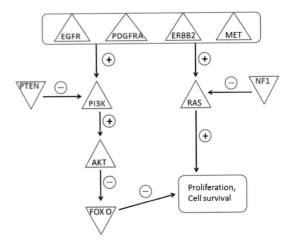

RTK/ PI3K signalling pathway

complex, which, when activated sets into action a series of genes with Akt (also called protein kinase B) first, followed by mTOR, which integrates several upstream signals into effector actions on multiple downstream targets involved in cell growth and division (Mao et al. 2012). The triggering stimulus for the cascade of events is the activation of receptor tyrosine kinase family members, most notably, EGFR, ERBB2, PDGFRA, c-MET, etc. Hence, gene activating alterations like gene amplification or activating mutation will lead to the cascade of events which enhance cell proliferation. However, genes like PTEN usually put a check on cell proliferation by inhibiting PI3K. Thus, an inactivating mutation or deletion of this gene will not limit the activation of PI3K, leading to aberrant cell proliferation (Cancer Genome Atlas Research Network 2008).

– **P53/MDM2/p14ARF pathway (altered in 87% glioblastomas** (Cancer Genome Atlas Research Network 2008)) (Fig. 2.9):

– P53, as described earlier, is a key tumor suppressor gene and also a broad transcription factor which regulates over 2500 genes involved in tumorigenesis and tumor invasion. An inactivating mutation in TP53 or negative regulation of TP53 results in tumorigenesis. MDM2 and MDM4 are essential negative regulators of TP53 gene. MDM2 may inactivate p53 through transcriptional inhibition by direct binding, and degradation through its E3 ligase activity. MDM4 inactivates p53 only through transcriptional inhibition. Thus, gene activating alterations in MDM2 and MDM4 such as amplifications inhibit p53 and contribute to oncogenesis. A gene CDKN2A (p14 ARF), which is further upstream to MDM2, inhibits regulation of p53 pathway by directly binding to MDM2 and subsequently inhibiting its E3 ubiquitin ligase activity (Toledo and Wahl 2007) (Kamijo et al. 1998),. Thus, an inactivating alteration in CDKN2A results in uninhibited action of MDM2 which in turn, inhibits p53. This pathway is altered in 87% of glioblastomas.

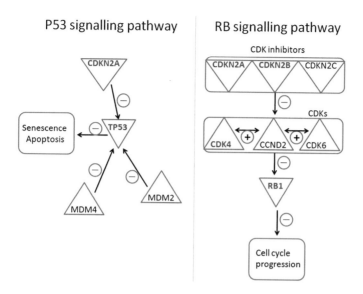

Fig. 2.10 Illustrates the RTK/PI3K pathway. Δ Indicates gene activating alterations like amplification and ∇ indicates gene inactivating alterations like deletion. The more commonly altered genes are highlighted in purple. Inhibition is indicated by – and activation is indicated by +

- **CDKN2A/CDK4/retinoblastoma protein pathway (altered in 78% glioblastomas** (Cancer Genome Atlas Research Network 2008)) (Fig. 2.10):

The RB gene codes for a tumor suppressor protein retinoblastoma (pRB) which plays a crucial role in inhibiting cell cycle progression by binding to and inhibiting transcription factors of the E2F family. Hence, an inactivating alteration of RB gene leads to uninhibited cell division. The RB gene is negatively regulated by the complex of cyclin-dependent kinases (CDKs), notably, CDK4, CCND2, CDK6. Thus, an activating alteration in these kinases accentuates the inhibition of RB gene, leading to excessive cell proliferation. These Cyclin Dependent kinases are normally inhibited by CDK inhibitors, CDKN2A, CDKN2B and CDKN2C. When these inhibitors suffer inactivating alterations, it would result in unchecked cyclin-dependent kinase activity and thus, exaggerated RB inhibition, thus leading to aberrant cell proliferation (Cancer Genome Atlas Research Network 2008; Mao et al. 2012).

2.6 Molecular Biology of Recurrence in Glioblastoma Tumors

Glioblastoma is notorious for its inevitable recurrence after maximal safe resection despite concomitant radiation and chemotherapy following surgery. The recurrent tumor tends to come back with a vengeance and is more resistant to therapy. Currently, there is no accepted standard therapy for recurrent glioblastoma. A select few patients derive benefit from a re-surgery with majority being left out in the proverbial cold due to lack of approved therapy with promising results. Strikingly, not many studies focus on recurrent glioblastoma. One major reason for this is that not all recurrent tumors are operable, limiting the access to the recurrent tumor tissue. Thus, paired tumor sample scarcity precludes any molecular studies on recurrent glioblastoma. As a result, research on recurrence has been mostly limited to documentation of clinical characteristics and very few clinical trials using angiogenesis inhibitors, etc. Our knowledge on recurrence mainly stems from a handful of studies. Recurrences are predominantly local (recurring within 2 cm margin of the original tumor) with only a small proportion coming back as distant recurrences(recurring distantly in a different lobe or in contralateral hemisphere). The genetic makeup of the local and distant recurrences when compared to their primary counterparts still remains largely unknown, though some recent studies have attempted to answer this question. The genetic landscape of local recurrences was thought be similar to the original tumor and the distant recurrences were argued to be possibly second primary tumors (Reis et al. 2001; Martinez et al. 2003). However, other researchers identified sufficient similarities between the primary and distant recurrent tumors to conclude that they were indeed remote recurrences rather than entirely new primary tumors (van Nifterik et al. 2006). In a recent study comparing the mutations in the local and distant recurrences with their original primary tumors, distant recurrences were found to share an average 25% of mutations with their primary tumors while local recurrences possessed an average of 70% of shared mutations (Kim et al. 2015).

The few studies which attempted to understand molecular profile of recurrent vs primary tumors, had compared only a few candidate genes and had a small sample size and none of them considered the intratumor heterogeneity (Campos et al. 2016). A summary of the studies is listed in Table 2.6.

Mounting evidence points towards definite alterations in recurrent glioblastoma, the nature of which depends on the profile of first tumor. For example, in conjunction with the above studies, other researchers have found evidence of tumor evolution possibly in response to radio-chemotherapy. For example, primary glioblastomas with MGMT promoter methylation were found to lose the methylation with higher MGMT expression in recurrent tumors (Christmann et al. 2010). Consequently, a series of clinical trials with dose-intensified treatment with Temozolomide came into effect, however, the results were not promising (Gilbert et al. 2013). Kim, et al., while analyzing 21 paired samples, found that one recurrent glioblastoma had a hypermutated phenotype and that was originally an IDH1 mutant. The authors suggested that IDH1, commonly associated with a hypermethylator phenotype may have suppressed MGMT and rendered the tumor more susceptible to temozolomide induced mutagenesis. Interesting to note is the fact that majority of the accumulated mutations were found to affect mismatch repair genes like PMS1 and MSH5 (Kim et al. 2015).

Evidence from several studies which assessed the possible effect of treatment modality on glioblastoma recurrence suggests that, altogether, glioblastomas undergo evolutionary change and selective pressures such as radio-chemotherapy and targeted therapies are likely to alter the molecular composition of these tumors

Table 2.6 Summary of genetic alterations studied so far in recurrent glioblastoma

Genes studied	Findings
MLH1, MSH2, MSH6	Expression lower in recurrence (Stark et al. 2010; Shinsato et al. 2013)
TP53 and PTEN mutation, EGFR amplification	One study found lower expression at recurrence (Stark et al. 2003). Another study identified two distinct patterns of accumulation of molecular alterations depending on the profile of the original tumor (Martinez et al. 2010).
Methylation of promoters of MGMT, CASP8, CASP3, CASP9, DCR1, DR4, DR5, TMS1, CDH1, CDH13, RASSF1A, BLU, CHFR, CASP8	More methylation observed at recurrence (Martinez et al. 2007)
miRNA-10b, miRNA-21, miRNA-181b, miRNA-181c, miRNA-195, miRNA-221, miRNA-222	No change observed at recurrence (Ilhan-Mutlu et al. 2013)

(Campos et al. 2016). However, the original tumor composition plays a significant role, of which, tumor heterogeneity is a major player. As discussed earlier, glioblastomas possess such heterogeneity as not seen in most other malignancies. Intertumor heterogeneity is clearly evidenced by histomorphology. But intratumor heterogeneity of glioblastoma is unmistakable when molecular profiling is done. For instance, Andor et al. have found as many as seven subclones within 100 mg of tumor tissue (Andor et al. 2014). This heterogeneity makes it difficult to predict which clonal subtype has re-emerged and hence, will respond to which type of agent. Though angiogenesis inhibitors like Bevacizumab have seen response in some patients, intratumor heterogeneity clearly explains its failure in other patients. The same group studied the effect of Temozolomide on the number of subclones in recurrent tumors, and showed that three types of changes may occur in this respect. A dominant subclone in primary tumor may shrink and disappear in recurrence or a dominant subclone may resist treatment and remain a dominant subclone or a smaller subclone may resist treatment and emerge as the dominant subclone in recurrence. Thus, future research focusing on understanding intratumor heterogeneity and predicting the possible molecular landscape of recurrent glioblastoma will greatly help in decision making in the treatment of recurrent glioblastoma.

Another line of research in recurrence has focused on the cancer stem cells present within the tumor which are relatively slow-dividing as compared to the fast-dividing glioblastoma cells (Lathia et al. 2011; Richichi et al. 2013). It is thought that through various cell to cell signaling methods, the therapy resistant, slow-growing cells are maintained in a quiescent state by the fast-growing neighboring cells. When these inhibitory signals are lost due to resection of the tumor, the remaining slow-growing cells regain their proliferative potential to cause recurrence. Cancer stem cells are resistant to therapy due to various properties analogous to normal stem cells, like overexpression of DNA-damage repair enzymes (Bao et al. 2006), metabolic traits which allow for their growth in hypoxic conditions (Li et al. 2009), their slow growth helping them escape the routine therapy which is targeted at proliferating cells, etc. Therefore, glioblastoma cancer stem cells play a role in recurrence.

Further research attempting to identify molecular patterns of recurrence in glioblastoma is direly needed to address the pressing issue of tumor recurrence and consequently poor survival in glioblastoma patients.

2.7 Summary

In view of the evolving molecular landscape of glioblastoma and the emphasis on arriving at a histomolecular diagnosis, one must bear in mind the following essentials:

(a) Two entities of Glioblastoma are now recognized- IDH wild type and IDH mutant.

(b) Clinicopathologically defined primary (de novo) glioblastoma is usually IDH wild type and clinicopathologically defined secondary glioblastoma corresponds to IDH mutant type.

(c) IDH mutant type has a significantly better prognosis than an IDH wild type glioblastoma.

(d) MGMT promoter methylation confers better prognosis to the patients with glioblastoma and is an independent prognostic factor.

(e) Pseudoprogression is commonly associated with MGMT methylated phenotype and resolves with steroids and Temozolomide therapy is continued.

(f) In MGMT unmethylated cases, pseudoprogression is usually rare and it is more likely to be recurrence rather than pseudoprogression. They are less likely to respond to Temozolomide therapy and other drugs may be required.

(g) Molecular sub-classification of glioblastoma may be of prognostic value with proneural type showing better prognosis which may, again be due to the fact that IDH mutations occur with high frequency in the proneural type.

(h) Most common molecular alterations conferring poor prognosis in glioblastoma are: EGFR amplification with EGFRvIII mutation, PTEN deletion, TERT promoter mutation.

2.8 Clinical Trials

Clinical trials using targeted drug therapies against IDH1, EGFRvIII, Tyrosine receptor kinases, etc., have been performed with mixed results. IDH1 R132H vaccine has been developed in the hope that they can be of use in IDH mutant glioblastomas (Schumacher et al. 2014). It has, so far, shown promising results in animal models (Dimitrov et al. 2015). Two clinical trials are currently in effect using IDH 1 and 2 mutant inhibitors.

Another molecular alteration that has successfully reached the clinical trial phase is the EGFR vIII mutant amplification (Taylor et al. 2012). Animal experiments have shown that tumors with this mutation are found to be sensitive to Cetuximab (Padfield et al. 2015). Several small molecule inhibitors, vaccines developed against various mutants have failed to show significance in the treatment of glioblastoma, the possible reason could be the extensive intratumor heterogeneity seen in glioblastoma.

2.9 Need of the Hour

As discussed above, the various exploratory studies carried out in glioblastoma have unearthed several mutations, epigenetic modifications, chromosomal aberrations, gene copy number changes, etc. But we are still a long way from developing a therapeutic strategy which will increase the longevity of the patients with good quality of life. The first hurdle towards achieving this is the incomplete understanding of the pathobiology of glioblastoma. Though the large scale 'omic' studies have made significant contribution towards this, there remain various missing links in the pathways and the holistic picture is lacking. The key areas of research currently in vogue in glioblastoma are aimed at understanding inter and intratumor heterogeneity, glioblastoma cancer stem cell biology, angiogenesis, tumor metabolism, resistance to therapeutic response, etc. However, a major aspect of glioblastoma, which is its invariable recurrence, has been relatively less studied and the treatment of patients with recurrence poses a dilemma to the treating clinicians. Limited number of hypotheses trying to explain the inevitable recurrence have been put forth, of which, the theory in vogue is that since the tumor cannot be completely resected due to its diffuse nature, tumor cells which escape resection may also resist radiation and chemotherapy and cause recurrence. Further research addressing this question is essential to help those patients who may have benefited from the primary treatment but presented with recurrence.

The initial excitement generated due to revelation of molecular landscape of glioblastoma had kick started the development of several inhibitors, vaccines, etc. for targeted therapy. Several of these molecules had passed the test in vitro and in animal models but failed to show significant results in the next phases. But the lesson learnt from this exercise is that the need for personalized treatment is paramount in glioblastoma due to its vastly varied features. Inter and intra tumor heterogeneity has to be fully understood if the hope for development of therapeutic strategies for glioblastoma is to be realized.

Though the data is plentiful and more is being generated this moment, there is need for further more fundamental research to understand the biological behavior of this tumor, which is the only way to handpick the right molecules which could serve as drug targets. The meaningful interpretation of the enormous data, prospective studies in the clinical setting and functional studies on the bench, building a bridge between the bedside and the bench are the need of the hour. After all, the end point to any disease related research is the benefit of the patient.

Acknowledgements The authors acknowledge the technical and scientific inputs from the Neurooncology team, NIMHANS, Mrs. Hemavathy U and Mr. K Manjunath, Department of Neuropathology, NIMHANS, for the assistance in IHC experiments and contributions towards compiling the images respectively. We are deeply indebted to NMITLI, CSIR and DBT COE programmes for their grants, supporting our research on glioblastoma.

References

Andor, N., J.V. Harness, S. Müller, H.W. Mewes, and C. Petritsch. 2014. EXPANDS: expanding ploidy and allele frequency on nested subpopulations. *Bioinformatics* 30: 50–60.

Arita, H., et al. 2013. Upregulating mutations in the TERT promoter commonly occur in adult malignant gliomas and are strongly associated with total 1p19q loss. *Acta Neuropathologica* 126: 267–276.

Bady, P., et al. 2012. MGMT methylation analysis of glioblastoma on the Infinium methylation BeadChip identifies two distinct CpG regions associated with gene silencing and outcome, yielding a prediction model for comparisons across datasets, tumor grades, and CIMP-status. *Acta Neuropathologica* 124: 547–560.

Bahuleyan, B., S. Robinson, A.R. Nair, J.L. Sivanandapanicker, and A.R. Cohen. 2013. Anatomic hemispherectomy: historical perspective. *World Neurosurgery* 80 (3–4): 396–398. <http://www.ncbi.nlm.nih.gov/pubmed/22480976>.

Bao, S., et al. 2006. Glioma stem cells promote radioresistance by preferential activation of the DNA damage response. *Nature* 444: 756–760.

Batzdorf, U., and N. Malamud. 1963. The problem of multicentric gliomas. *Journal of Neurosurgery* 20: 122–136.

Brennan, C.W., et al. 2013. The somatic genomic landscape of glioblastoma. *Cell* 155: 462–477.

Broniscer, A., et al. 2014. Clinical, radiological, histological and molecular characteristics of paediatric epithelioid glioblastoma. *Neuropathology and Applied Neurobiology* 40: 327–336.

Campos, B., L.R. Olsen, T. Urup, and H.S. Poulsen. 2016. A comprehensive profile of recurrent glioblastoma. *Oncogene*. doi:10.1038/onc.2016.85.

Cancer Genome Atlas Research Network. 2008. Comprehensive genomic characterization defines human glioblastoma genes and core pathways. *Nature* 455: 1061–1068.

Capper, D., H. Zentgraf, J. Balss, C. Hartmann, and A. von Deimling. 2009. Monoclonal antibody specific for IDH1 R132H mutation. *Acta Neuropathologica* 118: 599–601.

Christians, A., et al. 2012. Prognostic value of three different methods of MGMT promoter methylation analysis in a prospective trial on newly diagnosed glioblastoma. *PLoS One* 7: e33449.

Christmann, M., et al. 2010. MGMT activity, promoter methylation and immunohistochemistry of pretreatment and recurrent malignant gliomas: a comparative study on astrocytoma and glioblastoma. *International Journal of Cancer* 127: 2106–2118.

Dang, L., et al. 2010. Cancer-associated IDH1 mutations produce 2-hydroxyglutarate. *Nature* 465 (7300): 966. doi:10.1038/nature09132.

Dimitrov, L., C.S. Hong, C. Yang, Z. Zhuang, and J.D. Heiss. 2015. New developments in the pathogenesis and therapeutic targeting of the IDH1 mutation in glioma. *International Journal of Medical Sciences* 12: 201–213.

Ellison, D.W., B.K. Kleinschmidt-DeMasters, and S.-H. Park. 2016. Epithelioid glioblastoma. In *WHO classification of tumors of the central nervous system*, ed. Webster K. Cavenee, David N. Louis, Hiroko Ohgaki, and Otmar D. Wiestler, 4th ed., 50–51. France: International Agency for Research on Cancer (IARC).

Endersby, R., and S.J. Baker. 2008. PTEN signaling in brain: Neuropathology and tumorigenesis. *Oncogene* 27: 5416–5430.

Esteller, M., S.R. Hamilton, P.C. Burger, S.B. Baylin, and J.G. Herman. 1999. Inactivation of the DNA repair gene O6-methylguanine-DNA methyltransferase by promoter hypermethylation is a common event in primary human neoplasia. *Cancer Research* 59: 793–797.

Fan, Q.-W., et al. 2013. EGFR phosphorylates tumor-derived EGFRvIII driving STAT3/5 and progression in glioblastoma. *Cancer Cell* 24: 438–449.

Foote, M.B., et al. 2015. Genetic classification of gliomas: Refining histopathology. *Cancer Cell* 28: 9–11.

Gibbons, R.J., D.J. Picketts, L. Villard, and D.R. Higgs. 1995. Mutations in a putative global transcriptional regulator cause X-linked mental retardation with α-thalassemia (ATR-X syndrome). *Cell* 80: 837–845.

Gilbert, M.R., et al. 2013. Dose-dense temozolomide for newly diagnosed glioblastoma: a randomized phase III clinical trial. *Journal of Clinical Oncology* 31: 4085–4091.

Gillet, E., et al. 2014. TP53 and p53 statuses and their clinical impact in diffuse low grade gliomas. *Journal of Neuro-Oncology*. doi:10.1007/s11060-014-1407-4.

Goldberg, A.D., et al. 2010. Distinct factors control histone variant H3.3 localization at specific genomic regions. *Cell* 140: 678–691.

Haddad, S.F., S.A. Moore, R.L. Schelper, and J.A. Goeken. 1992. Vascular smooth muscle hyperplasia underlies the formation of glomeruloid vascular structures of glioblastoma multiforme. *Journal of Neuropathology and Experimental Neurology* 51: 488–492.

Hart, M., R. Grant, R. Garside, et al. 2011. Chemotherapy wafers for high grade glioma. *Cochrane Database of Systematic Reviews* 16: CD007294.

Hatanpaa, K.J., S. Burma, D. Zhao, and A.A. Habib. 2010. Epidermal growth factor receptor in glioma: signal transduction, neuropathology, imaging, and radioresistance. *Neoplasia* 12: 675–684.

He, J., et al. 2001. Glioblastomas with an oligodendroglial component: a pathological and molecular study. *Journal of Neuropathology and Experimental Neurology* 60: 863–871.

Hegi, M.E., et al. 2005. MGMT gene silencing and benefit from temozolomide in glioblastoma. *The New England Journal of Medicine* 352: 997–1003.

———. 2008. Correlation of O6-methylguanine methyltransferase (MGMT) promoter methylation with clinical outcomes in glioblastoma and clinical strategies to modulate MGMT activity. *Journal of Clinical Oncology* 26: 4189–4199.

Heimberger, A.B., et al. 2005. The natural history of EGFR and EGFRvIII in glioblastoma patients. *Journal of Translational Medicine* 3: 38.

Homma, T., et al. 2006. Correlation among pathology, genotype, and patient outcomes in glioblastoma. *Journal of Neuropathology and Experimental Neurology* 65: 846–854.

Horn, S., et al. 2013. TERT promoter mutations in familial and sporadic melanoma. *Science* 339: 959–961.

Hygino da Cruz, L.C., I. Rodriguez, R.C. Domingues, E.L. Gasparetto, and A.G. Sorensen. 2011. Pseudoprogression and pseudoresponse: Imaging challenges in the assessment of posttreatment glioma. *American Journal of Neuroradiology* 32: 1978–1985.

Ilhan-Mutlu, A., et al. 2013. Comparison of microRNA expression levels between initial and recurrent glioblastoma specimens. *Journal of Neuro-Oncology* 112: 347–354.

Inda, M.-M., et al. 2010. Tumor heterogeneity is an active process maintained by a mutant EGFR-induced cytokine circuit in glioblastoma. *Genes & Development* 24: 1731–1745.

Jänne, P.A., J.A. Engelman, and B.E. Johnson. 2005. Epidermal growth factor receptor mutations in non-small-cell lung cancer: implications for treatment and tumor biology. *Journal of Clinical Oncology* 23: 3227–3234.

Jansen, M., S. Yip, and D.N. Louis. 2010. Molecular pathology in adult gliomas: diagnostic, prognostic, and predictive markers. *Lancet Neurology* 9: 717–726.

Joseph, N.M., et al. 2013. Diagnostic implications of IDH1-R132H and OLIG2 expression patterns in rare and challenging glioblastoma variants. *Modern Pathology* 26: 315–326.

Kamijo, T., et al. 1998. Functional and physical interactions of the ARF tumor suppressor with p53 and Mdm2. *Proceedings of the National Academy of Sciences of the United States of America* 95: 8292–8297.

Kannan, K., et al. 2012. Whole-exome sequencing identifies ATRX mutation as a key molecular determinant in lower-grade glioma. *Oncotarget* 3: 1194–1203.

Killela, P.J., et al. 2013. TERT promoter mutations occur frequently in gliomas and a subset of tumors derived from cells with low rates of self-renewal. *Proceedings of the National Academy of Sciences of the United States of America* 110: 6021–6026.

Kim, J., et al. 2015. Spatiotemporal evolution of the primary glioblastoma genome. *Cancer Cell* 28: 318–328.

Kleinschmidt-DeMasters, B.K., D.L. Aisner, and N.K. Foreman. 2015. BRAF VE1 immunoreactivity patterns in epithelioid glioblastomas positive for BRAF V600E mutation. *The American Journal of Surgical Pathology* 39: 528–540.

Koelsche, C., et al. 2013. Distribution of TERT promoter mutations in pediatric and adult tumors of the nervous system. *Acta Neuropathologica* 126: 907–915.

Kumabe, T., Y. Sohma, T. Kayama, T. Yoshimoto, and T. Yamamoto. 1992. Overexpression and amplification of alpha-PDGF receptor gene lacking exons coding for a portion of the extracellular region in a malignant glioma. *The Tohoku Journal of Experimental Medicine* 168: 265–269.

Kwon, C.-H., et al. 2008. Pten haploinsufficiency accelerates formation of high-grade astrocytomas. *Cancer Research* 68: 3286–3294.

Lai, A., et al. 2011. Evidence for sequenced molecular evolution of IDH1 mutant glioblastoma from a distinct cell of origin. *Journal of Clinical Oncology* 29: 4482–4490.

Lathia, J.D., et al. 2011. Distribution of CD133 reveals glioma stem cells self-renew through symmetric and asymmetric cell divisions. *Cell Death & Disease* 2: e200.

Lee, J.C., et al. 2006. Epidermal growth factor receptor activation in glioblastoma through novel missense mutations in the extracellular domain. *PLoS Medicine* 3: e485.

Lewis, P.W., S.J. Elsaesser, K.-M. Noh, S.C. Stadler, and C.D. Allis. 2010. Daxx is an H3.3-specific histone chaperone and cooperates with ATRX in replication-independent chromatin assembly at telomeres. *Proceedings of the National Academy of Sciences of the United States of America* 107: 14075–14080.

Li, J., et al. 1997. PTEN, a putative protein tyrosine phosphatase gene mutated in human brain, breast, and prostate cancer. *Science* 275: 1943–1947.

Li, Z., et al. 2009. Hypoxia-inducible factors regulate tumorigenic capacity of glioma stem cells. *Cancer Cell* 15: 501–513.

Liu, X.-Y., et al. 2012. Frequent ATRX mutations and loss of expression in adult diffuse astrocytic tumors carrying IDH1/IDH2 and TP53 mutations. *Acta Neuropathologica* 124: 615–625.

Loenarz, C., and C.J. Schofield. 2008. Expanding chemical biology of 2-oxoglutarate oxygenases. *Nature Chemical Biology* 4: 152–156.

Louis, David N., Hiroko Ohgaki, Otmar D. Wiestler, Webster K. Cavenee, Peter C. Burger, Anne Jouvet, Bernd W. Scheithauer, and Paul Kleihues. 2007. The 2007 WHO Classification of tumours of the central nervous system. *Acta Neuropathologica.* doi:10.1007/s00401-007-0243-4.

Louis, David N., Arie Perry, Guido Reifenberger, Andreas von Deimling, Dominique Figarella-Branger, Webster K. Cavenee, Hiroko Ohgaki, Otmar D. Wiestler, Paul Kleihues, and David W. Ellison. 2016. The 2016 World Health Organization classification of tumors of the central nervous system: A summary. *Acta Neuropathologica* 131 (6): 803–820. doi:10.1007/s00401-016-1545-1.

Louis, D.N., et al. 2014. International society of neuropathology–haarlem consensus guidelines for nervous system tumor classification and grading. *Brain Pathology* 24: 429–435.

Louis, D.N., M.L. Suva, P.C. Burger, A. Perry, P. Kleihues, K.D. Aldape, D.J. Brat, et al. 2016. Glioblastoma, IDH-Wild Type. In *WHO classification of tumors of the central nervous system*, ed. Webster K. Cavenee, David N. Louis, Hiroko Ohgaki, and Otmar D. Wiestler, 4th ed., 28–45. France: International Agency for Research on Cancer (IARC).

Lu, Z., G. Jiang, P. Blume-Jensen, and T. Hunter. 2001. Epidermal growth factor-induced tumor cell invasion and metastasis initiated by dephosphorylation and downregulation of focal adhesion kinase. *Mol. Cell. Biol.* 21: 4016–4031.

Malmström, A., et al. 2012. Temozolomide versus standard 6-week radiotherapy versus hypofractionated radiotherapy in patients older than 60 years with glioblastoma: the Nordic randomised, phase 3 trial. *The Lancet Oncology* 13: 916–926.

Mao, H., D.G. Lebrun, J. Yang, V.F. Zhu, and M. Li. 2012. Deregulated signaling pathways in glioblastoma multiforme: molecular mechanisms and therapeutic targets. *Cancer Investigation* 30: 48–56.

Marko, N.F., and R.J. Weil. 2013. The molecular biology of WHO grade II gliomas. *Neurosurgical Focus* 34: E1.

Martinez, R., et al. 2003. Independent molecular development of metachronous glioblastomas with extended intervening recurrence-free interval. *Brain Pathology* 13: 598–607.

———. 2007. CpG island promoter hypermethylation of the pro-apoptotic gene caspase-8 is a common hallmark of relapsed glioblastoma multiforme. *Carcinogenesis* 28: 1264–1268.

Martinez, R., V. Rohde, and G. Schackert. 2010. Different molecular patterns in glioblastoma multiforme subtypes upon recurrence. *Journal of Neuro-Oncology* 96: 321–329.

Meyer-Puttlitz, B., et al. 1997. Molecular genetic analysis of giant cell glioblastomas. *The American Journal of Pathology* 151: 853–857.

Mikeska, T., C. Bock, H. Do, and A. Dobrovic. 2012. DNA methylation biomarkers in cancer: progress towards clinical implementation. *Expert Review of Molecular Diagnostics* 12: 473–487.

Miller, C.R., C.P. Dunham, B.W. Scheithauer, and A. Perry. 2006. Significance of necrosis in grading of oligodendroglial neoplasms: a clinicopathologic and genetic study of newly diagnosed high-grade gliomas. *Journal of Clinical Oncology* 24: 5419–5426.

Mosrati, M.A., et al. 2015. TERT promoter mutations and polymorphisms as prognostic factors in primary glioblastoma. *Oncotarget* 6: 16663–16673.

van Nifterik, K.A., et al. 2006. Genetic profiling of a distant second glioblastoma multiforme after radiotherapy: Recurrence or second primary tumor? *Journal of Neurosurgery* 105: 739–744.

Nishikawa, R., et al. 1994. A mutant epidermal growth factor receptor common in human glioma confers enhanced tumorigenicity. *Proceedings of the National Academy of Sciences of the United States of America* 91: 7727–7731.

Nobusawa, S., T. Watanabe, P. Kleihues, and H. Ohgaki. 2009. IDH1 mutations as molecular signature and predictive factor of secondary glioblastomas. *Clinical Cancer Research* 15: 6002–6007.

Nonoguchi, N., et al. 2013. TERT promoter mutations in primary and secondary glioblastomas. *Acta Neuropathologica* 126: 931–937.

Noushmehr, H., et al. 2010. Identification of a CpG island methylator phenotype that defines a distinct subgroup of glioma. *Cancer Cell* 17: 510–522.

Ohgaki, H.P., A. Kleihues, D.N. von Deimling, G. Reifenberger Louis, H. Yan, and M. Weller. 2016. Glioblastoma, IDH-Mutant. In *WHO classification of tumors of the central nervous system*, ed. Webster K. Cavenee, David N. Louis, Hiroko Ohgaki, and Otmar D. Wiestler. France: Revised 4t, 52 to 56. International Agency for Research on Cancer (IARC).

Padfield, E., H.P. Ellis, and K.M. Kurian. 2015. Current therapeutic advances targeting EGFR and EGFRvIII in glioblastoma. *Frontiers in Oncology* 5: 5.

Parsons, D.W., et al. 2008. An integrated genomic analysis of human glioblastoma multiforme. *Science* 321: 1807–1812.

Peltier, J., A. O'Neill, and D.V. Schaffer. 2007. PI3K/Akt and CREB regulate adult neural hippocampal progenitor proliferation and differentiation. *Developmental Neurobiology* 67: 1348–1361.

Phillips, H.S., et al. 2006. Molecular subclasses of high-grade glioma predict prognosis, delineate a pattern of disease progression, and resemble stages in neurogenesis. *Cancer Cell* 9 (3): 157–173. doi:10.1016/j.ccr.2006.02.019.

Phillips, J.J., et al. 2013. PDGFRA amplification is common in pediatric and adult high-grade astrocytomas and identifies a poor prognostic group in IDH1 mutant glioblastoma. *Brain Pathology* 23: 565–573.

Rao, Shilpa, Palavalasa Sravya, Chitra Chandran, Jitender Saini, Sampath Somanna, and Vani Santosh. 2017. Granular cells in oligodendroglioma suggest a neoplastic change rather than a reactive phenomenon: Case report with molecular characterisation. *Brain Tumor Pathology* 34 (1): 42–47. doi:10.1007/s10014-016-0273-5.

Reis, R.M., et al. 2001. Second primary glioblastoma. *Journal of Neuropathology and Experimental Neurology* 60: 208–215.

Richardson, W.D., N. Pringle, M.J. Mosley, B. Westermark, and M. Dubois-Dalcq. 1988. A role for platelet-derived growth factor in normal gliogenesis in the central nervous system. *Cell* 53: 309–319.

Richichi, C., P. Brescia, V. Alberizzi, L. Fornasari, and G. Pelicci. 2013. Marker-independent method for isolating slow-dividing cancer stem cells in human glioblastoma. *Neoplasia* 15: 840–847.

Scherer, H., and J. Structural. 1938. Development in gliomas. *The American Journal of Cancer* 34: 333–351.

Schumacher, T., et al. 2014. A vaccine targeting mutant IDH1 induces antitumour immunity. *Nature* 512: 324–327.

Schwartzentruber, J., et al. 2012. Driver mutations in histone H3.3 and chromatin remodelling genes in paediatric glioblastoma. *Nature* 482: 226–231.

Shih, A.H., and E.C. Holland. 2006. Platelet-derived growth factor (PDGF) and glial tumorigenesis. *Cancer Letters* 232: 139–147.

Shinojima, N., et al. 2003. Prognostic value of epidermal growth factor receptor in patients with glioblastoma multiforme. *Cancer Research* 63 (20): 6962–6970.

Shinsato, Y., et al. 2013. Reduction of MLH1 and PMS2 confers temozolomide resistance and is associated with recurrence of glioblastoma. *Oncotarget* 4: 2261–2270.

Song, X., et al. 2011. Glioblastoma with PNET-like components has a higher frequency of isocitrate dehydrogenase 1 (IDH1) mutation and likely a better prognosis than primary glioblastoma. *International Journal of Clinical and Experimental Pathology* 4: 651–660.

Spiegl-Kreinecker, S., et al. 2015. Prognostic quality of activating TERT promoter mutations in glioblastoma: interaction with the rs2853669 polymorphism and patient age at diagnosis. *Neuro-Oncology*. doi:10.1093/neuonc/nov010.

Srividya, M.R., et al. 2010. Age-dependent prognostic effects of EGFR/p53 alterations in glioblastoma: Study on a prospective cohort of 140 uniformly treated adult patients. *Journal of Clinical Pathology* 63: 687–691.

———. 2011. Homozygous 10q23/PTEN deletion and its impact on outcome in glioblastoma: A prospective translational study on a uniformly treated cohort of adult patients. *Neuropathology* 31: 376–383.

Stark, A.M., P. Witzel, R.J. Strege, H.-H. Hugo, and H.M. Mehdorn. 2003. p53, mdm2, EGFR, and msh2 expression in paired initial and recurrent glioblastoma multiforme. *Journal of Neurology, Neurosurgery, and Psychiatry* 74: 779–783.

Stark, A.M., A. Doukas, H.-H. Hugo, and H.M. Mehdorn. 2010. The expression of mismatch repair proteins MLH1, MSH2 and MSH6 correlates with the Ki67 proliferation index and survival in patients with recurrent glioblastoma. *Neurological Research* 32: 816–820.

Stupp, R., et al. 2009. Effects of radiotherapy with concomitant and adjuvant temozolomide versus radiotherapy alone on survival in glioblastoma in a randomised phase III study: 5-year analysis of the EORTC-NCIC trial. *The Lancet Oncology* 10: 459–466.

———. 2014. Cilengitide combined with standard treatment for patients with newly diagnosed glioblastoma with methylated MGMT promoter (CENTRIC EORTC 26071-22072 study): a multicentre, randomised, open-label, phase 3 trial. *The Lancet Oncology* 15: 1100–1108.

Switzeny, O.J., et al. 2016. MGMT promoter methylation determined by HRM in comparison to MSP and pyrosequencing for predicting high-grade glioma response. *Clinical Epigenetics* 8: 49.

Taylor, J.W., and D. Schiff. 2015. Treatment Considerations for MGMT-Unmethylated Glioblastoma. *Current Neurology and Neuroscience Reports* 15: 507.

Taylor, T.E., F.B. Furnari, and W.K. Cavenee. 2012. Targeting EGFR for treatment of glioblastoma: Molecular basis to overcome resistance. *Current Cancer Drug Targets* 12: 197–209.

Thota, B., et al. 2012. IDH1 mutations in diffusely infiltrating astrocytomas. *American Journal of Clinical Pathology* 138 (2): 177–184.

Toledo, F., and G.M. Wahl. 2007. MDM2 and MDM4: p53 regulators as targets in anticancer therapy. *The International Journal of Biochemistry & Cell Biology* 39: 1476–1482.

Turcan, S., et al. 2012. IDH1 mutation is sufficient to establish the glioma hypermethylator phenotype. *Nature* 483: 479–483.

Verhaak, R.G.W., et al. 2010. Integrated genomic analysis identifies clinically relevant subtypes of glioblastoma characterized by abnormalities in PDGFRA, IDH1, EGFR, and NF1. *Cancer Cell* 17: 98–110.

Vlassenbroeck, I., et al. 2008. Validation of real-time methylation-specific PCR to determine O6-methylguanine-DNA methyltransferase gene promoter methylation in glioma. *The Journal of Molecular Diagnostics* 10: 332–337.

Wang, Y., et al. 2012. Glioblastoma with an oligodendroglioma component: distinct clinical behavior, genetic alterations, and outcome. *Neuro-Oncology* 14: 518–525.

Watanabe, T., S. Nobusawa, P. Kleihues, and H. Ohgaki. 2009. IDH1 mutations are early events in the development of astrocytomas and oligodendrogliomas. *The American Journal of Pathology* 174 (4): 1149–1153.

Weller, M., et al. 2010. MGMT promoter methylation in malignant gliomas: ready for personalized medicine? *Nature Reviews. Neurology* 6: 39–51.

Weller, M., M. van den Bent, K. Hopkins, J.C. Tonn, R. Stupp, A. Falini, et al. 2014. EANO guideline for the diagnosis and treatment of anaplastic gliomas and glioblastoma. *The Lancet Oncology* 15 (9): 395–403.

Wick, W., et al. 2014. MGMT testing—the challenges for biomarker-based glioma treatment. *Nature Reviews. Neurology* 10: 372–385.

Wiestler, B., et al. 2013. ATRX loss refines the classification of anaplastic gliomas and identifies a subgroup of IDH mutant astrocytic tumors with better prognosis. *Acta Neuropathologica* 126: 443–451.

Xu, X., et al. 2004. Structures of human cytosolic NADP-dependent isocitrate dehydrogenase reveal a novel self-regulatory mechanism of activity. *The Journal of Biological Chemistry* 279: 33946–33957.

Yan, H., et al. 2009. IDH1 and IDH2 mutations in gliomas. *The New England Journal of Medicine* 360: 765–773.

Yuan, Y., et al. 2016. TERT mutation in glioma: Frequency, prognosis and risk. *Journal of Clinical Neuroscience* 26: 57–62.

Zhu, Y., et al. 2005. Early inactivation of p53 tumor suppressor gene cooperating with NF1 loss induces malignant astrocytoma. *Cancer Cell* 8: 119–130.

Chapter 3
Current Therapies and Future Directions in Treatment of Glioblastoma

Joshua L. Wang, Luke Mugge, Pierre Giglio, and Vinay K. Puduvalli

Abstract The current standard of care for initial treatment of adults with newly diagnosed glioblastoma (GBM) constitutes maximal safe resection followed by concurrent chemoradiation therapy and adjuvant chemotherapy with temozolomide; recent studies have shown improvement in survival benefit with the addition of tumor treatment fields (TTF) to this regimen. For recurrent disease, lomustine and bevacizumab yield benefit in progression-free survival but not in overall survival. Recent advances in the understanding of the biology of GBM have provided the basis for new therapeutic approaches against these tumors. However, the initial promise of agents targeted against specific pathways active in GBM failed to yield the expected improvement in outcome likely due to intra- and inter-tumoral heterogeneity. Current efforts are focused on immunotherapy, biological agents and combination targeted therapies to overcome these challenges. Additionally, ongoing research to better understand the basis of tumor heterogeneity is expected to provide new insights that can help broadly target GBMs that can translate into improved survival and quality of life for these patients. This review provides an outline of current treatments and examines the newer approaches that bear promise to provide a meaningful improvement in outcome of patients with GBM.

Keywords Glioblastoma • Targeted Agents • Antiangiogenic agents • Biological therapies • Immunotherapy

3.1 Introduction

Glioblastoma (GBM) is the most common primary brain tumor in adults and is associated with a dismal outcome. Several new therapeutic strategies have been developed over the past 4 decades that have provided new standards of care which have resulted in improvement in overall survival (OS). However, these improvements have

Joshua L. Wang and Luke Mugge contributed equally to this manuscript

J.L. Wang • L. Mugge • P. Giglio (✉) • V.K. Puduvalli, MD (✉)
Division of Neuro-oncology, The Ohio State University Comprehensive Cancer Center,
320 W 10th Ave Suite M410 Starling Loving Hall, 43210 Columbus, OH, USA
e-mail: Pierre.Giglio@osumc.edu; Vinay.Puduvalli@osumc.edu

© Springer International Publishing AG 2017
K. Somasundaram (ed.), *Advances in Biology and Treatment of Glioblastoma*,
Current Cancer Research, DOI 10.1007/978-3-319-56820-1_3

been only incremental in nature and no significant shifts in paradigms of care have yet emerged to provide the expected dramatic improvements in survival. There is a growing realization that new approaches to treatment are needed to address the complexity and heterogeneity of GBM; this in turn has led to exploring exciting new avenues of treatment including biological therapies, immunotherapies, nanotherapies, and technology-based treatment modalities. Ongoing clinical trials are expected to better characterize the relative efficacies of such approaches and identify the ones that may potentially provide the anticipated paradigm-shifting therapy that significant improves survival with good quality of life. This review provides a comprehensive outline of the rationale for current standards of care for newly diagnosed and recurrent GBM and examines the development of promising novel approaches to therapy against these tumors.

3.2 Newly Diagnosed Glioblastoma

Current treatment for patients with newly diagnosed GBM includes maximal safe resection followed by concurrent chemoradiation therapy and adjuvant chemotherapy (chemoRT) with temozolomide (TMZ), a monofunctional alkylating agent. This multimodal approach leads to a median OS of 15–17 months and notably improved 2- and 5-year survival compared to radiation therapy (RT) alone. New standards have also been established in elderly patients with GBM who have a good functional status. While these standards have provided a modest yet significant improvement in outcome for GBM patients, much remains to be achieved in further meaningfully improving survival and quality of life for these patients. Novel insights into genetic and epigenetic characteristics of GBM gained in recent years aim to provide new therapeutic strategies to bring a paradigm shift in treatment in these patients (Hegi et al. 2005) (Table 3.1).

Table 3.1 Selected phase III trials for newly diagnosed GBM

Regimen	Median PFS (months)	Median OS (months)	% OS at 2 years	Reference
TMZ + RT	6.9	14.6	26.5%	Stupp et al. (2005)
RT alone	5.0	12.1	10.4%	
DD TMZ (21/28 days)	6.7	14.9	33.9%	Gilbert et al. (2013)
TMZ	5.5	16.6	34.2%	
Bevacizumab + TMZ/RT	10.7	15.7	NR	Gilbert et al. (2014)
Placebo + TMZ/RT	7.3	16.1	NR	
Bevacizumab + TMZ/RT	10.6	16.8	33.9%	Chinot et al. (2014)
Placebo + TMZ/RT	6.2	16.7	30.1%	
TTFields + TMZ	7.1	20.5	43%	Stupp et al. (2015)
TMZ	4.0	15.6	29%	

GBM glioblastoma, *TMZ* temozolomide, *RT* radiation therapy, *DD* dose-dense, *TTFields* tumor treating fields (alternating electric fields), *PFS* progression free survival, *OS* overall survival, *NR* not reported

3.2.1 Surgical Resection

Surgical resection in patients with newly diagnosed GBM is aimed initially at providing sufficient tissue for histologic and molecular diagnosis, reducing mass effect, and relieving symptoms. Whether extent of resection can improve overall survival has been less clear due to the absence of level 1 evidence for the same. However, cumulative evidence from several studies has strongly supported the potential for survival benefit with a greater extent of surgical resection. In the first major study assessing the effect of extent of resection in patients with newly diagnosed GBM, Lacroix et al. reported a single center retrospective study of 416 patients which showed that increasing extent of resection of the enhancing portion of the tumor ≥89% provided improved survival for every unit increase in volumetric resection (Lacroix et al. 2001). A subsequent retrospective study of a series of 500 patients by Sanai et al. again supported this finding with benefit being seen even in patients who underwent a partial resection (≥78%) and improving in a stepwise manner with greater extent of resection (Sanai et al. 2011). In a more recent large retrospective study expanding on the analysis by Lacroix et al. from the same center, Li et al. not only confirmed improvement in survival resulting from maximal resection of the enhancing part of the tumor in 1229 patients with newly diagnosed GBM, but also reported that increasing the extent of resection to safely remove the non-enhancing hyperintense portion on fluid-attenuated inversion recovery (FLAIR) magnetic resonance imaging (MRI) yielded additional improvement in survival (Li et al. 2016). These results suggest that maximal safe resection of the enhancing and non-enhancing components of newly diagnosed GBM should be attempted in all patients who are surgical candidates. While these studies provide a proof-of-principle for maximal safe resection, it should be noted that these results may also be strongly influenced by the neurosurgeons' experience with brain tumor surgeries and the availability of high quality MRI techniques and of advanced neurosurgical instrumentation, which are not always readily available in the community when the patient initially presents with symptoms. The development of intraoperative tools such as fluorescence-guided surgery with 5-aminolevulinic acid (5-ALA), which allows visualization of residual tumor cells, and intraoperative MRI that allows monitoring of residual tumor during surgery have helped improve the extent of resection and thus contribute to survival outcomes (Stummer et al. 2006; Kubben et al. 2011). Further, to preserve neurologic function during aggressive surgeries, awake craniotomies can be performed with real-time intra-operative neurologic and language assessments with an option for local stimulation to detect and avoid functional areas when operating on tumors near eloquent areas. However, when gross total resection is not possible due to the location or extent of the tumor or the patient's clinical condition, subtotal resection or stereotactic biopsy may serve to relieve mass effect and to establish definitive histologic diagnosis.

3.2.2 First Line Therapy for Newly Diagnosed GBM

Given the infiltrative nature of GBM, maximal surgical resection has to be followed by adjuvant therapy to maximize tumor control and improve survival. The initial use of adjuvant whole brain radiation therapy (WBRT) in the late 1970s (Andersen 1978; Walker et al. 1978, 1980) was replaced by involved field radiation therapy (IFRT) to offer maximal treatment to the tumor while minimizing radiation to normal brain tissue, given that tumor recurrence following WBRT usually occurs within 2–3 cm of the original lesion (Wallner et al. 1989) and that less than 10% of patients develop multifocal recurrence (Choucair et al. 1986). Dose escalation studies failed to show any survival benefit for total doses above 60 Gy (Chan et al. 2002; Nelson et al. 1988). The current standards for radiotherapy consist of IFRT to the gross tumor volume with a 2–3 cm margin for the clinical target volume delivered with linear accelerators.

Chemoradiation Therapy In a landmark study that established the current standard of care, Stupp et al. reported a significant improvement in OS and progression free survival (PFS) in adults between the ages of 18 and 70 years of age with newly diagnosed GBM who received concurrent chemoRT compared with those who received radiation therapy (RT) alone (Stupp et al. 2005). The treatment constituted fractionated involved-field radiation (2 Gy per day, 5 days a week, for a total dose of 60 Gy) with concurrent TMZ (75 mg/m^2 of body surface area daily for 6 weeks) followed by six cycles of TMZ at 150–200 mg/m^2 for 5 days during each 28 day cycle. Median OS was 14.6 months with RT plus TMZ versus 12.1 months with RT alone (HR 0.63 [95% CI, 0.52 to 0.75; P < 0.001]). More strikingly, there was improvement in 2-year survival from 10.4% on RT alone to 26.5% with chemoRT.

   A companion retrospective study by Hegi et al. demonstrated the relevance of promoter methylation of *O-6 methyl-guanine DNA methyl-transferase* (MGMT), the protein product of which is involved in repair of DNA lesions induced by methylating agents such as temozolomide (Hegi et al. 2005). Of 206 evaluable patients, those with methylated MGMT promoter (44.7%) had a significantly better OS compared to those with unmethylated promoters, regardless of treatment (18.2 vs. 12.2 months, respectively; HR 0.45; 95% CI 0.32–0.61), supporting a prognostic role for this marker. Patients with MGMT promoter methylated tumors who received RT plus TMZ had an improved median survival (21.7 months [95% CI, 17.4–30.4]) compared to those who received RT alone (15.3 months [95% CI, 13.0–20.9]) (p = 0.007). In the promoter methylated cohort, the 2-year survival rate was 46% for the group treated with RT plus TMZ compared with 22.7% for those receiving RT only. A five-year analysis of the patient cohort in this study showed an OS of 27.2% at 2 years and 9.8% at 5 years for the RT plus TMZ arm compared with 10.9% and 1.9% with RT alone (hazard ratio 0.6, 95% CI 0.5–0.7; p < 0.0001) (Stupp et al. 2009). Patients with MGMT promoter methylated GBM had the best survival outcomes.

   Dose escalation of standard IFRT beyond 60 Gy has not yielded improved outcome and indeed has resulted in increased radiation toxicity (Chan et al. 2002;

Nelson et al. 1988). Alternative strategies such as brachytherapy, involving interstitial delivery of radioactive isotopes such as ^{125}Iodine (I-125), has been used as a local boost in conjunction with IFRT in the setting of newly diagnosed GBM and as treatment for recurrent GBM. However, the paucity of prospective randomized studies of brachytherapy and the confounding study designs and mixed results of nonrandomized prospective studies have resulted in this modality not being actively used against GBM (Barbarite et al. 2016). Similarly, stereotactic radiosurgery (SRS), which involves the precise delivery of high dose radiation to a specified lesion by either in a single fraction or as fractionated stereotactic radiotherapy (FSRT) used in the setting of deep-seated lesions or those abutting eloquent brain have not yielded definite survival benefit in GBM patients (Nwokedi et al. 2002; Souhami et al. 2004). Radioimmunotherapy, the use of radiolabeled antibodies to target cancer cells, has been most notably used to target tenascin, an extracellular glycoprotein highly expressed in GBM but not in normal brain tissue. In a phase II trial of a I-125-conjugated murine anti-tenascin monoclonal antibody delivered by direct injection into the resection cavity during surgery, Reardon et al. reported a median survival of 79.4 weeks, which exceeded that of historical controls. Given the promising outcomes and tolerable toxicity, a phase III study is currently being planned (Reardon et al. 2006; Zalutsky et al. 2008).

BCNU Wafers Interstitial biodegradable bis-chloroethyl-nitrosourea (BCNU, carmustine) wafers were developed as a way to initiate chemotherapy immediately after tumor resection and avoid the side-effects of systemic administration of BCNU. Using a biodegradable polymer containing 3.85% BCNU (Gliadel®, Arbor Pharmaceuticals, Atlanta, GA, USA) in a randomized trial of 240 patients with newly diagnosed high grade gliomas, Westphal et al. demonstrated the survival advantage of BCNU wafers compared to control (median OS 13.9 months vs. 11.6 months), which led to the FDA approval of Gliadel wafers for these patients (Westphal et al. 2003). Adverse events were similar to placebo although BCNU treated patients were more likely to experience cerebrospinal fluid leaks (5.0% vs. 0.8%) and intracranial hypertension (9.1% vs. 1.7%). The survival advantage remained consistent at long-term follow up 3 years following the initial analysis (Westphal et al. 2006). Despite these results, the use of BCNU wafers has declined in routine surgical practice since the advent of the current chemoRT regimen.

Dose intensification of chemotherapy Patients with MGMT promoter methylated GBM experience an improved outcome after treatment with temozolomide (Hegi et al. 2005; Esteller et al. 2000), which is believed to be due to their decreased ability to repair the O6-MG DNA lesion induced by TMZ therapy. These results suggested that MGMT-depletion could potentially sensitize GBMs to alkylating agents. Tolcher et al. found in two phase 1 trials that prolonged exposure to alkylating agents depleted intracellular MGMT in peripheral blood monocytes (Tolcher et al. 2003). Hypothesizing that a similar effect could be induced in tumor cells by dose intensification, Gilbert et al. conducted a multinational phase III trial (1173 patients registered, 833 randomized) comparing two schedules of adjuvant temozolomide: standard (5 days) or dose-dense (21 days) of a 28 day cycle, following concurrent chemoRT therapy in adults (≥18 years) with newly diagnosed GBM (Gilbert et al. 2013). However, the median survival in the dose-dense arm was not statistically different from that in the standard arm (16.6 months vs. 14.9 months, HR 1.03, p = 0.63); in addition, toxicity was also higher in the dose-dense schedule. The study did prospectively confirm the prognostic significance of MGMT promoter methylation in this patient population; MGMT promoter methylation was associated with improved median survival of 21.2 months versus 14 months in the unmethylated tumors (HR, 1.74; p < 0.001).

Alternating Electric Fields (Tumor Treatment Fields) Kirson et al. developed technology that hampered cell division through the application of electric fields that alternated at a frequency in the range of 150–200 Hz and induced a cytotoxic effect on tumor cells *in vitro* in a dose-dependent manner in relation to the field intensity (Kirson et al. 2009a). Exposure to these tumor treatment fields (TTF) resulted in mitotic abnormalities, most notably membrane blebbing during entry into anaphase, which in turn resulted in aberrant mitotic exit and cell death (Gera et al. 2015). TTF were found to be most effective against protein targets that have high dipole moments, and its chief targets were the mitotic septin complex and the α/β-tubulin monomeric subunit of tubulin (Wong et al. 2015). The effects observed *in vitro* were additionally characterized in animal tumor models and human cancers, including colon adenocarcinoma, melanoma, and Lewis lung carcinoma (Kirson et al. 2007, 2009b). This was commercialized in the form of NovoTTF-100A (Novocure Ltd., Jersey Isle), a device with electrodes that could be applied directly to the scalp and generates a 50-V field (>0.7 V/cm at the center of the brain) that alternates at a frequency of 200 Hz and was intended to be worn continuously for at least 18 hours a day. In a multinational phase III trial by Stupp et al., adults with newly diagnosed GBM were randomized after chemoRT to receive adjuvant temozolomide with (n = 210) or without (n = 105) TTF therapy (Stupp et al. 2015). The trial was halted after a planned interim analysis demonstrated a significant improvement of PFS (7.1 vs. 4.0 months, HR 0.62, p = 0.001), which was the primary end-point of the study. Based on the results of this study, the US FDA approved the NovoTTF-100A for use with adjuvant temozolomide in patients with newly diagnosed GBM. Use of the NovoTTF-100A device was not associated with systemic toxic effects or increase in seizures, but it was associated with higher incidence of scalp irritation, anxiety, confusion, insomnia, and headaches compared to the control arm. The widespread use of this modality has been limited due to the slow acceptance of the potential utility of TTF, the cosmetic issues associated with the application of electrodes for over 18 hours a day, and the weight of the device (>3 kg). A newer version of the device has been released incorporating several improvements in design and weighing ~1 kg. In light of a separate randomized trial that found that TTF performed equally as well as physician's choice chemotherapy in recurrent GBM (Stupp et al. 2012), the United States Food and Drug Administration (FDA) approved the device for use in patients with recurrent GBM.

Antiangiogenic strategies in initial therapy of GBM Based on encouraging results with the use of bevacizumab in the setting of recurrent disease, two large randomized phase III studies examined the benefit of adding bevacizumab to standard treatment for newly diagnosed GBM both in the chemoRT and adjuvant settings. One study by Gilbert et al. reported the results of a multicenter Radiation Therapy Oncology Group (RTOG) trial in which 637 patients were randomized to either bevacizumab (10 mg/kg) or placebo beginning week 4 of chemoRT therapy with temozolomide and treatment was continued for up to 12 cycles along with adjuvant chemotherapy (Gilbert et al. 2014). The study also assessed the net clinical benefit of the treatments (including neurocognitive assessments, patient reported outcomes (PRO), and health-related quality of life [HRQOL] measures). No significant difference in the median OS was seen between the bevacizumab group and the placebo groups (15.7 months vs 16.1 months, HR, 1.13). However, an improvement in PFS was seen in the bevacizumab group (10.7 months vs. 7.3 months; HR, 0.79) but did not reach the protocol specified threshold for significance. Despite this improvement in PFS, patients on the bevacizumab arm showed a decline in quality of life with increase in symptom burden and neurocognitive worsening compared with the placebo arm.

The other study (AVAglio) was a multinational trial which randomized 921 patients to either bevacizumab (n = 458) or to placebo (n = 463) (Chinot et al. 2014). In results that were strikingly similar to the RTOG study, no difference was seen in OS in the bevacizumab arm compared with the placebo arm (median OS 16.8 months vs 16.7 months, HR, 0.88; 95% CI, 0.76–1.02; p = 0.10), whereas an improvement in PFS was associated with bevacizumab treatment, which in this trial reached a pre-specified threshold for statistical significance (10.6 months vs 6.2 months; HR 0.64; 95% CI 0.55–0.74; p < 0.001). Both studies confirmed the value of MGMT promoter methylation as a prognostic marker associated with therapy in both arms. However, the two studies reported significant differences in HRQOL and PRO: results that remain to be fully understood. The AVAglio study showed an improvement in the quality of life measures associated with bevacizumab whereas the RTOG study showed a significant decline in both neurocognitive and PRO measures used in the study. A better understanding of the results of the two studies through an independent analysis will be critical in defining the significance of these net clinical benefit data.

3.3 Recurrent Glioblastoma

Despite aggressive initial therapy for newly diagnosed GBM, tumor recurrence is inevitable (Stupp et al. 2009). Recurrent GBM tend to be less sensitive to subsequent therapies due to development of emergent and adaptive resistance partly related to tumor heterogeneity. Several retrospective studies have shown that age and performance status at the time of recurrence were important independent prognostic factors for survival (Michaelsen et al. 2013). A small percentage of patients remain eligible for additional surgical resection (Weller et al. 2013). But for most patients, systemic therapies with agents such as bevacizumab, dose dense temozolomide, nitrosoureas or occasionally local therapies such as re-irradiation are required. This section provides a review of modalities used in patients with recurrent GBM.

Resection of Recurrent Glioma Surgical resection of recurrent tumor is often required for individual patients to relieve symptomatic mass effect, recover function, or prevent neurological deterioration. However, there is a paucity of evidence to support a consistent role for re-resection in patients with recurrent GBM. While some prospective studies reported better OS with gross total resection (Suchorska et al. 2016; Yong et al. 2014), others have reported improvement in neither PFS nor post-recurrence OS with reoperation. A major role for repeat surgery is to provide histologic confirmation of recurrence, to differentiate the true progression from radiation necrosis and to identify biomarkers that may be useful in tailoring chemotherapeutic regimens. However, stereotactic biopsy can be a viable option to realize these goals even for the majority of patients who are not candidates for resection (Weller et al. 2013). Additional prospective and adequately powered trials are needed to evaluate whether re-resection provides a survival benefit in patients with recurrent GBM; however, such trials may be challenging due to the influence of other treatments being given to the patient subsequent to surgery as well as the issues related to patient selection for such resections.

Bevacizumab Vascular proliferation and neoangiogenesis are hallmarks of GBM that are driven by its production of several angiogenesis promoting factors, especially vascular endothelial growth factor (VEGF). Bevacizumab, a monoclonal antibody that binds VEGF to inhibit angiogenesis, was first reported to show unexpected activity in terms of radiological responses in a small series of patients with high grade gliomas (Stark-Vance 2005). This led to a more systematic evaluation of bevacizumab both as a single agent and in combination with irinotecan in a phase II open-label trial focused on patients with recurrent GBM. Of the 167 patients randomized to receive bevacizumab alone (10 mg/kg, n = 85) or bevacizumab plus irinotecan (n = 82) every 2 weeks, the PFS-6 rates (primary end point) were 42.6% and 50.3%, respectively with ORR of 28.2% and 37.8%, respectively. Median OS was 9.2 months with bevacizumab alone and 8.7 months with the combination. Treatment on these two arms were associated with significant toxicity with ≥grade 3 toxicities of 46.4% for the bevacizumab alone arm and 65.8% in the combination arm. Intracranial hemorrhage was seen in 2.4% of the patient in the bevacizumab-alone arm and in 3.8% in the combination arm, addressing the concerns about intracranial bleeding from such antiangiogenic therapies.

A second study examined the use of single agent bevacizumab in 48 patients with recurrent GBM and added irinotecan to bevacizumab when patients progressed on single agent bevacizumab therapy (Kreisl et al. 2009). The study showed a PFS6 of 29%, ORR of 35% (by Macdonald criteria), median PFS of 16 weeks, median OS of 31 weeks and OS6 rate of 57%. In this study, a higher rate of treatment related complication was reported, with 6 of the patients being removed from the trial due to thromboembolic events or intestinal perforation. Other adverse events included hypertension (12.5%), hypophosphatemia (6%), and thrombocytopenia (6%). Patients who progressed on bevacizumab had no objective responses when irinotecan was added at progression; median PFS was 30 days. The results of these two studies provided reasonable evidence that bevacizumab had activity in patients with recurrent GBM without significant toxicities and led to accelerated approval of bevacizumab by the US FDA as a single agent for treatment of this patient population. Of note, the approval was based on objective response rates that were also found to be durable; partial responses were observed in 25.9% and 19.6% respectively in these two studies with median response duration of 4.2 months and 3.9 months respectively. Bevacizumab is now considered the standard of care for patients with recurrent GBM without contraindications for this agent.

Progression after Bevacizumab Treatment Patients developing progression after treatment with bevacizumab were clinically seen to have a possibly worse outcome and a lack of response to subsequent treatments, an issue which was addressed by several retrospective studies. Iwamoto et al. reported a median OS of 4.5 months for patients with GBM progressing after bevacizumab therapy; the subset of patients who received salvage chemotherapy after bevacizumab failure had a median PFS of 2 months, median OS of 5.2 months, and a PFS6 rate of 0% (Iwamoto et al. 2009). Similarly, in a similar population of patients, Lu-Emerson et al. reported a median PFS of 28 days, median OS of 78 days, and a PFS6 rate of 0%. These studies showed that outcome was dismal for patients who had progression after bevacizumab therapy and that salvage therapy in this setting was largely ineffective. In the absence of toxicity or progression, bevacizumab is often continued indefinitely, even after progression and often in combination with other agents due to concerns regarding tumor rebound seen in some patients with GBM and reported in patients with metastatic colorectal cancer (Bennouna et al. 2013). Quant et al. examined outcomes of patients who were continued on a bevacizumab containing regimen after progression on single agent bevacizumab therapy and reported a median PFS on the first regimen of 124 days and PFS6 rate of 33% and a median PFS on the second regimen of 37.5 days with a PFS6 of 2% (Quant et al. 2009). In another randomized phase II trial comparing bevacizumab with and without carboplatin, patient who progressed were randomized again to continue or cease bevacizumab; in this subset, there was no difference in median PFS (1.8 months vs 2.0 months) or median OS (3.4 months vs. 3.0 months) for those did or did not continue bevacizumab. There was also not definite evidence for a rebound effect (Hovey et al. 2015). Hence, the options for patients with bevacizumab failure remain limited prompting clinicians to postpone the use of this agent to the later stages of the disease.

Nitrosoureas Nitrosoureas such as BCNU (carmustine), CCNU (lomustine), nimustine, and fotemustine, as well as another alkylating agent, procarbazine, were used frequently for first line therapy for newly diagnosed GBM precluding its use in the recurrent setting. However, following the approval of temozolomide for newly diagnosed glioblastoma, nitrosoureas were once again utilized more frequently to treat recurrence. Two phase II trials evaluating the efficacy of BCNU monotherapy in recurrent GBM showed PFS6 rates of 17.5% and 24%, though the second trial grouped patients who received temozolomide and BCNU together (Brandes et al. 2004; van den Bent et al. 2009). The response to BCNU in both studies was similar to historical reports, but patients were much more likely to experience hematologic, hepatic, and/or pulmonary toxicity. Serious toxicities such as irreversible pneumonitis or pulmonary fibrosis, prolonged myelosuppression, myelodysplasia and delayed secondary malignancies can occur in a minority of patients, which limit the cumulative dose of these agents. Locoregional therapy with placement of BCNU wafers at the time of reoperation for recurrent GBM was developed to reduce such systemic toxicity and was associated with a significantly longer OS in a randomized phase III trial compared to placebo (31 vs. 23 weeks, HR = 0.67, p = 0.006), without increased CNS toxicity (Brem et al. 1995), leading to its regulatory approval in the US.

Concurrent CCNU and bevacizumab showed improved PFS and OS in patients with recurrent GBM compared with those treated with CCNU (n = 46) or bevacizumab (n = 50) alone in initial results of the randomized phase II BELOB trial (Taal et al. 2014). However, results from a recently completed phase III trial comparing bevacizumab plus CCNU to CCNU alone showed no improvement in OS in the combination therapy arm (HR 0.95 CI 0.74, 1.21, p = 0.650), whereas PFS was longer with the addition of bevacizumab to CCNU (HR 0.49 (CI 0.39, 0.61). Median efficacy outcomes were: OS 9.1 (8.1, 10.1) versus 8.6 (7.6, 10.4) months and PFS 4.2 (3.7, 4.3) versus 1.5 (1.5, 2.5) months in the combination arm versus the CCNU arm, respectively. Toxicity was in the expected range with more events in the combination arm being also longer on treatment. These data suggest clinically relevant activity of CCNU as a single agent and in combination with bevacizumab. However, treatment with CCNU resulted in frequent hematologic toxicity (up to 50% of patients affected), particularly in combination with bevacizumab, leading to a dose reduction for CCNU with bevacizumab. Further phase III trials are needed to expand on this body of data.

Fotemustine is used mainly in Italy and France, and several studies found similar survival outcomes compared to CCNU (Brandes et al. 2009a; Fabrini et al. 2009). Hematologic toxicity was also not insignificant with fotemustine. Despite their toxicity profiles, nitrosoureas will likely continue to be utilized in the clinic and in trials.

Re-irradiation Re-irradiation for recurrent GBM is most commonly considered in the setting of rapidly progressive symptomatic disease when there are few other treatment options available, but this decision has to be tempered by the potential risk of neurotoxicity from overlap of treatment fields with areas previously radiated. Since most recurrences occur within the target volume treated with IFRT, treatment planning needs to be adequately tailored to treat recurrence safely. Retrospective studies have suggested a potential benefit from re-irradiation with SRS or FSRT (typical doses 30–36 Gy) (Torok et al. 2011). Nevertheless, there is a lack of concordance in the literature regarding the time interval necessary from initial irradiation and a paucity of prospective and randomized trials to define properly the role of re-irradiation as monotherapy in the treatment of recurrent GBM (Seystahl et al. 2016). Combination therapy strategies have shown early promise; preliminary data regarding the use of SRS or FSRT with concurrent bevacizumab in recurrent GBM showed positive responses with minimal neurotoxicity (Gutin et al. 2009; Cabrera et al. 2013). The potential effects of this combination are hypothesized to be due to vascular normalization induced by bevacizumab that results in improved oxygenation of the tumor tissue and consequent increased radiation effect.

Laser-induced thermal therapy If maximal resection is not feasible, newer modalities of tumor ablation have been developed as alternatives. Laser induced (or interstitial) thermal therapy (LITT) is one such procedure which utilizes minimally invasive percutaneous insertion of an optical fiber into the tumor under intraoperative MR guidance and generates ablative heat, which induces targeted thermocoagulative necrosis of tumor cells, which may be particularly suitable for deep-seated brain lesions or lesions located in eloquent areas. A recent phase 1 trial of a commercial LITT device, NeuroBlate (Monteris Medical, Inc., Plymouth, MN, USA) in recurrent GBM demonstrated that LITT is a viable, safe option for treatment of GBM (Sloan et al. 2013). Additional trials are warranted to characterize fully the safety and efficacy profile of LITT systems in treatment of newly diagnosed GBM. Local thermal injury during intracranial use of LITT can result in serious neurologic morbidities or cerebrovascular complications. Further, the technique does not adequately address the extensive infiltrative disease usually seen in GBM.

3.4 Glioblastoma in Older Adults

The EORTC/NCIC trial established a new standard of care for adult patients between ages 18 and 70 years but did not provide information about patients >70 years with GBM (Stupp et al. 2005). Older age and poor performance status have been consistently shown to be associated with shorter survival (Buckner 2003). The median OS of patients age 65 and older with a new diagnosis of GBM is approximately six months (compared to 12–14 months in younger patients) (Paszat et al. 2001; Kita et al. 2009). However, this could be explained by differences in treatment administered, as older patients are less likely to be considered for more aggressive interventions (Paszat et al. 2001), and older adults were found to exhibit similar survival outcomes as younger adults when both groups receive the same treatments (Kita et al. 2009).

Current literature supports the role of maximal safe resection as an initial step in treatment of an older patient with newly diagnosed GBM, if the patient can tolerate the surgery. One prospective randomized trial reported significant benefits OS with maximal safe resection (n = 10) compared to biopsy alone (n = 13) in OS (171 vs. 85 days, respectively, p = 0.035), but no significant difference in PFS (105 vs. 72 days, respectively, p = 0.057) (Vuorinen et al. 2003). However if surgical resection is contraindicated, biopsy of the tumor is needed to establish histologic diagnosis and to assess molecular characteristics that can influence subsequent treatment (such as MGMT promoter methylation (Reifenberger et al. 2012)).

Two prospective trials demonstrated that postsurgical RT was safe and effective in older patients. A randomized phase III trial of 85 elderly patient with GBM by Keime-Guibert et al. reported that RT plus supportive care resulted in improved median survival compared with supportive care alone (29.1 weeks vs 16.9 weeks, HR 0.47, 95% CI 0.29–0.76, p = 0.002) with no significant differences in QOL and cognitive measures between the treatment groups (Keime-Guibert et al. 2007). To determine the optimal RT dose for elderly patients, Roa et al. conducted a phase III trial randomizing 98 patients ≥60 years of age with newly diagnosed GBM to either standard RT (60 Gy in 30 fractions over 6 weeks) or a shorter course of RT (40 Gy in 15 fractions over 3 weeks) and reported no significant difference in median OS between the two groups (5.1 months versus 5.6 months, log-rank test, p = 0.57), suggesting that the hypofractionated RT course may be reasonable for older patients with GBM (Roa et al. 2004).

The role of chemotherapy in this patient population was addressed in the Nordic study, a large multinational trial in which 291 patients aged ≥60 years were randomized to receive TMZ alone (200 mg/m^2 days 1–5 of a 28 day cycle for up to six cycles, n = 93), hypofractionated RT (34 Gy over 2 weeks, n = 98), or standard RT (60 Gy over 6 weeks, n = 100), and an additional 51 were randomized to either TMZ alone (n = 26) or hypofractionated RT (n = 25) (Malmstrom et al. 2012). The study reported that treatment with TMZ alone yielded a longer median OS compared with standard RT (8.3 months vs 6 months, HR 0.70, p = 0.01), but not with hypofractionated RT (7.5 months vs 6 months, HR 0.85, p = 0.24). Overall survival was similar for patients who received TMZ (n = 119) or hypofractionated RT (n = 123), (8.4 months vs 7.4 months; HR 0.82, p = 0.12). However, in the subset of patients ≥70 years, better survival was noted with TMZ alone (HR 0.35, p < 0.0001) or with hypofractionated RT (HR 0.59, p = 0.02) compared with standard RT. In addition, in the subgroup receiving TMZ alone, patients with MGMT promoter methylation had significantly longer survival compared with those an unmethylated MGMT promoter (9.7 months vs 6.8 months; HR 0.56, p = 0.02), an improvement that was not seen in patients treated with RT (HR 0.97; p = 0.81). These results suggested that TMZ or hypofractionated RT may be considered as standard treatment options in elderly patients with GBM with MGMT promoter methylation status as a predictive marker for TMZ. This trial did not test the role of concurrent chemoRT in this population.

In an attempt to ascertain if dose intensification of TMZ may provide a greater benefit, the NOA-08 study compared the efficacy of RT versus dose dense TMZ in elderly patients (≥65 years) with good functional status with GBM or anaplastic astrocytoma. Patients were randomized to TMZ (100 mg/m^2 daily on a week on week off schedule, n = 195) or standard RT (60 Gy in 30 fractions, n = 178) in a non-inferiority design. Median OS was 8.6 months in the TMZ group versus 9.6 months in the RT group (HR 1.09, $p_{non-inferiority}$ = 0.033). The majority of patients had GBM (n = 331) and the rest anaplastic astrocytoma (n = 40) but there were no significant difference in survival based on histology (HR 0.69, p = 0.20). *MGMT* promoter methylation was associated with longer OS than was unmethylated status (11.9 months *vs* 8.2 months, HR 0.62, p = 0.014). Dose intensive temozolomide was found to be non-inferior to radiotherapy alone in elderly patients with malignant astrocytoma but was associated with increased toxicity.

Building on earlier studies of chemoRT using temozolomide, which suggested that this treatment was well tolerated in elderly patients with good functional status (Combs et al. 2008; Brandes et al. 2009b; Minniti et al. 2015), and to address whether the addition of TMZ to RT improves survival in elderly patients, a recent phase III trial enrolled 562 patients over 65 years old with newly diagnosed GBM and good functional status (ECOG 0-2) and randomized them to receive RT alone (40 Gy in 15 fractions, n=281) or RT (40 Gy in 15 fractions) with 3 weeks of concomitant TMZ plus monthly adjuvant TMZ (n=281) until progression or 12 cycles (Perry et al. 2016). RT combined with TMZ significantly improved OS over RT alone (median 9.3 months vs 7.6 months, HR 0.67, 95%CI 0.56-0.80, p<0.0001), a benefit that was seen in both MGMT methylated (OS 13.5 months and 7.7 months, respectively, HR: 0.53, p=0.0001) and MGMT unmethylated patients (OS 10.0 months vs 7.9 months, respectively, HR 0.75, p=0.055). The treatment was noted to be well tolerated, and patients with MGMT methylated tumors benefited the most from chemoRT with near doubling of median OS. This regimen is hence now considered the standard of care for elderly patients with a good functional status.

At the time of submission, no data exist specific to treatment of older patients with GBM recurrence. There are several ongoing trials investigating bevacizumab in this patient population.

In summary, although age remains a significant prognostic factor, age alone need not be the basis of exclusion for standard therapies in treatment of GBM in elderly patients with good functional status. However in some cases dose reduction may decrease toxicity while providing similar clinical benefits, particularly in combination chemoRT and in hypofractionated radiotherapy.

3.5 Gliomatosis Cerebrii

Gliomatosis cerebri (GC) is an uncommon, highly infiltrative presentation of gliomas first described in 1938 (Nevin 1938). Diagnosis requires histology demonstrating a glial-origin neoplasm and radiological evidence of involvement of more than two lobes of the brain on T2-weighted/FLAIR MRI. There is considerable variation in published literature regarding the prognostic factors and course of disease with varied reports of poor prognosis in some studies and promising outcomes compared to GBM. Given that GC is defined radiologically, the histology can vary from low grade infiltrative gliomas to GBM. These differences in reported interpretation and managements of patients with GC have made treatment decisions challenging in clinical practice. Given the diffuse nature of the disease, surgical resection is not indicated even in the presence of enhancing foci; instead, histological diagnosis is made by stereotactic or open biopsy often focusing on regions of enhancement if present to obtain the most accurate diagnosis. Radiation therapy is often the first line treatment with IFRT being used in cases where the cancer is more localized, and a focal boost given to contrast-enhancing lesion if present (e.g. total dose 50.4 Gy without a focal lesion, 45 Gy plus a 14.4 Gy boost in case of a focal lesion) although there is no standardized schedule. However, in many instances, the extent of the lesion may warrant the use of WBRT despite the risks of neurologic sequelae (Cozad et al. 1996). Although median survival ranges from 11 to 24 months following radiotherapy, a retrospective study found no difference in survival between patients receiving or not receiving radiotherapy (Herrlinger 2012). In contrast, the use of chemotherapy was a highly significant prognostic factor in an analysis of 296 patients with GC (Taillibert et al. 2006). The PCV regimen is most commonly used for these patients comprising of lomustine (110 mg/m^2 on day 1), procarbazine (60 mg/m^2 daily for days 8–21 of a 42-day schedule), and vincristine (1.4 mg/m^2 on days 8 and 29). Since vincristine does not penetrate the blood-brain barrier, it is only used in patients with a focal contrast-enhancing lesion. Given the higher risks of toxicity associated with PCV, temozolomide has often been used as a substitute and has yielded similar survival. Overall, the scarcity of data regarding the natural progression of this disease and its response to multimodal therapy has resulted treatment being often directed to the histological nature of the tumor and has limited the ability to develop evidence-based treatment guidelines or prospective clinical trials for patients with GC.

3.6 Targeted Agents in Treatment of GBM

Insights into the specific signaling pathways in glioblastoma growth, invasion and angiogenesis, coupled with the development of technology platforms allowing for testing of the genetic mutations and proteins associated with these pathways has created enormous opportunity for the development of new therapeutics in this disease. The best studied of these targets are the Epidermal Growth Factor Receptor (EGFR) and its ligand (EGF), the angiogenic pathway best exemplified by the activity of the Vascular Endothelial Growth Factor (VEGF) and its receptor (VEGFR), and the phosphoinositide 3-kinase (PI3K)/mammalian target of rapamycin (mTOR) signaling pathway.

3.6.1 EGFR Inhibitors

The majority of glioblastomas have a mutation, amplification, or deletion in at least one receptor tyrosine kinase, with mutations in epidermal growth factor receptor (EGFR) accounting for over half of these (Brennan et al. 2013). Roughly half of the patients who have EGFR amplification also have a specific deletion of the extracellular domain (exons 2–7): a genotype variant referred to as EGFRvIII (Pelloski et al. 2007; Del Vecchio et al. 2013). Numerous attempts have been made to capitalize on the deregulated expression and activity of EGFR in glioblastoma using small molecule inhibitors of EGFR (e.g. erlotinib and gefitinib) and monoclonal antibodies (e.g. cetuximab and nimotuzumab), though none have been particularly successful.

A phase II multi-center trial in newly diagnosed GBM by the North Central Cancer Treatment Group reported in 2008 that treatment of 97 patients with erlotinib 1 week prior to and concurrent with the standard Stupp protocol resulted in mean OS that was similar to TMZ era controls (median survival 15.3 months) (Brown et al. 2008). None of the tested genetic/molecular alterations were associated with survival, including EGFR amplification, combination EGFR and PTEN, and EGFRvIII (p > 0.05). In recurrent glioblastoma, a multi-center phase II trial randomized 110 patients to receive either erlotinib in the experimental arm or single agent temozolomide or BCNU if previously treated with TMZ as the control arm (van den Bent et al. 2009). The PFS at six months was 11.4% in the erlotinib arm and 24% in the control arm. EGFR expression, amplification, mutation in exons 18, 19, and 21, and EGFRvIII were not significant predictors of survival, though low levels of p-Akt was a borderline predictor of improved survival (p = 0.048).

Nimotuzumab, a monoclonal antibody against EGFR, was tested for newly diagnosed glioblastoma in a multi-center open label phase III trial that randomized 149 patients to receive either standard of care (Stupp regimen) or nimotuzumab in addition to the Stupp protocol (Westphal et al. 2015). The study found that 12 month PFS was 25.6% in the experimental arm, compared to 20.3% in the control arm (p = 0.53, Fisher's exact test), with median OS at 22.3 and 19.6 months (p = 0.49, log-rank test), respectively. EGFR amplification was not associated with outcome (p = 0.88). Multiple phase II trials have failed to find significant benefit of cetuximab (monoclonal antibody to EGFR) in newly diagnosed and recurrent GBM.

3.6.2 PI3K and mTOR Inhibitors

The phosphoinositide 3-kinase (PI3K)/mammalian target of rapamycin (mTOR) signaling pathway plays a central role in cellular processes including cell growth, survival, and motility (Engelman 2009). Derangements in the PI3K/mTOR pathway are common in glioblastoma and can promote oncogenic activity (Choe et al. 2003). Such dysregulations can occur upstream (e.g. EGFR amplification or EGFRvIII leading to constitutive activation of PI3K), within PI3K (e.g. mutation or amplification of PI3K components), or in inhibitory regulatory processes (e.g. loss of phosphatase and tensin homolog [PTEN], a tumor suppressor) (Pitz et al. 2015; Wen et al. 2015). mTOR is a potential target for anti-cancer therapies, given its deregulation and role in cell growth in cancers.

In the only multi-center randomized controlled trial studying inhibition of the PI3K/mTOR pathway in glioblastoma, Wick and colleagues compared temozolomide to temsirolimus (an mTOR inhibitor) in newly diagnosed GBM (Wick et al. 2016). The investigators randomized 111 MGMT promoter unmethylated patients to receive either standard of care (Stupp regimen) or radiotherapy with weekly temsirolimus. Median PFS in the temsirolimus arm was 5.4 months versus 6.0 months in the control group. Median OS in patients treated with temsirolimus was 14.8 months, compared to 16.0 months in the control arm.

Two phase II single-arm trials investigating single-agent temsirolimus in recurrent glioblastoma reported did not find a survival benefit (Galanis et al. 2005; Chang et al. 2005). Galanis and colleagues found that in 65 patients treated with 250 mg of temsirolimus intravenously, PFS at 6 months was 7.8%. Chang and colleagues found that in 43 patients treated with 250 mg of temsirolimus (or 170 mg for those not on EIAED), PFS at 6 months was 2.4%.

Other phase II single-arm trials examining temsirolimus and everolimus (another mTOR inhibitor) in combination with chemotherapy and radiation sorafenib, and bevacizumab failed to find significant survival benefit of these mTOR inhibitors in both newly diagnosed and recurrent glioblastoma.

3.6.3   VEGF and VEGFR Inhibitors

Bevacizumab, a monoclonal antibody against VEGF, is FDA approved for single-agent treatment of recurrent glioblastoma patients.

To examine the strategy of pan-VEGFR inhibition to inhibit angiogenesis, the 'Recentin in GBM alone and with lomustine' (REGAL) trial studied the efficacy of cediranib, a potent orally bioavailable VEGFR inhibitor given singly or in combination with lomustine with a lomustine alone arm as control in a randomized phase III, placebo-controlled, trial in adults with recurrent glioblastoma who had failed radiation and temozolomide (Batchelor et al. 2013). The study randomized 325 patients to one of three arms: cediranib alone, cediranib plus lomustine or lomustine plus placebo in a 2:2:1 ratio. The final results of the study showed that there was no difference in PFS, the primary endpoint, for cediranib alone (median PFS 92 days, HR 1.05, p = 0.90) or cediranib plus lomustine (median PFS 125 days, HR 0.76, p = 0.16) compared with lomustine plus placebo (median PFS 82 days). Similarly, no improvement in median OS, the secondary endpoint, was seen for cediranib alone (8 months, HR 1.43, p = 0.10) or cediranib plus lomustine (9.4 months, HR 1.15 p = 0.50) compared with lomustine (9.8 months). The PFS6 was also not significantly different in the cediranib alone (16%) or cediranib plus lomustine (35%) arms compared with the lomustine arm (25%). Correlative studies showed that treatment on either of the cediranib arms showed sustained decreases in median serum soluble VEGFR2 (sVEGFR2) levels whereas treatment with lomustine alone was not associated with significant change in median sVEGFR2 levels; these results suggest that cediranib was able to hit its target at least in serum (although inhibition of tumor VEGFR remains unknown) but still lacked activity against recurrent GBM.

A multicenter open label phase III trial examined the efficacy of enzastaurin, an oral serine/threonine kinase inhibitor, which targets both protein kinase Cβ that mediates VEGF driven angiogenesis, and the PI3K/AKT pathways which drives proliferation in glioblastoma (Wick et al. 2010). The trial was designed to randomize 397 patients to enzastaurin or lomustine in a 2:1 ratio; however, the accrual was halted early after enrolling 266 patients (enzastaurin, n = 174; lomustine, n = 92) based on a planned interim futility analysis which showed no significant differences in median PFS (1.5 vs. 1.6 months; HR 1.28), median OS (6.6 vs. 7.1 months; HR 1.20), or PFS6 rate (11.1% vs. 19.0% p = 0.13) between the enzastaurin and lomustine arms.

3.7 Biological Agents in Clinical Trials Against Glioblastoma

3.7.1 Virus-Based Therapies

Viruses have been employed in clinical research for malignant glioma therapy for quite a few years with two main virus modifications made as follows: a) replication-deficient viral vectors which are used to deliver genes with therapeutic activity to the tumor environment and b) replication competent oncolytic viruses which function by infecting and replicating within a tumor cell, eventually causing tumor cell death and infecting other tumor cells. Broadly speaking, there are two main strategies underlying virus-based therapies in gliomas: The first is delivery of specific genes to modify the biology of the tumor and exert their antitumor effects; replication-deficient viruses such as the herpes simplex virus type I thymidine kinase (HSV-TK) construct are typically employed for therapy delivery. The second strategy is by replication of the virus within the glioma cell resulting in destruction of glioma cells after infection (oncolysis); this is achieved by use of oncolytic viruses which are replication (Table 3.2). Additionally, both virus

Table 3.2 Virus types and therapeutic strategies in the management of malignant gliomas

Virus type	Strategy	Specific example
Replication-deficient viral vectors: deliver genes with therapeutic activity to the tumor environment	Suicide gene transfer: genes for enzymes with ability to convert prodrugs to cytotoxic agents Immune response to tumor	Herpes simplex virus type I thymidine kinase (HSV-TK) construct: activates ganciclovir (GCV) into its toxic nucleotide metabolites which incorporate into DNA (Yang et al. 1998)
Replication-competent oncolytic viruses (OVs): infect cancer cells, destroy them and disseminate in the tumor	Oncolysis Immune response to tumor Virally encoded therapeutic genes	DNX-2401 oncolytic adenovirus; Recombinant herpes simplex viruses with deletions of the ICP34.5 gene (McKie et al. 1996)

categories of have the added benefit of immune activation, resulting in glioma cell destruction through secondary immune effects. Tables 3.2 and 3.3 highlight some of the completed and ongoing virus trials in high grade gliomas. Research in virus based therapies have yielded several valuable insights into this novel therapeutic approach

- Virus therapies studied have so far been shown to be safe but not conclusively effective.
- The most commonly studied gene therapy approach in gliomas has been that of suicide gene transfer; basically transfer of a gene encoding for enzymes with therapeutic activity. Thus, the herpes simplex type I – thymidine kinase construct (HSV-TK) allows for (systemically administered) ganciclovir to be converted to nucleotides that are incorporated into and are toxic to glioma cell DNA. Table 3.3 illustrates trials employing this strategy that have been completed.
- Viruses must be engineered to be safe through genetic modifications that prevent normal cell infection. An example of such modification is the recombinant herpes simplex virus with deletions of both viral copies of the ICP34.5 gene. This modification removes virulence but allows the virus to destroy infected glioma cells.
- Viruses can be genetically engineered and maintain replication competence. The ideal virus is one that is not virulent to normal cells, specifically infects gliomas cells and replicates within them, ultimately causing cell death (oncolysis), release of daughter virus particles and infection of neighboring glioma cells. The release of tumor and virus antigens stimulates an immune response causing further tumor cell destruction. DNX-2401, a replication competent oncolytic adenovirus engineered to exploit the interaction between the virus and the retinoblastoma (Rb) protein pathway has shown early promise in phase I and II trials in patients with recurrent GBM with long term control of disease in some patients; this virus replicates in cells with an impaired Rb pathway (seen in >80% of GBM cells) but not in those with an intact Rb pathway (normal brain cells). Oncolysis by this virus can trigger an immune response which is being now exploited by immune stimulants such as interferon-γ or pembrolizumab, a PD1 inhibitor.
- Viruses can also be engineered to have a gene payload with therapeutic potential. An example of a virus construct that combines these qualities is Toca 511, a genetically engineered retrovirus that is replication competent and carries the gene for yeast cytosine deaminase (Ostertag et al. 2012). This enzyme converts 5-flucytosine (administered to patients orally) to 5-flurouracil, a chemotherapeutic agent that thus gets produced within the infected tumor cells where it exerts a chemotherapeutic effect and also diffuses to surrounding tumor cells. This is therefore another example of suicide gene therapy but has the potential added benefit of more efficient dissemination within the tumor due to virus replication and chemotherapy diffusion currently being tested in several trials (NCT01470794, NCT01156584).
- Table 3.4 illustrates other examples of ongoing and completed clinical trials that employ replication competent viruses for the treatment of malignant gliomas.

Table 3.3 Examples of High Grade Glioma Trials Employing Replication-Deficient Viral Vectors

Diagnosis	Trial design	Treatment arms	Viral construct	Delivery	Drug	MS	PFS	Ref	Comments
Newly Diagnosed Glioblastoma	Randomized open-label Phase III	Standard therapy				354 days	183 days	Rainov (2000)	Safe but no improvement in median or progression free survival
		standard therapy + adjuvant gene therapy during surgery	HSV-TK–expressing retroviral vector	PA317 producer cells	Ganciclovir	365 days	180 days		
Newly Diagnosed & Recurrent Malignant Glioma	Phase I	Control (transduced with lacZ marker gene 4–5 days before tumor resection)				8.3 months		Sandmair et al. (2000)	Mean survival time in adenovirus group was significantly prolonged to 15.0 months and treatment was well tolerated
		Retroviral vector-producing cells	HSV-TK	Retrovirus-packaging cells	Ganciclovir over 14 days	7.4 months	PFS3: 0%		
		Plaque-forming units of adenoviral vector injected peritumorally	AdV-HSV-TK		Ganciclovir over 14 days	15 months	PFS3: 42.85%		
Primary or Recurrent Malignant Glioma (n = 36)	Randomized controlled	Control (radiation)				37.7 days		Immonen et al. (2004)	AdvHSV-TK treatment produced a clinically and statistically significant increase in mean survival
		AdvHSV-TK gene therapy	AdV-HSV-TK		Ganciclovir over 14 days	62.4 days			
Newly Diagnosed Malignant Glioma (n = 13)	Phase IB	AdvHSV-TK gene therapy Radiation within 9 days after AdV-tk injection. Temozolomide administered after completing valacyclovir treatment.	AdV-HSV-TK		Vala-cyclovir for 14 days			Chiocca et al. (2011)	2-year survival: 33% 3 year survival: 25%. Three patients with MGMT unmethylated GBM survived 6.5, 8.7, and 46.4 months.

Table 3.4 Examples of completed and ongoing high grade glioma trials employing replication-competent oncolytic viruses (OVs)

Diagnosis (N)	Trial design	Treatment arm(s)	Viral construct	Delivery	Median survival	Progression free survival	Reference	Comments
Completed trials								
Recurrent malignant glioma (N = 9)	Phase I	Experimental only	HSV1716: ICP34.5-deleted HSV	Virus injection into tumor cavity	Not reported	4 alive 14–24 months after treatment	Rampling et al. (2000)	no induction of encephalitis, no adverse clinical symptoms, and no reactivation of latent HSV
Recurrent glioma (N = 12)	Phase I	Experimental only	HSV1716: ICP34.5-deleted HSV	Virus injection into tumor cavity	Not reported		Harrow et al. (2004)	
Recurrent or Newly Diagnosed (N = 12)	Phase I	Experimental only	HSV1716: ICP34.5-deleted HSV	Virus injection into tumor cavity	Not reported	3 patients alive and clinically stable at 15, 18 and 22 months after treatment.	Paparastassiou et al. (2002)	No toxicity
(N = 21)	Phase I	Experimental only	G207 (ICP34.5-deleted HSV with additional deletion of ICP6 gene)	Virus injection into tumor cavity	Not reported		Markert et al. (2000)	
Recurrent malignant glioma (N = 24)	Phase I	Experimental only	ONYX-015		6.2 months	46 days	Chiocca et al. (2004)	

Ongoing trials

Recurrent Malignant Glioma (N = 37)	Phase I	Experimental only	DNX-2401 (oncolytic virus with Delta-24 mutation: makes virus replication specific to cells defective in the retinoblastoma protein tumor suppressor).	Virus injection into tumor	Results pending	Results pending	NCT00805376, Pol et al. (2013)	Preliminary results indicate activity: >50% with stable disease, partial response or complete response)
Recurrent Glioblastoma (N = 20)	Phase I/II	Experimental only	DNX-2401 (Ref Walker et al. 1979) for additional details)	Convection-enhanced delivery	Results pending	Results pending	(NCT01582516)	
Recurrent Glioblastoma (N = 65)	Phase I	Experimental only	Poliovirus PVS-RIPO (Poliovirus vaccine engineered towards non-neurovirulence due to chimera with human rhinovirus and glioblastoma cell specificity due to nectin-5 receptor specificity)	Convection-enhanced delivery	Results pending	Results pending	Pol et al. (2013)	Three objective tumor responses noted on follow up

3.7.2 Immunotherapies

Given the immune system's role in human protection from infections and malignancy, the development of cancer could be viewed as a failure of this system. Additionally, once cancer develops it is associated with further immune suppression through effects of the tumor on immune system components. The strategy of immune therapy in central nervous system tumors was late in gaining acceptance compared to other cancers, mainly because of a perceived "immune privilege" of the central nervous system compared to other organ systems. However, clinical observations have shown that the immune system is activated specifically in response to central nervous system infections (meningitis and meningoencephalitis) and is in fact pivotal to the development and perpetuation of central nervous system pathologies (e.g. demyelinating disease). It is now known that intracranial malignancies do stimulate a T-cell response and that brain tumors, like systemic malignancies, do suppress the immune system in a variety of ways (Vauleon et al. 2010; Wilson et al. 2010). The following provides a brief overview of the most commonly employed strategies in currently ongoing clinical research in malignant gliomas.

Vaccine therapy The most traditional way to stimulate an immune response is through the use of vaccines which may include cell-based or non-cell based approaches.

(a) Cell-based vaccines:

Dendritic-cell vaccines: Dendritic cells are immune cells with very efficient antigen-presenting properties. In glioblastoma trials these cells are obtained from the patient and exposed to the tumor tissue obtained at surgery. DCVax-L® is an example of a dendritic-cell-based vaccine. The vaccine is a lysate consisting of peripheral blood mononuclear cells (PBMC) from the patient mixed with tumor tissue. The PBMC mature to dendritic cells a process that is encouraged by exposure to granulocyte-macrophage colony-stimulating factor (GM-CSF) and IL-4. A Phase I trial showed this treatment to be safe and showed a promising overall survival of almost 32 months (Prins et al. 2011), leading to Phase III trial (NCT00045968). This study is ongoing although not currently recruiting patients.

Autologous vaccine: The strategy of autologous vaccination employs modification of the tumor cells or of immune cells (usually T-lymphocytes) and introduction of the altered cells into the patient to induce immune responses. An example of this strategy is the use of autologous formalin-fixed tumor vaccines in which T-cells are sensitized to the tumor. A recent study by Muragaki et al. employed this vaccine in newly diagnosed glioblastoma patients during radiation therapy (Muragaki et al. 2011). The median duration of overall survival was 19.8 months and the actuarial 2-year survival rate was 40%. The median duration of progression-free survival was 7.6 months leading the investigators to conclude that further clinical testing was warranted.

(b) Non-cell based vaccines:

Peptide vaccines: EGFRvIII is a constitutively active mutant form of the epidermal growth factor receptor. It is present in about a third of glioblastoma specimens (Wong et al. 1992). A peptide-based vaccine was developed to induce a response to EGFR-VIII positive glioblastoma. A phase II trial examined the progression-free survival (PFS), and overall survival (OS) in patients with newly diagnosed glioblastoma who received the vaccine after ascertaining EGFR-VIII expression in the tumor specimen (Sampson et al. 2010). There were a total of eighteen patients enrolled and the median PFS and OS were 14.2 and 26 months for those receiving the vaccine. This compared very favorably with a PFS of 6.3 months and an OS of 15 months for the unvaccinated controls. However, a phase III trial to confirm these results did not show any difference in survival between treated patients and the placebo group, leading the independent Data Safety and Monitoring Board (DSMB) to recommend study discontinuation (Celldex 2016).

Heat-shock protein vaccines: Heat-shock proteins are considered to be crucial to the survival of cancers such as glioblastoma due to their key roles in stabilizing proteins, facilitating protein conformational change, protein trafficking and breakdown as well as control of apoptosis (Powers et al. 2010). They are activated by the "stress" environment found in tumor beds and consisting mainly of hypoxia and inflammation (Young et al. 2004). It is therefore not surprising that they would be considered targets in an immune strategy for treatment of glioblastoma. A Phase I study of 12 patients with recurrent glioblastoma was designed to test the hypothesis that since heat shock protein peptide complexes (HSPPCs) carry tumor-specific antigenic proteins and facilitate immune responses, peptides bound to a 96 kD chaperone protein (HSP-96) from brain tissue containing glioblastoma can be used to immunize patients with recurrent disease (Crane et al. 2013) The study showed that this could be done safely; testing of peripheral blood leukocytes before and after vaccination showing a significant peripheral immune response specific for the peptides bound to HSP-96, in almost all (11 of the 12) patients treated. The study also included correlative brain biopsies of immune responders after vaccination showing focal CD4, CD8, and CD56 IFNγ positive cell infiltrates, consistent with tumor site specific immune responses. The immune responders had a median survival of 47 weeks after surgery and vaccination, compared with 16 weeks for one patient who did not show a response. The following Phase II trial was also promising with patients having a total resection of recurrent glioblastoma and then receiving vaccine with HSPPC-96 (Bloch et al. 2014). The median PFS of this cohort was 19.1 weeks with a median OS of 42.6 weeks. There is an ongoing randomized Phase II study examining this vaccine strategy with bevacizumab and comparing it bevacizumab alone [NCT01814813].

3.7.2.1   Immune Checkpoint Inhibitors

The immune system employs a system of checks and balances that include "checkpoints', essentially proteins that down regulate the immune response to prevent damage to self. CTLA-4 controls T-cell activity and is a protein found on cytotoxic T-cells (CD8+) and subsets of helper (CD4+) T cells (Schwartz 1992; Rudd et al. 2009). Activation of the protein through ligand binding causes a reduction in IL-2 production, reduced IL-2 receptor expression, lymphocyte cell division (Alegre et al. 2001) and enhancement of T suppressor cell function (Wing et al. 2008; Peggs et al. 2009). The development of an antibody to CTLA-4, ipilimumab holds promise for inhibition of this checkpoint and has been approved for melanoma. Similarly, PD-1 is a protein expressed by T-cells, including regulatory T-cells (T_{regs}) (Francisco et al. 2009), B-cells and NK cells (Velu et al. 2009). Its expression serves as a "brake" on the immune response and it binds to PD-L1, a ligand that seems to be associated with derangements in the PI3K–Akt signaling pathway (Parsa et al. 2007) Nivolumab is a PD-1 antibody. There is an ongoing phase III trial (NCT02017717) comparing the efficacy of nivolumab with bevacizumab in patients with recurrent glioblastoma. There is also a phase I trial comparing ipilimumab, nivolumab, and the combination in patients with newly diagnosed glioblastoma (NCT02311920) and a randomized phase III open label study of nivolumab versus bevacizumab and multiple phase I safety cohorts of nivolumab or nivolumab in combination with ipilimumab (NCT02017717).

3.7.2.2   Genetically Engineered T-cells

The development of chimeric antigen receptor (CAR) technology has opened yet another door to the immune therapy possibilities in cancer. T-cells are engineered to recognize antigens on tumors by fusing an extracellular binding domain to the intracellular signaling domain of the T cell receptor (Eshhar et al. 1993). The extracellular domain is derived from an antibody to a tumor-associated antigen. CARs have been developed for HER2, IL-13Rα2, and EGFRvIII. The preclinical activity demonstrated by these cells led to clinical trial testing and these efforts have been comprehensively reviewed in recent publications (Thaci et al. 2014). CAR technology offers important advantages when compared to other immune therapies, including cytotoxicity that is independent of MHC class I expression. Given the variability of this expression in glioblastoma this may represent a significant therapeutic advantage. Additionally, CARs may have better penetration into blood vessel walls and tumor than other non-genetically engineered components of the immune system (Miao et al. 2014).

3.8 Conclusions

In contrast to the several decades of therapeutic strategies against GBMs during which only incremental advances in our knowledge of glioblastoma had been achieved, the past few years have seen an veritable explosion of knowledge of the basic biology of glioma and generated a high degree of enthusiasm and optimism in the field that we are closer to effective treatments that will dramatically improve outcomes of patients with GBM. In addition, the wealth of knowledge gained in modulation of the human immune system and the harnessing of biological therapies that are active regardless of tumor heterogeneity promise to transform therapeutic strategies against these aggressive tumors. These factors combined with the advances in technology and basic research are set to potentially shift the paradigm in therapeutic approaches for patients with GBM.

References

Alegre, M.L., K.A. Frauwirth, and C.B. Thompson. 2001. T-cell regulation by CD28 and CTLA-4. *Nature Reviews. Immunology* 1(3): 220–228. doi:10.1038/35105024.

Andersen, A.P. 1978. Postoperative irradiation of glioblastomas. Results in a randomized series. *Acta Radiologica: Oncology, Radiation, Physics, Biology* 17 (6): 475–484.

Barbarite, E., J.T. Sick, E. Berchmans, A. Bregy, A.H. Shah, N. Elsayyad, and R.J. Komotar. 2016. The role of brachytherapy in the treatment of glioblastoma multiforme. *Neurosurgical Review* 40 (2): 195–211. doi:10.1007/s10143-016-0727-6.

Batchelor, T.T., P. Mulholland, B. Neyns, L.B. Nabors, M. Campone, A. Wick, et al. 2013. Phase III randomized trial comparing the efficacy of cediranib as monotherapy, and in combination with lomustine, versus lomustine alone in patients with recurrent glioblastoma. *Journal of Clinical Oncology* 31 (26): 3212–3218. doi:10.1200/JCO.2012.47.2464.

Bennouna, J., J. Sastre, D. Arnold, P. Osterlund, R. Greil, E. Van Cutsem, et al. 2013. Continuation of bevacizumab after first progression in metastatic colorectal cancer (ML18147): A randomised phase 3 trial. *The Lancet Oncology* 14 (1): 29–37. doi:10.1016/S1470-2045(12)70477-1.

van den Bent, M.J., A.A. Brandes, R. Rampling, M.C. Kouwenhoven, J.M. Kros, A.F. Carpentier, et al. 2009. Randomized phase II trial of erlotinib versus temozolomide or carmustine in recurrent glioblastoma: EORTC brain tumor group study 26034. *Journal of Clinical Oncology* 27 (8): 1268–1274. doi:10.1200/JCO.2008.17.5984.

Bloch, O., C.A. Crane, Y. Fuks, R. Kaur, M.K. Aghi, M.S. Berger, et al. 2014. Heat-shock protein peptide complex-96 vaccination for recurrent glioblastoma: A phase II, single-arm trial. *Neuro-Oncology* 16: 274–910.1093. doi:10.1093/neuonc/not203.

Brandes, A.A., A. Tosoni, P. Amista, L. Nicolardi, D. Grosso, F. Berti, et al. 2004. How effective is BCNU in recurrent glioblastoma in the modern era? A phase II trial. *Neurology* 63 (7): 1281–1284.

Brandes, A.A., A. Tosoni, E. Franceschi, V. Blatt, A. Santoro, M. Faedi, et al. 2009a. Fotemustine as second-line treatment for recurrent or progressive glioblastoma after concomitant and/or adjuvant temozolomide: A phase II trial of Gruppo Italiano Cooperativo di Neuro-Oncologia (GICNO). *Cancer Chemotherapy and Pharmacology* 64 (4): 769–775. doi:10.1007/s00280-009-0926-8.

Brandes, A.A., E. Franceschi, A. Tosoni, F. Benevento, L. Scopece, V. Mazzocchi, et al. 2009b. Temozolomide concomitant and adjuvant to radiotherapy in elderly patients with glioblastoma: Correlation with MGMT promoter methylation status. *Cancer* 115 (15): 3512–3518. doi:10.1002/cncr.24406.

Brem, H., S. Piantadosi, P.C. Burger, M. Walker, R. Selker, N.A. Vick, et al. 1995. Placebo-controlled trial of safety and efficacy of intraoperative controlled delivery by biodegradable polymers of chemotherapy for recurrent gliomas. *The Polymer-brain Tumor Treatment Group. Lancet.* 345 (8956): 1008–1012.

Brennan, C.W., R.G. Verhaak, A. McKenna, B. Campos, H. Noushmehr, S.R. Salama, et al. 2013. The somatic genomic landscape of glioblastoma. *Cell* 155 (2): 462–477. doi:10.1016/j.cell.2013.09.034.

Brown, P.D., S. Krishnan, J.N. Sarkaria, W. Wu, K.A. Jaeckle, J.H. Uhm, et al. 2008. Phase I/II trial of erlotinib and temozolomide with radiation therapy in the treatment of newly diagnosed glioblastoma multiforme: North Central Cancer Treatment Group Study N0177. *Journal of Clinical Oncology* 26 (34): 5603–5609. doi:10.1200/JCO.2008.18.0612.

Buckner, J.C. 2003. Factors influencing survival in high-grade gliomas. *Seminars in Oncology* 30 (6 Suppl 19): 10–14.

Cabrera, A.R., K.C. Cuneo, A. Desjardins, J.H. Sampson, F. McSherry, J.E. Herndon 2nd, et al. 2013. Concurrent stereotactic radiosurgery and bevacizumab in recurrent malignant gliomas: A prospective trial. *International Journal of Radiation Oncology, Biology, Physics* 86 (5): 873–879. doi:10.1016/j.ijrobp.2013.04.029.

Celldex, Public Communication. 2016. http://ir.celldex.com/releasedetail.cfm?ReleaseID=959021.

Chan, J.L., S.W. Lee, B.A. Fraass, D.P. Normolle, H.S. Greenberg, L.R. Junck, et al. 2002. Survival and failure patterns of high-grade gliomas after three-dimensional conformal radiotherapy. *Journal of Clinical Oncology* 20 (6): 1635–1642.

Chang, S.M., P. Wen, T. Cloughesy, H. Greenberg, D. Schiff, C. Conrad, et al. 2005. Phase II study of CCI-779 in patients with recurrent glioblastoma multiforme. *Investigational New Drugs* 23 (4): 357–361. doi:10.1007/s10637-005-1444-0.

Chinot, O.L., W. Wick, W. Mason, R. Henriksson, F. Saran, R. Nishikawa, et al. 2014. Bevacizumab plus radiotherapy-temozolomide for newly diagnosed glioblastoma. *The New England Journal of Medicine* 370 (8): 709–722. doi:10.1056/NEJMoa1308345.

Chiocca, E.A., K.M. Abbed, S. Tatter, et al. 2004. A phase I open-label, dose-escalation, multi-institutional trial of injection with an E1B-attenuated adenovirus, ONYX-015, into the peritumoral region of recurrent malignant gliomas, in the adjuvant setting. *Molecular Therapy* 10: 958–966.

Chiocca, E.A., L.K. Aguilar, S.D. Bell, et al. 2011. Phase IB study of gene-mediated cytotoxic immunotherapy adjuvant to up-front surgery and intensive timing radiation for malignant glioma. *Journal of Clinical Oncology* 29: 3611–3619.

Choe, G., S. Horvath, T.F. Cloughesy, K. Crosby, D. Seligson, A. Palotie, et al. 2003. Analysis of the phosphatidylinositol 3'-kinase signaling pathway in glioblastoma patients in vivo. *Cancer Research* 63 (11): 2742–2746.

Choucair, A.K., V.A. Levin, P.H. Gutin, R.L. Davis, P. Silver, M.S. Edwards, et al. 1986. Development of multiple lesions during radiation therapy and chemotherapy in patients with gliomas. *Journal of Neurosurgery* 65 (5): 654–658. doi:10.3171/jns.1986.65.5.0654.

Combs, S.E., J. Wagner, M. Bischof, T. Welzel, F. Wagner, J. Debus, et al. 2008. Postoperative treatment of primary glioblastoma multiforme with radiation and concomitant temozolomide in elderly patients. *International Journal of Radiation Oncology, Biology, Physics* 70 (4): 987–992. doi:10.1016/j.ijrobp.2007.07.2368.

Cozad, S.C., P. Townsend, R.A. Morantz, A.B. Jenny, J.J. Kepes, and S.R. Smalley. 1996. Gliomatosis cerebri. Results with radiation therapy. *Cancer* 78 (8): 1789–1793.

Crane, C.A., S.J. Han, B. Ahn, J. Oehlke, V. Kivett, A. Fedoroff, et al. 2013. Individual patient-specific immunity against high-grade glioma after vaccination with autologous tumor derived peptides bound to the 96 KD chaperone protein. *Clinical Cancer Research* 19: 205–214. doi:10.1158/1078-0432.ccr-11-3358.

Del Vecchio, C.A., C.P. Giacomini, H. Vogel, K.C. Jensen, T. Florio, A. Merlo, et al. 2013. EGFRvIII gene rearrangement is an early event in glioblastoma tumorigenesis and expression defines a hierarchy modulated by epigenetic mechanisms. *Oncogene* 32 (21): 2670–2681. doi:10.1038/onc.2012.280.

Engelman, J.A. 2009. Targeting PI3K signalling in cancer: Opportunities, challenges and limitations. *Nature Reviews. Cancer* 9 (8): 550–562. doi:10.1038/nrc2664.

Eshhar, Z., T. Waks, G. Gross, and D.G. Schindler. 1993. Specific activation and targeting of cytotoxic lymphocytes through chimeric single chains consisting of antibody-binding domains and the gamma or zeta subunits of the immunoglobulin and T-cell receptors. *Proceedings of the National Academy of Sciences of the United States of America* 90: 720–410.

Esteller, M., J. Garcia-Foncillas, E. Andion, S.N. Goodman, Hidalgo OF, V. Vanaclocha, et al. 2000. Inactivation of the DNA-repair gene MGMT and the clinical response of gliomas to alkylating agents. *The New England Journal of Medicine* 343 (19): 1350–1354. doi:10.1056/NEJM200011093431901.

Fabrini, M.G., G. Silvano, I. Lolli, F. Perrone, A. Marsella, V. Scotti, et al. 2009. A multi-institutional phase II study on second-line Fotemustine chemotherapy in recurrent glioblastoma. *Journal of Neuro-Oncology* 92 (1): 79–86. doi:10.1007/s11060-008-9739-6.

Francisco, L.M., V.H. Salinas, K.E. Brown, V.K. Vanguri, G.J. Freeman, V.K. Kuchroo, et al. 2009. PD-L1 regulates the development, maintenance, and function of induced regulatory T cells. *The Journal of Experimental Medicine* 206: 3015–3029. doi:10.1084/jem.20090847.

Galanis, E., J.C. Buckner, M.J. Maurer, J.I. Kreisberg, K. Ballman, J. Boni, et al. 2005. Phase II trial of temsirolimus (CCI-779) in recurrent glioblastoma multiforme: A North Central Cancer Treatment Group Study. *Journal of Clinical Oncology* 23 (23): 5294–5304. doi:10.1200/JCO.2005.23.622.

Gera, N., A. Yang, T.S. Holtzman, S.X. Lee, E.T. Wong, and K.D. Swanson. 2015. Tumor treating fields perturb the localization of septins and cause aberrant mitotic exit. *PLoS One.* 10 (5): e0125269. doi:10.1371/journal.pone.0125269.

Gilbert, M.R., M. Wang, K.D. Aldape, R. Stupp, M.E. Hegi, K.A. Jaeckle, et al. 2013. Dose-dense temozolomide for newly diagnosed glioblastoma: A randomized phase III clinical trial. *Journal of Clinical Oncology* 31 (32): 4085–4091. doi:10.1200/JCO.2013.49.6968.

Gilbert, M.R., J.J. Dignam, T.S. Armstrong, J.S. Wefel, D.T. Blumenthal, M.A. Vogelbaum, et al. 2014. A randomized trial of bevacizumab for newly diagnosed glioblastoma. *The New England Journal of Medicine* 370 (8): 699–708. doi:10.1056/NEJMoa1308573.

Gutin, P.H., F.M. Iwamoto, K. Beal, N.A. Mohile, S. Karimi, B.L. Hou, et al. 2009. Safety and efficacy of bevacizumab with hypofractionated stereotactic irradiation for recurrent malignant gliomas. *International Journal of Radiation Oncology, Biology, Physics* 75 (1): 156–163. doi:10.1016/j.ijrobp.2008.10.043.

Harrow, S., V. Papanastassiou, J. Harland, et al. 2004. HSV1716 injection into the brain adjacent to tumour following surgical resection of high-grade glioma: Safety data and long-term survival. *Gene Therapy* 11: 1648–1658. doi:10.1038/sj.gt.3302289.

Hegi, M.E., A.C. Diserens, T. Gorlia, M.F. Hamou, N. de Tribolet, M. Weller, et al. 2005. MGMT gene silencing and benefit from temozolomide in glioblastoma. *The New England Journal of Medicine* 352 (10): 997–1003. doi:10.1056/NEJMoa043331.

Herrlinger, U. 2012. Gliomatosis cerebri. *Handbook of Clinical Neurology* 105: 507–515. doi:10.1016/B978-0-444-53502-3.00005-7.

Hovey, E., J., Field, K., M., Rosenthal, M., Nowak, A., K., Cher, L., Wheeler, H. et al. 2015. Continuing or ceasing bevacizumab at disease progression: Results from the CABARET study, a prospective randomized phase II trial in patients with recurrent glioblastoma. *2015 ASCO Annual Meeting: American Society of Clinical Oncology.*

Immonen, A., M. Vapalahti, K. Tyynela, et al. 2004. AdvHSV-tk gene therapy with intravenous ganciclovir improves survival in human malignant glioma: A randomised, controlled study. *Molecular Therapy* 10: 967–972. doi:10.1016/j.ymthe.2004.08.002.

84

J.L. Wang et al.

Iwamoto, F.M., L.E. Abrey, K. Beal, P.H. Gutin, M.K. Rosenblum, V.E. Reuter, L.M. DeAngelis, and A.B. Lassman. 2009. Patterns of relapse and prognosis after bevacizumab failure in recurrent glioblastoma. *Neurology* 73 (15): 1200–1206. doi:10.1212/WNL.0b013e3181bc0184.

Keime-Guibert, F., O. Chinot, L. Taillandier, S. Cartalat-Carel, M. Frenay, G. Kantor, et al. 2007. Radiotherapy for glioblastoma in the elderly. *The New England Journal of Medicine* 356 (15): 1527–1535. doi:10.1056/NEJMoa065901.

Kirson, E.D., V. Dbaly, F. Tovarys, J. Vymazal, J.F. Soustiel, A. Itzhaki, et al. 2007. Alternating electric fields arrest cell proliferation in animal tumor models and human brain tumors. *Proceedings of the National Academy of Sciences of the United States of America* 104 (24): 10152–10157. doi:10.1073/pnas.0702916104.

Kirson, E.D., R.S. Schneiderman, V. Dbaly, F. Tovarys, J. Vymazal, A. Itzhaki, et al. 2009a. Chemotherapeutic treatment efficacy and sensitivity are increased by adjuvant alternating electric fields (TTFields). *BMC Medical Physics* 9: 1. doi:10.1186/1756-6649-9-1.

Kirson, E.D., M. Giladi, Z. Gurvich, A. Itzhaki, D. Mordechovich, R.S. Schneiderman, et al. 2009b. Alternating electric fields (TTFields) inhibit metastatic spread of solid tumors to the lungs. *Clinical & Experimental Metastasis* 26 (7): 633–640. doi:10.1007/s10585-009-9262-y.

Kita, D., I.F. Ciernik, S. Vaccarella, S. Franceschi, P. Kleihues, U.M. Lutolf, et al. 2009. Age as a predictive factor in glioblastomas: Population-based study. *Neuroepidemiology* 33 (1): 17–22. doi:10.1159/000210017.

Kreisl, T.N., L. Kim, K. Moore, P. Duic, C. Royce, I. Stroud, et al. 2009. Phase II trial of single-agent bevacizumab followed by bevacizumab plus irinotecan at tumor progression in recurrent glioblastoma. *Journal of Clinical Oncology* 27 (5): 740–745. doi:10.1200/JCO.2008.16.3055.

Kubben, P.L., K.J. ter Meulen, O.E. Schijns, M.P. ter Laak-Poort, J.J. van Overbeeke, and H. van Santbrink. 2011. Intraoperative MRI-guided resection of glioblastoma multiforme: A systematic review. *The Lancet Oncology* 12 (11): 1062–1070. doi:10.1016/S1470-2045(11)70130-9.

Lacroix, M., D. Abi-Said, D.R. Fourney, Z.L. Gokaslan, W. Shi, F. DeMonte, F.F. Lang, I.E. McCutcheon, S.J. Hassenbusch, E. Holland, K. Hess, C. Michael, D. Miller, and R. Sawaya. 2001. A multivariate analysis of 416 patients with glioblastoma multiforme: prognosis, extent of resection, and survival. *Journal of Neurosurgery* 95 (2): 190–198. doi:10.3171/jns.2001.95.2.0190.

Li, Y.M., D. Suki, K. Hess, and R. Sawaya. 2016. The influence of maximum safe resection of glioblastoma on survival in 1229 patients: Can we do better than gross-total resection? *Journal of Neurosurgery* 124 (4): 977–988. doi:10.3171/2015.5.JNS142087.

Malmstrom, A., B.H. Gronberg, C. Marosi, R. Stupp, D. Frappaz, H. Schultz, et al. 2012. Temozolomide versus standard 6-week radiotherapy versus hypofractionated radiotherapy in patients older than 60 years with glioblastoma: The Nordic randomised, phase 3 trial. *The Lancet Oncology* 13 (9): 916–926. doi:10.1016/S1470-2045(12)70265-6.

Markert, J.M., M.D. Medlock, S.D. Rabkin, et al. 2000. Conditionally replicating herpes simplex virus mutant, G207 for the treatment of malignant glioma: Results of a phase I trial. *Gene Therapy* 7: 867–874. doi:10.1038/sj.gt.3301205.

McKie, E.A., A.R. MacLean, A.D. Lewis, et al. 1996. Selective in vitro replication of herpes simplex virus type 1 (HSV-1) ICP34.5 null mutants in primary human CNS tumours—evaluation of a potentially effective clinical therapy. *British Journal of Cancer* 74: 745–752.

Miao, H., B.D. Choi, C.M. Suryadevara, L. Sanchez-Perez, S. Yang, G. De Leon, et al. 2014. EGFRvIII-specific chimeric antigen receptor T cells migrate to and kill tumor deposits infiltrating the brain parenchyma in an invasive xenograft model of glioblastoma. *PLoS One* 9 (4): e94281. doi:10.1371/journal.pone.0094281.

Michaelsen, S.R., I.J. Christensen, K. Grunnet, M.T. Stockhausen, H. Broholm, M. Kosteljanetz, et al. 2013. Clinical variables serve as prognostic factors in a model for survival from glioblastoma multiforme: An observational study of a cohort of consecutive non-selected patients from a single institution. *BMC Cancer* 13: 402. doi:10.1186/1471-2407-13-402.

Minniti, G., C. Scaringi, G. Lanzetta, I. Terrenato, V. Esposito, A. Arcella, et al. 2015. Standard (60 Gy) or short-course (40 Gy) irradiation plus concomitant and adjuvant temozolomide for elderly patients with glioblastoma: A propensity-matched analysis. *International Journal of Radiation Oncology, Biology, Physics* 91 (1): 109–115. doi:10.1016/j.ijrobp.2014.09.013.

Muragaki, Y., T. Maruyama, H. Iseki, M. Tanaka, C. Shinohara, K. Takakura, et al. 2011. Phase I/IIa trial of autologous formalin-fixed tumor vaccine concomitant with fractionated radiotherapy for newly diagnosed glioblastoma. *Journal of Neurosurgery* 115: 248–255. doi:10.3171/2011.4.JNS10377.

NCT00805376. https://clinicaltrials.gov/ct2/show/NCT00805376?term=NCT00805376&rank=1.

NCT01582516. https://clinicaltrials.gov/ct2/show/NCT01582516?term=NCT01582516&rank=1.

Nelson, D.F., M. Diener-West, J. Horton, C.H. Chang, D. Schoenfeld, and J.S. Nelson. 1988. Combined modality approach to treatment of malignant gliomas--re-evaluation of RTOG 7401/ECOG 1374 with long-term follow-up: A joint study of the Radiation Therapy Oncology Group and the Eastern Cooperative Oncology Group. *NCI Monographs* 6: 279–284.

Nevin, S. 1938. Gliomatosis cerebri. *Brain* 61: 170–191.

Nwokedi, E.C., S.J. DiBiase, S. Jabbour, J. Herman, P. Amin, and L.S. Chin. 2002. Gamma knife stereotactic radiosurgery for patients with glioblastoma multiforme. *Neurosurgery* 50 (1): 41–46. discussion 46–7.

Ostertag, D., K.K. Amundson, F. Lopez Espinoza, B. Martin, T. Buckley, A.P. Galvao da Silva, A.H. Lin, D.T. Valenta, O.D. Perez, C.E. Ibanez, C.I. Chen, P.L. Pettersson, R. Burnett, V. Daublebsky, J. Hlavaty, W. Gunzburg, N. Kasahara, H.E. Gruber, D.J. Jolly, and J.M. Robbins. 2012. Brain tumor eradication and prolonged survival from intratumoral conversion of 5-fluorocytosine to 5-fluorouracil using a nonlytic retroviral replicating vector. *Neuro-Oncology* 14 (2): 145–159. doi:10.1093/neuonc/nor199.

Papanastassiou, V., R. Rampling, M. Fraser, et al. 2002. The potential for efficacy of the modified (ICP 34.5(−)) herpes simplex virus HSV1716 following intratumoural injection into human malignant glioma: A proof of principle study. *Gene Therapy* 9(6): 398–406. doi:10.1038/sj.gt.3301664.

Parsa, A.T., J.S. Waldron, A. Panner, C.A. Crane, I.F. Parney, J.J. Barry, et al. 2007. Loss of tumor suppressor PTEN function increases B7-H1 expression and immunoresistance in glioma. *Nature Medicine* 13: 84–88. doi:10.1038/nm1517.

Paszat, L., N. Laperriere, P. Groome, K. Schulze, W. Mackillop, and E. Holowaty. 2001. A population-based study of glioblastoma multiforme. *International Journal of Radiation Oncology, Biology, Physics* 51 (1): 100–107.

Peggs, K.S., S.A. Quezada, C.A. Chambers, A.J. Korman, and J.P. Allison. 2009. Blockade of CTLA-4 on both effector and regulatory T cell compartments contributes to the antitumor activity of anti-CTLA-4 antibodies. *The Journal of Experimental Medicine* 206: 1717–1725. doi:10.1084/jem.20082492.

Pelloski, C.E., K.V. Ballman, A.F. Furth, L. Zhang, E. Lin, E.P. Sulman, et al. 2007. Epidermal growth factor receptor variant III status defines clinically distinct subtypes of glioblastoma. *Journal of Clinical Oncology* 25 (16): 2288–2294. doi:10.1200/JCO.2006.08.0705.

Perry, J.R., N. Laperriere, C.J. O'Callaghan, A.A. Brandes, J. Menten, C. Phillips, M.F. Fay, R. Nishikawa, J.G. Cairncross, W. Roa, D. Osoba, A. Sahgal, H.W. Hirte, W. Wick, F. Laigle-Donadey, E. Franceschi, O.L. Chinot, C. Winch, K. Ding, and W.P. Mason. 2016. A phase III randomized controlled trial of short-course radiotherapy with or without concomitant and adjuvant temozolomide in elderly patients with glioblastoma (CCTG CE.6, EORTC 26062-22061, TROG 08.02, NCT00482677). *Journal of Clinical Oncology* 34 (15, supplement (2016 ASCO Annual Meeting)):LBA2.

Pitz, M.W., E.A. Eisenhauer, M.V. MacNeil, B. Thiessen, J.C. Easaw, D.R. Macdonald, et al. 2015. Phase II study of PX-866 in recurrent glioblastoma. *Neuro-Oncology* 17 (9): 1270–1274. doi:10.1093/neuonc/nou365.

Pol, J.G., M. Marguerie, R. Arulanandam, et al. 2013. Panorama from the oncolytic virotherapy summit. *Molecular Therapy* 21: 1814–1818. doi:10.1038/mt.2013.207.

Powers, M.V., K. Jones, C. Barillari, I. Westwood, R.L. van Montfort, and P. Workman. 2010. Targeting HSP70: the second potentially druggable heat shock protein and molecular chaperone? *Cell Cycle* 9: 1542–1550. doi:10.4161/cc.9.8.11204.

Prins, R.M., H. Soto, Odesa S.K. KonkankitV, A. Eskin, W.H. Yong, et al. 2011. Gene expression profile correlates with T-cell infiltration and relative survival in glioblastoma patients vaccinated with dendritic cell immunotherapy. *Clinical Cancer Research* 17(6): 1603–1615. doi:10.1158/1078-0432.ccr-10-2563.

Quant, E.C., A.D. Norden, J. Drappatz, A. Muzikansky, L. Doherty, D. Lafrankie, A. Ciampa, S. Kesari, and P.Y. Wen. 2009. Role of a second chemotherapy in recurrent malignant glioma patients who progress on bevacizumab. *Neuro-Oncology* 11 (5): 550–555. doi:10.1215/15228517-2009-006.

Rainov, N.G. 2000. A phase III clinical evaluation of herpes simplex virus type 1 thymidine kinase and ganciclovir gene therapy as an adjuvant to surgical resection and radiation in adults with previously untreated glioblastoma multiforme. *Human Gene Therapy* 11(17): 2389–2401. doi:10.1089/104303400750038499.

Rampling, R., G. Cruickshank, V. Papanastassiou, ct al. 2000. Toxicity evaluation of replication-competent herpes simplex virus (ICP 34.5 null mutant 1716) in patients with recurrent malignant glioma. *Gene Therapy* 7: 859–866.

Reardon, D.A., G. Akabani, R.E. Coleman, A.H. Friedman, H.S. Friedman, J.E. Herndon 2nd, et al.2006. Salvage radioimmunotherapy with murine iodine-131-labeled antitenascin monoclonal antibody 81C6 for patients with recurrent primary and metastatic malignant brain tumors: Phase II study results. *Journal of Clinical Oncology* 24 (1): 115–122. doi:10.1200/JCO.2005.03.4082.

Reifenberger, G., B. Hentschel, J. Felsberg, G. Schackert, M. Simon, O. Schnell, et al. 2012. Predictive impact of MGMT promoter methylation in glioblastoma of the elderly. *International Journal of Cancer* 131 (6): 1342–1350. doi:10.1002/ijc.27385.

Roa, W., P.M. Brasher, G. Bauman, M. Anthes, E. Bruera, A. Chan, et al. 2004. Abbreviated course of radiation therapy in older patients with glioblastoma multiforme: a prospective randomized clinical trial. *Journal of Clinical Oncology* 22 (9): 1583–1588. doi:10.1200/JCO.2004.06.082.

Rudd, C.E., A. Taylor, and H. Schneider. 2009. CD28 and CTLA-4 coreceptor expression and signaltransduction.*ImmunologicalReviews*229:12–26.doi:10.1111/j.1600-065X.2009.00770.x.

Sampson, J.H., A.B. Heimberger, G.E. Archer, K.D. Aldape, A.H. Friedman, H.S. Friedman, et al. 2010. Immunologic escape after prolonged progression-free survival with epidermal growth factor receptor variant III peptide vaccination in patients with newly diagnosed glioblastoma. *Journal of Clinical Oncology* 28: 4722–4729. doi:10.1200/jco.2010.28.6963.

Sanai, N., M.Y. Polley, M.W. McDermott, A.T. Parsa, and M.S. Berger. 2011. An extent of resection threshold for newly diagnosed glioblastomas. *Journal of Neurosurgery* 115 (1): 3–8. doi:1 0.3171/2011.2.JNS10998.

Sandmair, A.M., S. Loimas, P. Puranen, et al. 2000. Thymidine kinase gene therapy for human malignant glioma, using replication-deficient retroviruses or adenoviruses. *Human Gene Therapy* 11(16): 2197–2205. doi:10.1089/104303400750035726.

Schwartz, R.H. 1992. Costimulation of T lymphocytes: The role of CD28, CTLA-4, and B7/ BB1 in interleukin-2 production and immunotherapy. *Cell* 71: 1065–1068.

Seystahl, K., W. Wick, and M. Weller. 2016. Therapeutic options in recurrent glioblastoma–An update. *Critical Reviews in Oncology/Hematology* 99: 389–408. doi:10.1016/j. critrevonc.2016.01.018.

Sloan, A.E., M.S. Ahluwalia, J. Valerio-Pascua, S. Manjila, M.G. Torchia, S.E. Jones, et al. 2013. Results of the NeuroBlate System first-in-humans Phase I clinical trial for recurrent glioblastoma: Clinical article. *Journal of Neurosurgery* 118 (6): 1202–1219. doi:10.3171/2 013.1.JNS1291.

Souhami, L., W. Seiferheld, D. Brachman, E.B. Podgorsak, M. Werner-Wasik, R. Lustig, et al. 2004. Randomized comparison of stereotactic radiosurgery followed by conventional radio-therapy with carmustine to conventional radiotherapy with carmustine for patients with glioblastoma multiforme: Report of Radiation Therapy Oncology Group 93-05 protocol. *International Journal of Radiation Oncology, Biology, Physics* 60 (3): 853–860. doi:10.1016/j. ijrobp.2004.04.011.

Stark-Vance, V. 2005. Bevacizumab and CPT-11 in the treatment of relapsed malignant glioma. *Neuro-Oncology* 7: 369.

Stummer, W., U. Pichlmeier, T. Meinel, O.D. Wiestler, F. Zanella, H.J. Reulen, et al. 2006. Fluorescence-guided surgery with 5-aminolevulinic acid for resection of malignant glioma: A randomised controlled multicentre phase III trial. *The Lancet Oncology* 7 (5): 392–401. doi:10.1016/S1470-2045(06)70665-9.

Stupp, R., W.P. Mason, M.J. van den Bent, M. Weller, B. Fisher, M.J. Taphoorn, et al. 2005. Radiotherapy plus concomitant and adjuvant temozolomide for glioblastoma. *The New England Journal of Medicine* 352 (10): 987–996. doi:10.1056/NEJMoa043330.

Stupp, R., M.E. Hegi, W.P. Mason, M.J. van den Bent, M.J. Taphoorn, R.C. Janzer, et al. 2009. Effects of radiotherapy with concomitant and adjuvant temozolomide versus radiotherapy alone on survival in glioblastoma in a randomised phase III study: 5-year analysis of the EORTC-NCIC trial. *The Lancet Oncology* 10 (5): 459–466. doi:10.1016/S1470-2045(09)70025-7.

Stupp, R., E.T. Wong, A.A. Kanner, D. Steinberg, H. Engelhard, V. Heidecke, et al. 2012. NovoTTF-100A versus physician's choice chemotherapy in recurrent glioblastoma: A randomised phase III trial of a novel treatment modality. *European Journal of Cancer* 48 (14): 2192–2202. doi:10.1016/j.ejca.2012.04.011.

Stupp, R., S. Taillibert, A.A. Kanner, S. Kesari, D.M. Steinberg, S.A. Toms, et al. 2015. Maintenance therapy with tumor-treating fields plus temozolomide vs temozolomide alone for glioblastoma: A randomized clinical trial. *Journal of the American Medical Association* 314 (23): 2535–2543. doi:10.1001/jama.2015.16669.

Suchorska, B., M. Weller, G. Tabatabai, C. Senft, P. Hau, M.C. Sabel, et al. 2016. Complete resection of contrast-enhancing tumor volume is associated with improved survival in recurrent glioblastoma-results from the DIRECTOR trial. *Neuro-Oncology* 18 (4): 549–556. doi:10.1093/neuonc/nov326.

Taal, W., H.M. Oosterkamp, A.M. Walenkamp, H.J. Dubbink, L.V. Beerepoot, M.C. Hanse, et al. 2014. Single-agent bevacizumab or lomustine versus a combination of bevacizumab plus lomustine in patients with recurrent glioblastoma (BELOB trial): A randomised controlled phase 2 trial. *The Lancet Oncology* 15 (9): 943–953. doi:10.1016/S1470-2045(14)70314-6.

Taillibert, S., C. Chodkiewicz, F. Laigle-Donadey, M. Napolitano, S. Cartalat-Carel, and M. Sanson. 2006. Gliomatosis cerebri: A review of 296 cases from the ANOCEF database and the literature. *Journal of Neuro-Oncology* 76 (2): 201–205. doi:10.1007/s11060-005-5263-0.

Thaci, B., C.E. Brown, E. Binello, K. Werbaneth, P. Sampath, and S. Sengupta. 2014. Significance of interleukin-13 receptor alpha 2-targeted glioblastoma therapy. *Neuro-Oncology* 16 (10): 1304–1312.

Tolcher, A.W., S.L. Gerson, L. Denis, C. Geyer, L.A. Hammond, A. Patnaik, et al. 2003. Marked inactivation of O6-alkylguanine-DNA alkyltransferase activity with protracted temozolomide schedules. *British Journal of Cancer* 88 (7): 1004–1011. doi:10.1038/sj.bjc.6600827.

Torok, J.A., R.E. Wegner, A.H. Mintz, D.E. Heron, and S.A. Burton. 2011. Re-irradiation with radiosurgery for recurrent glioblastoma multiforme. *Technology in Cancer Research & Treatment* 10 (3): 253–258.

Vauleon, E., T. Avril, B. Collet, J. Mosser, and V. Quillien. 2010. Overview of cellular immunotherapy for patients with glioblastoma. *Clinical & Developmental Immunology* 2010: 689171. doi:10.1155/2010/689171.

Velu, V., K. Titanji, B. Zhu, S. Husain, A. Pladevega, L. Lai, et al. 2009. Enhancing SIV-specific immunity in vivo by PD-1 blockade. *Nature* 458(7235): 206–210. doi:10.1038/nature07662.

Vuorinen, V., S. Hinkka, M. Farkkila, and J. Jaaskelainen. 2003. Debulking or biopsy of malignant glioma in elderly people – a randomised study. *Acta Neurochirurgica* 145 (1): 5–10. doi:10.1007/s00701-002-1030-6.

Walker, M.D., E. Alexander Jr., W.E. Hunt, C.S. MacCarty, M.S. Mahaley Jr., J. Mealey Jr., et al. 1978. Evaluation of BCNU and/or radiotherapy in the treatment of anaplastic gliomas. A cooperative clinical trial. *Journal of Neurosurgery* 49 (3): 333–343. doi:10.3171/jns.1978.49.3.0333.

Walker, M.D., S.B. Green, D.P. Byar, E. Alexander Jr., U. Batzdorf, W.H. Brooks, et al. 1980. Randomized comparisons of radiotherapy and nitrosoureas for the treatment of malignant glioma after surgery. *The New England Journal of Medicine* 303 (23): 1323–1329. doi:10.1056/NEJM198012043032303.

Wallner, K.E., J.H. Galicich, G. Krol, E. Arbit, and M.G. Malkin. 1989. Patterns of failure following treatment for glioblastoma multiforme and anaplastic astrocytoma. *International Journal of Radiation Oncology, Biology, Physics* 16 (6): 1405–1409.

Weller, M., T. Cloughesy, J.R. Perry, and W. Wick. 2013. Standards of care for treatment of recurrent glioblastoma–are we there yet? *Neuro-Oncology* 15 (1): 4–27. doi:10.1093/neuonc/nos273.

Wen, P.Y., A. Omuro, M.S. Ahluwalia, H.M. Fathallah-Shaykh, N. Mohile, J.J. Lager, et al. 2015. Phase I dose-escalation study of the PI3K/mTOR inhibitor voxtalisib (SAR245409, XL765) plus temozolomide with or without radiotherapy in patients with high-grade glioma. *Neuro-Oncology* 17 (9): 1275–1283. doi:10.1093/neuonc/nov083.

Westphal, M., D.C. Hilt, E. Bortey, P. Delavault, R. Olivares, P.C. Warnke, et al. 2003. A phase 3 trial of local chemotherapy with biodegradable carmustine (BCNU) wafers (Gliadel wafers) in patients with primary malignant glioma. *Neuro-Oncology* 5 (2): 79–88. doi:10.1215/S1522-8517-02-00023-6.

Westphal, M., Z. Ram, V. Riddle, D. Hilt, E. Bortey, and Executive Committee of the Gliadel Study G. 2006. Gliadel wafer in initial surgery for malignant glioma: Long-term follow-up of a multicenter controlled trial. *Acta Neurochirurgica* 148 (3): 269–275. doi:10.1007/s00701-005-0707-z.discussion 275

Westphal, M., O. Heese, J.P. Steinbach, O. Schnell, G. Schackert, M. Mehdorn, et al. 2015. A randomised, open label phase III trial with nimotuzumab, an anti-epidermal growth factor receptor monoclonal antibody in the treatment of newly diagnosed adult glioblastoma. *European Journal of Cancer* 51 (4): 522–532. doi:10.1016/j.ejca.2014.12.019.

Wick, W., V.K. Puduvalli, M.C. Chamberlain, M.J. van den Bent, A.F. Carpentier, L.M. Cher, et al. 2010. Phase III study of enzastaurin compared with lomustine in the treatment of recurrent intracranial glioblastoma. *Journal of Clinical Oncology* 28 (7): 1168–1174. doi:10.1200/JCO.2009.23.2595.

Wick, W., T. Gorlia, P. Bady, M. Platten, M.J. van den Bent, M.J. Taphoorn, et al. 2016. Phase II study of radiotherapy and temsirolimus versus radiochemotherapy with temozolomide in patients with newly diagnosed glioblastoma without MGMT promoter hypermethylation (EORTC 26082). *Clinical Cancer Research*. doi:10.1158/1078-0432.CCR-15-3153.

Wilson, E.H., W. Weninger, and C.A. Hunter. 2010. Trafficking of immune cells in the central nervous system. *The Journal of Clinical Investigation* 120: 1368–1379. doi:10.1172/jci41911.

Wing, K., Y. Onishi, P. Prieto-Martin, T. Yamaguchi, M. Miyara, Z. Fehervari, et al. 2008. CTLA-4 control over Foxp3+ regulatory T cell function. *Science* 322 (5899): 271–275. doi:10.1126/science.1160062.

Wong, A.J., J.M. Ruppert, S.H. Bigner, C.H. Grzeschik, P.A. Humphrey, D.S. Bigner, et al. 1992. Structural alterations of the epidermal growth factor receptor gene in human gliomas. *Proceedings of the National Academy of Sciences of the United States of America* 89: 2965–2969. doi:10.1073/pnas.89.7.2965.

Wong, E.T., E. Lok, and K.D. Swanson. 2015. An evidence-based review of alternating electric fields therapy for malignant gliomas. *Current Treatment Options in Oncology* 16 (8): 40. doi:10.1007/s11864-015-0353-5.

Yang, L., R. Hwang, Y. Chiang, et al. 1998. Mechanisms for ganciclovir resistance in gastrointestinal tumor cells transduced with a retroviral vector containing the herpes simplex virus thymidine kinase gene. *Clinical Cancer Research* 4: 731–741.

Yong, R.L., T. Wu, N. Mihatov, M.J. Shen, M.A. Brown, K.A. Zaghloul, et al. 2014. Residual tumor volume and patient survival following reoperation for recurrent glioblastoma. *Journal of Neurosurgery* 121 (4): 802–809. doi:10.3171/2014.6.JNS132038.

Young, J.C., V.R. Agashe, K. Siegers, and F.U. Hartl. 2004. Pathways of chaperone-mediated protein folding in the cytosol. *Nature Reviews. Molecular Cell Biology* 5 (10): 781–791. doi:10.1038/nrm1492.

Zalutsky, M.R., D.A. Reardon, G. Akabani, R.E. Coleman, A.H. Friedman, H.S. Friedman, et al. 2008. Clinical experience with alpha-particle emitting 211At: Treatment of recurrent brain tumor patients with 211At-labeled chimeric antitenascin monoclonal antibody 81C6. *Journal of Nuclear Medicine* 49 (1): 30–38. doi:10.2967/jnumed.107.046938.

Chapter 4
Recent Advances for Targeted Therapies in Glioblastoma

Michael Youssef, Jacob Mandel, Sajeel Chowdhary, and Santosh Kesari

Abstract Glioblastoma (GBM) is the most common primary brain tumors in adults. Despite aggressive multimodality therapies, GBM unfortunately remains among the most resistant cancers to treatment. In the past, traditional chemotherapy which works by impeding DNA synthesis or cell metabolism has been used to try and slow the progression of GBM with little success. Recently, research has become more focused into the development of targeted therapies in which drugs (small molecules or antibodies) effect specific molecular and genetic alterations in GBM attempting to inhibit and deregulate cell signaling pathways. The Cancer Genome Atlas (TCGA) GBM project has provided an in depth description of the distinct molecular and genetic alterations in GBM stimulating interest in the development of targeted molecular therapies. While the results of targeted therapy studies to date have failed to improve the overall survival of GBM patients, there continues to be enthusiasm in this approach with numerous clinical trials currently underway. Hopefully, knowledge from the previous failed trials will help provide further insight and assist future clinicians in designing new novel targeted treatments to overcome these barriers.

Keywords Glioblastoma • targeted therapy • The Cancer Genome Atlas • Retinoblastoma pathway • p53 pathway • Receptor tyrosine kinase pathway

M. Youssef, MD
Department of Neurology at Baylor College of Medicine,
7200 Cambridge Ave, Suite 9A, Houston, TX 77030, USA

J. Mandel, MD
Neurology and Neurosurgery at Baylor College of Medicine,
7200 Cambridge Ave, Suite 9A, Houston, TX 77030, USA
e-mail: Jacob.mandel@bcm.edu

S. Chowdhary, MD
Lynn Cancer Institute, Marcus Neuroscience Institute,
800 Meadows Road, 1st Floor, Boca Raton, FL 33486, USA
e-mail: SChowdhary@brrh.com

S. Kesari, MD, PhD (✉)
Department of Translational Neurosciences and Neurotherapeutics, John Wayne Cancer Institute and Pacific Neuroscience Institute at Providence Saint John's Health Center,
2200 Santa Monica Blvd, Santa Monica, CA 90404, USA
e-mail: kesaris@jwci.org

© Springer International Publishing AG 2017
K. Somasundaram (ed.), *Advances in Biology and Treatment of Glioblastoma*,
Current Cancer Research, DOI 10.1007/978-3-319-56820-1_4

91

4.1   Recent Advances for Targeted Therapies in Glioblastoma

Gliobastoma multiforme (GBM) is the most common malignant primary brain tumor in adults (Davis et al. 2001; Cloughesy et al. 2014). Currently, 10,000 new cases of GBM are diagnosed each year in the United States, and approximately 100,000 new cases are diagnosed yearly worldwide (Davis et al. 2001; Cloughesy et al. 2014; Porter et al. 2010; Ohgaki and Kleihues 2005). Patients often initially undergo surgical resection to provide symptomatic relief and confirm a pathologic diagnosis. However, surgery is not curative as the tumor cells invade surrounding normal brain tissue rendering a complete resection of the tumor impossible (Cloughesy et al. 2014). Following a maximal safe resection, the standard of care treatment for newly diagnosed GBM consists of cytotoxic chemotherapy with daily temozolomide and concurrent radiation therapy for 6 weeks, followed by 6–12 cycles of adjuvant temozolomide (Masui et al. 2012; Stupp et al. 2005). Despite aggressive multimodality therapies, GBM unfortunately remains among the most resistant cancers to treatment leading to a median survival of around 16 months (Stupp et al. 2005). Several potential reasons have been proposed to explain GBMs resistance to treatment including the genetic heterogeneity of the tumor, elaborate signaling pathways, and difficulties with designing drugs capable of crossing the blood brain barrier (Tanaka et al. 2013). In the past, traditional chemotherapy which works by impeding DNA synthesis or cell metabolism has been most often used to try and slow the progression of GBM with little success. Recently, research has become more focused into the development of targeted therapies in which drugs (small molecules or antibodies) effect specific molecular and genetic alterations in GBM attempting to inhibit and deregulate cell signaling pathways. This chapter will explore current targeted therapies and how they relate to the aberrant signaling pathways in GBM.

4.2   The Cancer Genome Atlas

GBM was one of the first cancers studied by The Cancer Genome Atlas (TCGA) Research Network, a collaboration between the National Cancer Institute (NCI) and National Human Genome Research Institute (NHGRI). The TCGAs key aims were to identify changes in each cancer's genome and understand how these changes interact to drive the disease, thereby laying the foundation for improved cancer prevention, early detection, and treatment (Cancer Genome Atlas Research Network 2008; Bredel et al. 2011; Parsons et al. 2008; Verhaak et al. 2010). The TCGA GBM project was conducted in two phases and developed a genome wide map of the genetic, epigenetic, and transcriptomic changes, as well as proteomic changes in over 500 GBM samples (Cancer Genome Atlas Research Network 2008; Brennan et al. 2013). Based on molecular typing and gene expression profiles, four distinct subtypes of GBM were found which are the classical, mesenchymal, neural, and proneural aubtypes (Freije et al. 2004; Gravendeel et al. 2009; Li et al. 2009; Nigro et al. 2005; Vitucci et al. 2011; Jue and McDonald 2016). The Classical subtype is associated with Endothelial growth factor receptor (EGFR) amplification, concomitant chromosome 7 amplification and chromosome 10 loss, and focal deletions of 9p encompassing cyclin-dependent kinase Inhibitor 2A (CDKN2A) . Tumor protein p53 (TP53) mutations, while common in GBM, are not seen in the classical subtype (Jue and McDonald 2016). The Mesenchymal subtype is characterized by deletions and mutations in Neurofibromin 1 (NF1) and Phosphatase and tensin homolog (PTEN) genes (Jue and McDonald 2016). The Neural subtype exhibits expression of neuronal markers and displays various mutations and copy number alterations including amplification of EGFR and deletion of PTEN (Jue and McDonald 2016). The Proneural subtype exhibits an oliogodendrocytic expression signature and features mutations of the isocitrate dehydrogenase 1(IDH 1) gene (Jue and McDonald 2016). The proneural subtype is associated with younger age and prolonged survival time, given the IDH1 mutation, as IDH1 mutations are frequently seen in lower grade gliomas and secondary gliomas (Verhaak et al. 2010; Jue and McDonald 2016). The TCGA analysis further identified three key molecular pathways for tumorigenesis: the p53 tumor suppressor and Retinoblastoma (RB) pathways, and the receptor tyrosine kinases (RTKs) signaling pathway (Fig. 4.1).

4.3   Tumor Protein P53 Signaling Pathway

Tumor protein p53 is a well-known tumor suppressor gene and transcription factor involved in the coordination of cell responses that are involved in processes such as apoptosis, DNA repair, neovascularization, and metabolism (Bogler et al. 1995; Matlashewski et al. 1984; May and May 1999). p53 has been found mutated in 37.5% and 58% of untreated and treated GBM samples, according to the TCGA (Cancer Genome Atlas Research Network 2008). Disruptions in the p53 pathway are achieved by disruptions in genes that regulate its function, including Mouse double minute homolog (MDM) 2/4 and the tumor suppressor protein alternate reading frame (ARF) in 70% of GBM samples (Cancer Genome Atlas Research Network 2008). A complex that can suppress p53 function is the MDM2-MDM4 heterocomplex through the exertion of degradative control. MDM2-MDM4 protein amplification may represent a possible mechanism that gliomas escape p53 restricted growth (Herman et al. 2011; Reifenberger et al. 1993; Riemenschneider et al. 1999). Inactivation of CDKN2a can also dysregulate the p53 signaling pathway. CDKN2a encodes two proteins (p16INK4a and p14ARF) which are tumor suppressors and are negative regulators of the cell cycle (Ruas and Peters 1998). p16INK4a and p14ARF are deleted in approximately 55% of GBMs (Cancer Genome Atlas Research Network 2008; Schmidt et al. 1994). An encoded protein product, p14ARF, was found to promote degradation of the p53 repressor and lead to stabilization and accumulation of p53. Loss of p14ARF results in suppression of p53 and provides a mechanism for tumorigenesis (Kamijo et al. 1997, 1998; Zhang et al. 1998). CDKN2a also encodes for p16INK4a which is a protein that inhibits CDK4/6

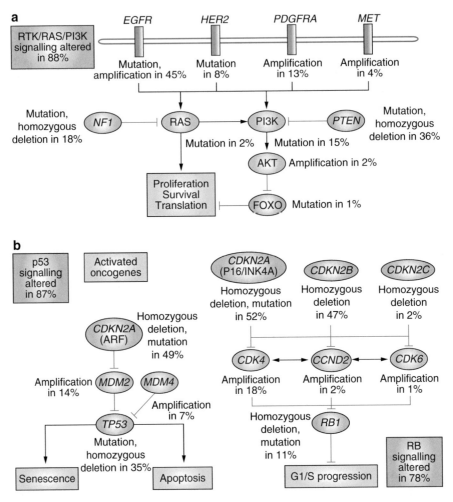

Fig. 4.1 Critical signaling pathways altered in malignant gliomas. Primary sequence alterations and significant copy number changes for components of the (**a**) RTK/RAS/PI3K, (**b**) p53 and (**c**) Rb signalling pathways are shown. *Red* indicates activating genetic alterations. Conversely, *blue* indicates inactivating alterations. For each altered component of a particular pathway, the nature of the alteration and the percentage of tumours affected are indicated. Boxes contain the final percentages of glioblastomas with alterations in at least one known component gene of the designated pathway. Abbreviation: *RTK* receptor tyrosine kinase (Permission obtained from Nature Publishing Group © The Cancer Genome Atlas Research Network (2008))

association with cyclin D. When associated, this forms a complex that promotes G1/S transition through activation of downstream mediators. This process is involved in phosphorylating retinoblastoma protein and facilitating the release of bound E2F, a G1/S transcription factor. If p16INK4a is lost, then CDK4/6 and cyclin D can associate and the G1/S transition occurs freely. In patients with wild-type pRB, CDK4/6 is a target for inhibition (Bastien et al. 2015).

4.4   Retinoblastoma (Rb) Pathway

The Rb protein is encoded by the Rb gene located on chromosome 13q14.1-q14.2. The function of the protein is to prevent unwanted cell growth by inhibiting cell cycle progression until the cell is to undergo mitosis, and at that point the Rb protein becomes phosphorylated by Cyclin D, CDK4, and CDK6, which inactivates it and allows for cell cycle progression (Murphree and Benedict 1984). Typically what occurs is a homozygous deletion of CDKN2A which produces a loss of p16INK4a, a suppressor of CDK4. This leads to a dysregulation of Rb signaling (Murphree and Benedict 1984; Ohgaki and Kleihues 2009; Lin et al. 2013).

4.5   Receptor Tyrosine Kinases Pathway

Recurring molecular alterations have recently been identified in GBM, leading to a better understanding of the pathways that become disrupted in this disease. Frequently seen are gene amplifications and deletions, with deletions most often in chromosomes 1, 9, and 10 and amplifications in chromosomes 7 and 12 (Bello et al. 1994; James et al. 1991; Reifenberger et al. 1995; Rey et al. 1987). Amplifications of a gene can cause an upregulation of various oncogenes while deletions can target tumor suppressors (Purow and Schiff 2009). These are mediated by receptor tyrosine kinases (RTKs), which are also key targets for deregulation in cancers (Zwick et al. 2001). Examples of RTKs in GBM include vascular endothelial growth factor (VEGFR), EGFR, Platelet-derived growth factor receptor (PDGFR), and hepatocyte growth factor receptor (MET) (Blume-Jensen and Hunter 2001). Mutations in these receptors act to relieve auto-inhibitory constraints to prevent degradation (Blume-Jensen and Hunter 2001). Growth factors and RTKs are typically strong candidates for therapeutic targets because mutations here are driver mutations critical for oncogenesis and because kinase receptors are targets for inhibitors that block kinase activation. Moreover, there has been success in other solid tumors (such as erlotinib in lung cancer) and in utilizing RTKs as a target.

4.5.1   VEGFR

A feature of high grade gliomas is angiogenesis, which may be attributed to high levels of VEGF-A in and around the tumor. Bevacizumab is a humanized monoclonal antibody which functions to bind VEGF-A ligand and alter binding to endothelial cells (Ferrara et al. 2005). Studies of bevacizumab have shown high radiographic response rate, prolonged progression-free survival (PFS), and reduced glucocorticoid requirements, all of which led to approval by the Food and Drug administration for patients with GBM (Gilbert et al. 2014). However, several phase III studies have indicated that despite the improved radiographic response, as well as PFS, there is no significant overall survival benefit (Gilbert et al. 2014; Chinot et al. 2014). Both of these studies showed a prolonged PFS with bevacizumab, however the Avaglio trial indicated that health-related quality of life was stable prior to progression while the RTOG-0825 indicated overall quality of life based on symptom burden was significantly worse in some domains with bevacizumab (Gilbert et al. 2014; Chinot et al. 2014). A post-hoc subgroup analysis of the Avaglio study identified a 4.3 month potential increase in median survival with the addition of bevacizumab for IDH1 wild-type GBM in the proneural subgroup (Sandmann et al. 2015). Phase III studies have not demonstrated a survival benefit in recurrent GBM for bevacizumab. The phase II BELOB trial initially suggested a benefit with combined bevacizumab and lomustine, however the phase III trial EORTC 26101 recently underwent an interim analysis and found no overall survival benefit with the addition of bevacizumab to lomustine compared to lomustine alone for recurrent GBM (Taal et al. 2014). Cediranib, another anti-angiogenic agent whose mechanism of action is as a VEGF receptor tyrosine kinase inhibitor, has been tested in phase III trials with GBM and were found to be ineffective in altering overall outcome (Swartz et al. 2014). Additionally, other VEGF inhibitors such as Pazopanib, Sorafenib, Nintedanib, Sunitib, Vandetanib, Aflibercept, Vatalanib, and Cabozantinib have also failed to improve survival in glioblastoma patients (Table 4.1).

4.5.2 EGFR

In GBM there is evidence EGFR plays an important role in oncogenesis and tumor biology (Swartz et al. 2014). EGFR is amplified in approximately 50% of GBM samples and is associated with an active, mutant form of the EGFRvIIIL receptor, which when overexpressed enhances GBM cell growth and contributes to GBM pathogenesis (Jaros et al. 1992; Nishikawa et al. 1994; Schlegel et al. 1994). EGFRvIII, has been identified in 30% of newly diagnosed GBM and is characterized by deletion of exons 2–7 (Gan et al. 2009). The receptor is rendered active and thereby enhances the tumorigenicity by promoting tumor cell migration, conferring protection from radiation and temozolomide, and secreting EGFRvIII-bound oncosomes onto plasma membranes of neighboring cells (Prados et al. 2015).

Furthermore, EGFR can stimulate increased signaling through the RAS, RAF, MEK, MAP, and mTOR pathways, as well as downregulating cell cycle inhibitor proteins (Mao et al. 2012; Nishikawa et al. 2004). A set of studies found that increased levels of EGFR and EGFRvIII co-activates the RTK MET which leads to ligand-independent activation of the EGFR receptor (Huang et al. 2007; Jo et al. 2000; Stommel et al. 2007). This suggests that a mechanism for tumor cells to reduce dependence on either RTK for downstream signaling exists due to the interaction between the c-MET and EGFR/EGFRvIII signaling pathways. Studies have suggested that RTK MET overexpression may correlate with a shorter median survival time (Kong et al. 2009; Koochekpour et al. 1997; Lamszus et al. 1999).

Table 4.1 Targeted therapies in clinical trials for glioblastoma

Therapy	Target/s	Trial phase	Time of treatment -newly diagnosed (N) or recurrent (R) disease	Mono therapy (M), combination therapy or both (B)	If combination, which other therapies used
Bevacizumab	VEGF-A	II	R	B	Irinotecan (Cohen et al. 2009; Friedman et al. 2009; Kreisl et al. 2009a)
Bevacizumab	VEGF-A	III	N	C	Radiation/Temozolomide, Temozolomide (Gilbert et al. 2014; Chinot et al. 2014)
Bevacizumab	VEGF-A	II,III	R	B	Lomustine (Taal et al. 2014; ClinicalTrialsgov)
Bevacizumab	VEGF-A	II	R	C	Fotemustine (Soffietti et al. 2014)
Bevacizumab	VEGF-A	II	R	C	Carboplatin (Field et al. 2015)
Cediranib	VEGFR-1, VEGFR-2, VEGFR-3, PDGFR-α/β, FGFR-1, c-Kit	II	R	M (Batchelor et al. 2010)	
Cediranib	VEGFR-1, VEGFR-2, VEGFR-3, PDGFR-α/β, FGFR-1, c-Kit	III	R	B	Lomustine (Batchelor et al. 2013)
Pazopanib	VEGFR, c-KIT, FGFR, and PDGFR	II	R	M (Iwamoto et al. 2010)	
Pazopanib	VEGFR, c-KIT, FGFR, and PDGFR	I/II	R	C	Lapatinib (Reardon et al. 2013)
Sorafenib	VEGFR-2, Raf, PDGFR, c-KIT, Flt-3	II	N	C	Radiation/Temozolomide, Temozolomide (Hainsworth et al. 2010)
Sorafenib	VEGFR-2, Raf, PDGFR, c-KIT, Flt-3	II	R	C	Temozolomide (Reardon et al. 2011a)
Sorafenib	VEGFR-2, Raf, PDGFR, c-KIT, Flt-3	II	R	C	Bevacizumab (Galanis et al. 2013)

(continued)

Table 4.1 (continued)

Therapy	Target/s	Trial phase	Time of treatment -newly diagnosed (N) or recurrent (R) disease	Mono therapy (M), combination therapy or both (B)	If combination, which other therapies used
Sorafenib	VEGFR-2, Raf, PDGFR, c-KIT, Flt-3	II	R	C	Erlotinib (Peereboom et al. 2013)
Sorafenib	VEGFR-2, Raf, PDGFR, c-KIT, Flt-3	I/II	R	C	Temsirolimus (Lee et al. 2012)
Nintedanib	VEGFR 1–3, FGFR 1–3, PDGFR-α/β	II	R	B	Bevacizumab (Muhic et al. 2013)
Vandetanib	VEFGR-2,EGFR	I/II	R	M (Kreisl et al. 2012)	
Vandetanib	VEGFR-2,EGFR	I	R	C	Sirolimus (Chheda et al. 2015)
Sunitinib	VEGFR2, PDGFR-α, and c-KIT	II	R	M (Neyns et al. 2011; Pan et al. 2012; Kreisl et al. 2013)	
Sunitinib	VEGFR2, PDGFR-α, and c-KIT	I	R	C	Irinotecan (Reardon et al. 2011b)
Aflibercept	VEGF and PlGF	II	R	M (de Groot et al. 2011)	
Vatalanib	VEGFR, PDGFR, and c-kit	I	N	C	Radiation/Temozolomide, Temozolomide (Gerstner et al. 2011)
Vatalanib	VEGFR, PDGFR, and c-kit	I	N	C	Imatinib and Hydroxyurea (Reardon et al. 2009b)
Vatalanib	VEGFR, PDGFR, and c-kit	I/II	N	C	Radiation/Temozolomide, Temozolomide (Brandes et al. 2010)
Cabozantinib	VEGFR-2, MET, and RET	II	R	M (Wen et al. 2010)	
Gefitinib	EGFR	II	N	M (Uhm et al. 2011)	
Gefitinib	EGFR	I/II	N	C	Radiation/Temozolomide, Temozolomide (Chakravarti et al. 2013)
Gefitinib	EGFR	II	R	M (Franceschi et al. 2007; Rich et al. 2004)	

Drug	Target	Phase	Status	Evidence	Combination/Reference
Gefitinib	EGFR	I	R	C	Sirolimus (Reardon et al. 2006)
Gefitinib	EGFR	I	R	C	Everolimus (Kreisl et al. 2009b)
Erlotinib	EGFR	II	R	M (Yung et al. 2010)	
Erlotinib	EGFR	II	R,N	M (Raizer et al. 2010)	
Erlotinib	EGFR	II,II,I/II,I	N	C	Radiation/Temozolomide, Temozolomide (Brown et al. 2008; Krishnan et al. 2006; Peereboom et al. 2010; Prados et al. 2009)
Erlotinib	EGFR	I	R	B	Temozolomide (Prados et al. 2006)
Erlotinib	EGFR	II	R	C	Carboplatin (de Groot et al. 2008)
Erlotinib	EGFR	II	R	C	Bevacizumab (Sathornsumetee et al. 2010)
Erlotinib	EGFR	I,II	R	C	Sirolimus (Nghiemphu et al. 2012; Reardon et al. 2010)
Cetuximab	EGFR	II	R	M (Neyns et al. 2009)	
Cetuximab	EGFR	II	R	C	Bevacizumab and Irinotecan (Hasselbalch et al. 2010)
Lapatinib	EGFR and HER2	I/II	R	M (Thiessen et al. 2010)	
Lapatinib	EGFR and HER2	I/II	R	C	Pazopanib (Reardon et al. 2013)
Lapatinib	EGFR and HER2	I	R	C	Temozolomide (Karavasilis et al. 2013)
Nimotuzumab	EGFR	I/II	N	M (Solomon et al. 2013)	
Imatinib	PDGFR, Bcr-Abl, and c-Kit	I/II	R	M (Wen et al. 2006)	
Imatinib	PDGFR, Bcr-Abl, and c-Kit	II	N,R	M (Razis et al. 2009)	
Imatinib	PDGFR, Bcr-Abl, and c-Kit	II	R	C	Hydroxyurea (Reardon et al. 2005, 2009a; Dresemann et al. 2010)
Dasatinib	PDGFR, Src, Bcr-Abl, c-Kit, and EphA2	II	R	M (Lassman et al. 2015)	
Enzastaurin	protein kinase C, PI3K, and Akt	II	N	C	Radiation/Temozolomide, Temozolomide (Butowski et al. 2011; Wick et al. 2013)

(continued)

Table 4.1 (continued)

Therapy	Target/s	Trial phase	Time of treatment -newly diagnosed (N) or recurrent (R) disease	Mono therapy (M), combination therapy or both (B)	If combination, which other therapies used
Enzastaurin	protein kinase C, PI3K, and Akt	II	R	M (Kreisl et al. 2010; Wick et al. 2010)	
Everolimus	mTOR	II	R	M (Cloughesy et al. 2011)	
Everolimus	mTOR	II	N	C	Radiation/Temozolomide, Temozolomide (Ma et al. 2015)
Everolimus	mTOR	II	N	C	Radiation/Temozolomide/ Bevacizumab, Bevacizumab (Hainsworth et al. 2012)
Temsirolimus	mTOR	II	R	M (Chang et al. 2005; Galanis et al. 2005)	
Temsirolimus	mTOR	II	N	C	Radiation/Temozolomide, Temozolomide (Sarkaria et al. 2010)
Temsirolimus	mTOR	II	R	C	Bevacizumab (Lassen et al. 2013)
Sirolimus	mTOR	I	R	C	Vandetanib (Chheda et al. 2015)
Sirolimus	mTOR	I	R	C	Gefitinib (Reardon et al. 2006)
Sirolimus	mTOR	I,II	R	C	Erlotinib (Nghiemphu et al. 2012; Reardon et al. 2010)
Tipifarnib	Ras	I	N	C	Radiation/Temozolomide, Temozolomide (Nghiemphu et al. 2011)
Tipifarnib	Ras	II	R	M (Cloughesy et al. 2006)	
Lonafarnib	Ras	II	R	M (Desjardins et al. 2011)	
Lonafarnib	Ras	I	R	C	Temozolomide (Yust-Katz et al. 2013)

EGFR remains an elusive target for therapy in GBM as initial studies have suggested activity of some EGFR inhibitors in molecular subsets of GBM but larger studies failed to replicate these results (Haas-Kogan et al. 2005; Mellinghoff et al. 2005; Reardon et al. 2014).

Rindopepimut is a tumor vaccine which is a conjugate of peptides that span the EGFRvIII mutation site with an immunogenic carrier protein keyhole limpet hemocyanin. Phase I and II trials in newly diagnosed GBM patients treated with rindopepimut along with temozolomide indicated a PFS of 10–15 months and overall survival of 22–26 months, which was improved compared to historical controls of 6 and 15 months respectively (Swartz et al. 2014). Another multi-center trial with rindopepimut in newly diagnosed GBM, the ACTIVATE trial, demonstrated an immune response after vaccination. In ACTIVATE, 43% of those treated had a positive humoral response, and the majority of patients with relapse had lost all of the EGFRvIII expression, a phenomenon known as antigen escape which suggested that the immune system successfully targeted EGFRvIII-expressing cells (Swartz et al. 2014). Furthermore a similar response in recurrent disease was noted in the ReACT trial, where rindopepimut reportedly caused an immune response and significantly prolonged survival when administered with bevacizumab (Phillips et al. 2016). However, in the phase III study ACT IV, rindopepimut combined with temozolomide did not increase overall survival in newly diagnosed EGFRvIII-positive GBM (Reardon et al. 2015; Inman 2016).

Therapy remains ongoing to identify new targets and mechanisms, such as ABT-414, which is a conjugate of a potent microtubule inhibitor and a monoclonal antibody against a tumor-selective EGFR epitope found in EGFR wild-type-overexpressing tumors and EGFRvIII mutant-expressing tumors. Preclinical studies have indicated that ABT-414 is selective and a phase I study, as well as a phase III study are ongoing (Gan et al. 2015; Phillips et al. 2016). Unfortunately, other EGFR inhibitors such as Gefitinib, Erlotinib, Cetuximab, Nimotuzumab, and Lapatinib, have similarly failed to improve survival in glioblastoma patients (Table 4.1).

4.5.3 PDGFR

Platelet derived growth factor receptors (PDGFR) are cell surface receptors for members of the platelet derived growth factor family and signal through the alpha and beta platelet derived growth factor receptor tyrosine kinases (Matsui et al. 1989). Chromosome 7p22 contains the PDGFR alpha gene which is amplified in approximately 13% of GBM samples (Cancer Genome Atlas Research Network 2008; Stenman et al. 1992). Multiple aberrations in expression of PDGFR have been observed, including overexpression, amplification, mutations, and truncations, however point mutations are exclusively seen in GBM (Alentorn et al. 2012).

An inhibitor of PDGFR is Imatinib mesylate, which also functions to inhibit bcr-abl and c-kit tyrosine kinases and is beneficial in the treatment of CML and in GI stromal tumors (Buchdunger et al. 2000; Druker et al. 2001; Demetri et al. 2002). Imatinib however has shown minimal activity in recurrent gliomas as well as newly diagnosed GBM (Wen et al. 2006; Razis et al. 2009). Others studies have been performed looking at the addition of hydroxyurea to imatinib in recurrent malignant gliomas and found that it failed to show any meaningful anti-tumor activity (Reardon et al. 2005, 2009a; Dresemann et al. 2010; Desjardins et al. 2007).

Another drug that has been studied is dastinib, which is an inhibitor of PDGFR, SRC, bcr-abl, c-Kit, and EphA2 receptors. The study was conducted in patients with recurrent GBM and found that dastinib was ineffective with no radiographic responses (Lassman et al. 2015). Another phase 1 trial of dastinib in combination with CCNU found hematological toxicities, which limited the amount of exposure available for both therapeutic agents, in contrast to a trial with dastinib and erlotinib which was much better tolerated (Reardon et al. 2012; Franceschi et al. 2012).

4.5.4 PI3K/AKT/PTEN/mTOR

Stimulation of the PI3K/AKT/PTEN/mTOR pathway enhances growth via activation of receptor tyrosine kinases. This occurs via the regulation of cell division, proliferation, differentiation, metabolism, and survival (Carnero et al. 2008; Morgensztern and McLeod 2005). Several genomic alterations in GBM activate this pathway, most often of which is the amplification of EGFR (Peraud et al. 1997; Watanabe et al. 1996; Wong et al. 1992). Other alterations leading to activation of this pathway include lesions in PIK3R1/PIK3CA and mutations or deletions of AKT, which occur in 84% of GBM cell lines and/or PTEN mutations, which occur in 30–44% of high-grade gliomas (Wang et al. 1997, 2004; Tohma et al. 1998; Teng et al. 1997; Koul 2008). PTEN typically inhibits the AKT pathway, therefore deletion of PTEN leads to activation of this pathway (Liu et al. 1997; Li et al. 1997; Stambolic et al. 1998). PTEN also facilitates the degradation of EGFR, which leads to termination of EGFR signaling, leading to an explanation for why PTEN confers resistance to epidermal growth factor inhibitors in vitro (Vivanco et al. 2010; Bianco et al. 2003).

mTOR is a master nutrient and energy sensor which regulates processes including transcription, protein synthesis, as well as other cellular functions including proliferation, cell motility survival, and anabolism (Hay and Sonenberg 2004; Kim et al. 2002; Sarbassov et al. 2004, 2005; Facchinetti et al. 2008; Ikenoue et al. 2008). mTOR is made of two different complexes—mammalian target of rapamycin complex 1 mTORC1 and mTORC2—and acts as a regulator of PI3K upstream and as its effector downstream (Akhavan et al. 2010). Inhibitors of mTOR have been developed, including Sirolimus, a mTORC1 inhibitor, which leads to reduced expression of neural stem cell progenitor markers and neurosphere formation in GBM (Sami and Karsy 2013; Sunayama et al. 2010). Another mTOR inhibitor, Dactolisib, a potent dual PI3K-mTOR inhibitor has shown potential benefit as a radiosensitizer for

GBMs in preclinical studies (Fan et al. 2010; Mukherjee et al. 2012). Regrettably, mTOR inhibitors examined to date including Sirolimus, Everolimus and Temsirolimus have not prolonged overall survival in glioblastoma patients (Table 4.1).

4.5.5 RAS/RAF/MEK/MAP (ERK) Kinase

The RAS/RAF/MEK/MAP kinase pathway mediates cellular responses via growth, migration, apoptosis, proliferation, differentiation, and cell survival. This pathway can be activated by EGFR and PDGFR via signal transmission through indirect associations with cytosolic mediator proteins growth factor receptor-bound protein 2 (GRB2) and son of sevenless (SOS) to RAS. RAS then stimulates RAF, which activates MAPK and MEK (Moodie et al. 1993; Thomas et al. 1992).

RAS has been found to be upregulated in GBM samples, and activation is typically through loss of the NF-1 gene, which encodes a tumor suppressor protein and is a negative regulator of RAS and mTOR signaling in astrocytes (Banerjee et al. 2011; Nissan et al. 2014; Dasgupta et al. 2005). NF-1 mutation has been implicated in prior studies in glioma tumorigenesis, specifically noting that the homozygous loss of NF-1 in glial cells has been shown to develop fully malignant astrocytomas with a p53-null background (Alcantara Llaguno et al. 2009; Zhu et al. 2005; Kwon et al. 2008). Hyper activation of protein kinase C also causes increased degradation of NF-1, which also puts patients at an increased risk of developing gliomas (McGillicuddy et al. 2009). NF-1 mutations are a defining feature of the mesenchymal GBM subtype, and therefore this subgroup may potentially be good candidates for agents that target NF-1 driven pathways (Cancer Genome Atlas Research Network 2008; Phillips et al. 2006). Loss of NF-1 function leads to enhanced RAS activity, which will lead to increased RAS/RAF/MEK/MAPK pathway activation, leading to the hypothesis that MEK inhibitors were good therapeutic targets. Two MEK inhibitors, PD0325901 and AZD6244, both appeared effective against NF-1 deficient GBM cells dependent on RAF/MEK signaling in preclinical studies (See et al. 2012). Furthermore, this study showed that MEK inhibitor-resistant NF-1 deficient cells could be re-sensitized to MEK inhibitors with the co-application of dual PI3K-mOTR inhibitor PI-103, also suggesting that NF-1 deficient GBM patients may respond to a MEK inhibitor based chemotherapy (See et al. 2012). Drugs that have been tested that target RAS specifically (Tipifarnib, Lonafarnib) have not shown any improvement in overall survival for GBM patients (Table 4.1).

4.6 IDH1/IDH2 Mutations

The identifications of mutations in the metabolic enzymes IDH 1 and 2 is one of the most important discoveries that has led to a remodeling of our understanding of gliomas, including GBMS (Parsons et al. 2008). The majority of tumor samples in this study bore this mutation and were classified as secondary GBMs, suggesting that IDH 1 and IDH 2 mutations can serve as a genetic marker for this type of GBM. When IDH 1 and 2 were mutated, the result was enzymes with a neomorphic function, meaning that the mutant enzymes acquired the ability to catalyze the NADPH-dependent reduction of alpha-KG to the R-enantiomer of 2-hydroxyglutarate (2-HG) (Dang et al. 2010). This study showed that IDH 1 and 2 mutants had high levels of 2-HG, which is also found in primary IDH 1 mutant gliomas, and is also found in AML patients (Gross et al. 2010; Ward et al. 2010). IDH 1 and 2 mutant expression results in inhibition of alpha-KG-dependent dioxygenases by 2-HG. The enzymes that are dependent on this regulate physiological processes including hypoxia sensing, histone demethylation, and changes in DNA methylation (Loenarz and Schofield 2008). The glioma CpG island methylator phenotype (C-CIMP) is a distinctive and nearly invariable feature of IDH 1 and 2 mutant gliomas that has been studied to indicate that gliomas with this mutant expression are correlated with better prognosis (Baysan et al. 2012; Noushmehr et al. 2010). IDH 1 and 2 mutant gliomas are detected with the IDH-R132H antibody as well as with DNA sequencing of antibody-negative cases, which provides more accurate diagnosis and prediction of patient outcomes and prognosis.

IDH 1 and 2 mutational status also provides a prognostic marker in patients with lower grade gliomas and GBMs, as well as providing insights about the origin of gliomas (Parsons et al. 2008; Hartmann et al. 2009; Sanson et al. 2009; Weller et al. 2009; Yan et al. 2009). IDH 1 and 2 wild-type GBMs typically exhibit a characteristic pattern of genetic changes associated with primary GBMs such as a gain of chromosome 7, loss of chromosome 10, and amplification of EGFR which are not seen in IDH 1 and 2 mutant GBMs.

The importance of IDH mutation is eminent as the new 2016 WHO Classification of tumors of the central nervous system now defines glioblastoma based upon IDH status (Louis et al. 2016). Currently, several phase I studies examining IDH mutation inhibitors in advanced malignancies including glioblastoma are underway. However, as IDH is thought to be an early driver mutation in glioma, it remains unknown the potential impact of its inhibition in recurrent glioblastoma (Watanabe et al. 2009; Mandel et al. 2016).

4.7   Discussion

The Cancer Genome Atlas analysis revealed multiple molecular pathways and potential therapeutic genetic targets ushering in a new era for glioblastoma treatment. Bevacizumab, an anti-VEGF agent, has displayed an increased time to progression and improved imaging response but disappointingly has been unsuccessful in increasing patient overall survival. Furthermore, it remains an area of debate whether bevacizumab has any anti-tumor benefit (Kruser et al. 2016). Despite our increased knowledge of these tumors, our ability to divide them into molecular subgroups, and several promising therapeutic targets, every targeted therapy examined to date unfortunately has failed to demonstrate any benefit in overall survival.

Several possible explanations for this lack of success have been proposed including lack of tumor dependence on the pathway targeted, inadequate CNS penetration of the drug, intratumoral heterogeneity, and clonal evolution.

In regards to lack of pathway dependence, evidence suggests that tumors may be able upregulate a different pathway when another pathway is inhibited. This has been seen in the use of EGFR inhibitors, where treatment has demonstrated the lack of ability to change targets downstream like Akt and can even upregulate the PI3K/Akt pathway (Hegi et al. 2011; Chakravarti et al. 2002). Another possible area of concern is that many of the mutations targeted are essential for early tumor development and may be subsequently superseded by secondary pathways of tumor growth (Lee et al. 2012). Additionally, mutations present in a tumor on initial presentation may change or no longer be expressed on disease recurrence (van den Bent et al. 2015).

Drug penetrance is also major concern as it is frequently difficult to determine how well therapeutic agents cross the blood brain barrier in brain tumor patients. Due to the eloquent location, it is often unfeasible to obtain tissue samples at recurrence making it impossible to assess how much of a chemotherapeutic agent is being delivered to its intended target. It is also possible that a targeted agent may fail, not due to being a poor genetic target, but rather because the drug is not reaching that target in adequate quantity to cause the desired or intended treatment effect.

Additionally, tumor heterogeneity and clonal evolution is an issue that may affect targeted therapies. GBM's are heterogenous in nature, and it is possible that when one cell group is inhibited via a targeted therapy to one pathway, another is left to proliferate unabated as their development is uninhibited.

While the results of targeted therapy studies to date in glioblastoma have been disappointing, there continues to be enthusiasm in this approach with numerous clinical trials currently underway. Hopefully, knowledge from the previous failed trials will help provide further insight and assist future clinicians in designing new novel targeted treatments to overcome these barriers.

References

Akhavan, D., T.F. Cloughesy, and P.S. Mischel. 2010. mTOR signaling in glioblastoma: Lessons learned from bench to bedside. *Neuro-Oncology* 12: 882–889.

Alcantara Llaguno, S., J. Chen, C.H. Kwon, et al. 2009. Malignant astrocytomas originate from neural stem/progenitor cells in a somatic tumor suppressor mouse model. *Cancer Cell* 15: 45–56.

Alentorn, A., Y. Marie, C. Carpentier, et al. 2012. Prevalence, clinico-pathological value, and co-occurrence of PDGFRA abnormalities in diffuse gliomas. *Neuro-Oncology* 14: 1393–1403.

Banerjee, S., N.R. Crouse, R.J. Emnett, S.M. Gianino, and D.H. Gutmann. 2011. Neurofibromatosis-1 regulates mTOR-mediated astrocyte growth and glioma formation in a TSC/Rheb-independent manner. *Proceedings of the National Academy of Sciences of the United States of America* 108: 15996–16001.

Bastien, J.I., K.A. McNeill, and H.A. Fine. 2015. Molecular characterizations of glioblastoma, targeted therapy, and clinical results to date. *Cancer* 121: 502–516.

Batchelor, T.T., D.G. Duda, E. di Tomaso, et al. 2010. Phase II study of cediranib, an oral pan-vascular endothelial growth factor receptor tyrosine kinase inhibitor, in patients with recurrent glioblastoma. *Journal of Clinical Oncology* 28: 2817–2823.

Batchelor, T.T., P. Mulholland, B. Neyns, et al. 2013. Phase III randomized trial comparing the efficacy of cediranib as monotherapy, and in combination with lomustine, versus lomustine alone in patients with recurrent glioblastoma. *Journal of Clinical Oncology* 31: 3212–3218.

Baysan, M., S. Bozdag, M.C. Cam, et al. 2012. G-cimp status prediction of glioblastoma samples using mRNA expression data. *PLoS One* 7: e47839.

Bello, M.J., J. Vaquero, J.M. de Campos, et al. 1994. Molecular analysis of chromosome 1 abnormalities in human gliomas reveals frequent loss of 1p in oligodendroglial tumors. *International Journal of Cancer* 57: 172–175.

Bianco, R., I. Shin, C.A. Ritter, et al. 2003. Loss of PTEN/MMAC1/TEP in EGF receptor-expressing tumor cells counteracts the antitumor action of EGFR tyrosine kinase inhibitors. *Oncogene* 22: 2812–2822.

Blume-Jensen, P., and T. Hunter. 2001. Oncogenic kinase signalling. *Nature* 411: 355–365.

Bogler, O., H.J. Huang, P. Kleihues, and W.K. Cavenee. 1995. The p53 gene and its role in human brain tumors. *Glia* 15: 308–327.

Brandes, A.A., R. Stupp, P. Hau, et al. 2010. EORTC study 26041-22041: phase I/II study on concomitant and adjuvant temozolomide (TMZ) and radiotherapy (RT) with PTK787/ZK222584 (PTK/ZK) in newly diagnosed glioblastoma. *European Journal of Cancer* 46: 348–354.

Bredel, M., D.M. Scholtens, A.K. Yadav, et al. 2011. NFKBIA deletion in glioblastomas. *The New England Journal of Medicine* 364: 627–637.

Brennan, C.W., R.G. Verhaak, A. McKenna, et al. 2013. The somatic genomic landscape of glioblastoma. *Cell* 155: 462–477.

Brown, P.D., S. Krishnan, J.N. Sarkaria, et al. 2008. Phase I/II trial of erlotinib and temozolomide with radiation therapy in the treatment of newly diagnosed glioblastoma multiforme: North Central Cancer Treatment Group Study N0177. *Journal of Clinical Oncology* 26: 5603–5609.

Buchdunger, E., C.L. Cioffi, N. Law, et al. 2000. Abl protein-tyrosine kinase inhibitor STI571 inhibits in vitro signal transduction mediated by c-kit and platelet-derived growth factor receptors. *The Journal of Pharmacology and Experimental Therapeutics* 295: 139–145.

Butowski, N., S.M. Chang, K.R. Lamborn, et al. 2011. Phase II and pharmacogenomics study of enzastaurin plus temozolomide during and following radiation therapy in patients with newly diagnosed glioblastoma multiforme and gliosarcoma. *Neuro-Oncology* 13: 1331–1338.

Cancer Genome Atlas Research Network. 2008. Comprehensive genomic characterization defines human glioblastoma genes and core pathways. *Nature* 455: 1061–1068.

Carnero, A., C. Blanco-Aparicio, O. Renner, W. Link, and J.F. Leal. 2008. The PTEN/PI3K/AKT signalling pathway in cancer, therapeutic implications. *Current Cancer Drug Targets* 8: 187–198.

Chakravarti, A., J.S. Loeffler, and N.J. Dyson. 2002. Insulin-like growth factor receptor I mediates resistance to anti-epidermal growth factor receptor therapy in primary human glioblastoma cells through continued activation of phosphoinositide 3-kinase signaling. *Cancer Research* 62: 200–207.

Chakravarti, A., M. Wang, H.I. Robins, et al. 2013. RTOG 0211: A phase 1/2 study of radiation therapy with concurrent gefitinib for newly diagnosed glioblastoma patients. *International Journal of Radiation Oncology, Biology, Physics* 85: 1206–1211.

Chang, S.M., P. Wen, T. Cloughesy, et al. 2005. Phase II study of CCI-779 in patients with recurrent glioblastoma multiforme. *Investigational New Drugs* 23: 357–361.

Chheda, M.G., P.Y. Wen, F.H. Hochberg, et al. 2015. Vandetanib plus sirolimus in adults with recurrent glioblastoma: Results of a phase I and dose expansion cohort study. *Journal of Neuro-Oncology* 121: 627–634.

Chinot, O.L., W. Wick, W. Mason, et al. 2014. Bevacizumab plus radiotherapy-temozolomide for newly diagnosed glioblastoma. *The New England Journal of Medicine* 370: 709–722.

ClinicalTrialsgov. 2016. Bevacizumab and Lomustine for Recurrent GBM. Identifier: NCT01290939.

Cloughesy, T.F., P.Y. Wen, H.I. Robins, et al. 2006. Phase II trial of tipifarnib in patients with recurrent malignant glioma either receiving or not receiving enzyme-inducing antiepileptic drugs: A North American Brain Tumor Consortium Study. *Journal of Clinical Oncology* 24: 3651–3656.

Cloughesy, T.R.J., J. Drappatz, et al. 2011. A phase II trial of everolimus in patients with recurrent glioblastoma multiforme. *Neuro-Oncology* 13: 42–43.

Cloughesy, T.F., W.K. Cavenee, and P.S. Mischel. 2014. Glioblastoma: From molecular pathology to targeted treatment. *Annual Review of Pathology* 9: 1–25.

Cohen, M.H., Y.L. Shen, P. Keegan, and R. Pazdur. 2009. FDA drug approval summary: Bevacizumab (Avastin) as treatment of recurrent glioblastoma multiforme. *The Oncologist* 14: 1131–1138.

Dang, L., S. Jin, and S.M. Su. 2010. IDH mutations in glioma and acute myeloid leukemia. *Trends in Molecular Medicine* 16: 387–397.

Dasgupta, B., W. Li, A. Perry, and D.H. Gutmann. 2005. Glioma formation in neurofibromatosis 1 reflects preferential activation of K-RAS in astrocytes. *Cancer Research* 65: 236–245.

Davis, F.G., V. Kupelian, S. Freels, B. McCarthy, and T. Surawicz. 2001. Prevalence estimates for primary brain tumors in the United States by behavior and major histology groups. *Neuro-Oncology* 3: 152–158.

de Groot, J.F., M.R. Gilbert, K. Aldape, et al. 2008. Phase II study of carboplatin and erlotinib (Tarceva, OSI-774) in patients with recurrent glioblastoma. *Journal of Neuro-Oncology* 90: 89–97.

de Groot, J.F., K.R. Lamborn, S.M. Chang, et al. 2011. Phase II study of aflibercept in recurrent malignant glioma: A North American Brain Tumor Consortium study. *Journal of Clinical Oncology* 29: 2689–2695.

Demetri, G.D., M. von Mehren, C.D. Blanke, et al. 2002. Efficacy and safety of imatinib mesylate in advanced gastrointestinal stromal tumors. *The New England Journal of Medicine* 347: 472–480.

Desjardins, A., J.A. Quinn, J.J. Vredenburgh, et al. 2007. Phase II study of imatinib mesylate and hydroxyurea for recurrent grade III malignant gliomas. *Journal of Neuro-Oncology* 83: 53–60.

Desjardins, A., D.A. Reardon, K.B. Peters, et al. 2011. A phase I trial of the farnesyl transferase inhibitor, SCH 66336, with temozolomide for patients with malignant glioma. *Journal of Neuro-Oncology* 105: 601–606.

Dresemann, G., M. Weller, M.A. Rosenthal, et al. 2010. Imatinib in combination with hydroxyurea versus hydroxyurea alone as oral therapy in patients with progressive pretreated glioblastoma resistant to standard dose temozolomide. *Journal of Neuro-Oncology* 96: 393–402.

Druker, B.J., M. Talpaz, D.J. Resta, et al. 2001. Efficacy and safety of a specific inhibitor of the BCR-ABL tyrosine kinase in chronic myeloid leukemia. *The New England Journal of Medicine* 344: 1031–1037.

Facchinetti, V., W. Ouyang, H. Wei, et al. 2008. The mammalian target of rapamycin complex 2 controls folding and stability of Akt and protein kinase C. *The EMBO Journal* 27: 1932–1943.

Fan, Q.W., C. Cheng, C. Hackett, et al. 2010. Akt and autophagy cooperate to promote survival of drug-resistant glioma. *Science Signaling* 3: ra81.

Ferrara, N., K.J. Hillan, and W. Novotny. 2005. Bevacizumab (Avastin), a humanized anti-VEGF monoclonal antibody for cancer therapy. *Biochemical and Biophysical Research Communications* 333: 328–335.

Field, K.M., J. Simes, A.K. Nowak, et al. 2015. Randomized phase 2 study of carboplatin and bevacizumab in recurrent glioblastoma. *Neuro-Oncology* 17: 1504–1513.

Franceschi, E., G. Cavallo, S. Lonardi, et al. 2007. Gefitinib in patients with progressive high-grade gliomas: A multicentre phase II study by Gruppo Italiano Cooperativo di Neuro-Oncologia (GICNO). *British Journal of Cancer* 96: 1047–1051.

Franceschi, E., R. Stupp, M.J. van den Bent, et al. 2012. EORTC 26083 phase I/II trial of dasatinib in combination with CCNU in patients with recurrent glioblastoma. *Neuro-Oncology* 14: 1503–1510.

Freije, W.A., F.E. Castro-Vargas, Z. Fang, et al. 2004. Gene expression profiling of gliomas strongly predicts survival. *Cancer Research* 64: 6503–6510.

Friedman, H.S., M.D. Prados, P.Y. Wen, et al. 2009. Bevacizumab alone and in combination with irinotecan in recurrent glioblastoma. *Journal of Clinical Oncology* 27: 4733–4740.

Galanis, E., J.C. Buckner, M.J. Maurer, et al. 2005. Phase II trial of temsirolimus (CCI-779) in recurrent glioblastoma multiforme: A North Central Cancer Treatment Group Study. *Journal of Clinical Oncology* 23: 5294–5304.

Galanis, E., S.K. Anderson, J.M. Lafky, et al. 2013. Phase II study of bevacizumab in combination with sorafenib in recurrent glioblastoma (N0776): A north central cancer treatment group trial. *Clinical Cancer Research* 19: 4816–4823.

Gan, H.K., A.H. Kaye, and R.B. Luwor. 2009. The EGFRvIII variant in glioblastoma multiforme. *Journal of Clinical Neuroscience* 16: 748–754.

Gan, H.K., P. Kumthekar, A.B. Lassman, et al. 2015. ATNT-01ABT-414 MONO- OR COMBINATION THERAPY WITH TEMOZOLOMIDE (TMZ) RECHALLENGE IN PATIENTS WITH RECURRENT GLIOBLASTOMA (GBM) AND AMPLIFIED EPIDERMAL GROWTH FACTOR RECEPTOR (EGFR): A PHASE I STUDY. *Neuro-Oncology* 17: v10.

Gerstner, E.R., A.F. Eichler, S.R. Plotkin, et al. 2011. Phase I trial with biomarker studies of vatalanib (PTK787) in patients with newly diagnosed glioblastoma treated with enzyme inducing anti-epileptic drugs and standard radiation and temozolomide. *Journal of Neuro-Oncology* 103: 325–332.

Gilbert, M.R., J.J. Dignam, T.S. Armstrong, et al. 2014. A randomized trial of bevacizumab for newly diagnosed glioblastoma. *The New England Journal of Medicine* 370: 699–708.

Gravendeel, L.A., M.C. Kouwenhoven, O. Gevaert, et al. 2009. Intrinsic gene expression profiles of gliomas are a better predictor of survival than histology. *Cancer Research* 69: 9065–9072.

Gross, S., R.A. Cairns, M.D. Minden, et al. 2010. Cancer-associated metabolite 2-hydroxyglutarate accumulates in acute myelogenous leukemia with isocitrate dehydrogenase 1 and 2 mutations. *The Journal of Experimental Medicine* 207: 339–344.

Haas-Kogan, D.A., M.D. Prados, T. Tihan, et al. 2005. Epidermal growth factor receptor, protein kinase B/Akt, and glioma response to erlotinib. *Journal of the National Cancer Institute* 97: 880–887.

Hainsworth, J.D., T. Ervin, E. Friedman, et al. 2010. Concurrent radiotherapy and temozolomide followed by temozolomide and sorafenib in the first-line treatment of patients with glioblastoma multiforme. *Cancer* 116: 3663–3669.

Hainsworth, J.D., K.C. Shih, G.C. Shepard, G.W. Tillinghast, B.T. Brinker, and D.R. Spigel. 2012. Phase II study of concurrent radiation therapy, temozolomide, and bevacizumab followed by bevacizumab/everolimus as first-line treatment for patients with glioblastoma. *Clinical Advances in Hematology & Oncology* 10: 240–246.

Hartmann, C., J. Meyer, J. Balss, et al. 2009. Type and frequency of IDH1 and IDH2 mutations are related to astrocytic and oligodendroglial differentiation and age: a study of 1,010 diffuse gliomas. *Acta Neuropathologica* 118: 469–474.

Hasselbalch, B., U. Lassen, S. Hansen, et al. 2010. Cetuximab, bevacizumab, and irinotecan for patients with primary glioblastoma and progression after radiation therapy and temozolomide: A phase II trial. *Neuro-Oncology* 12: 508–516.

Hay, N., and N. Sonenberg. 2004. Upstream and downstream of mTOR. *Genes & Development* 18: 1926–1945.

Hegi, M.E., A.C. Diserens, P. Bady, et al. 2011. Pathway analysis of glioblastoma tissue after preoperative treatment with the EGFR tyrosine kinase inhibitor gefitinib – A phase II trial. *Molecular Cancer Therapeutics* 10: 1102–1112.

Herman, A.G., M. Hayano, M.V. Poyurovsky, et al. 2011. Discovery of Mdm2-MdmX E3 ligase inhibitors using a cell-based ubiquitination assay. *Cancer Discovery* 1: 312–325.

Huang, P.H., A. Mukasa, R. Bonavia, et al. 2007. Quantitative analysis of EGFRvIII cellular signaling networks reveals a combinatorial therapeutic strategy for glioblastoma. *Proceedings of the National Academy of Sciences of the United States of America* 104: 12867–12872.

Ikenoue, T., K. Inoki, Q. Yang, X. Zhou, and K.L. Guan. 2008. Essential function of TORC2 in PKC and Akt turn motif phosphorylation, maturation and signalling. *The EMBO Journal* 27: 1919–1931.

Inman S. 2016. Rindopepimut misses OS endpoint in phase III glioblastoma trial. *OncLive*. http://www.onclive.com/web-exclusives/rindopepimut-misses-os-endpoint-in-phase-iii-glioblastoma-trial.

Iwamoto, F.M., K.R. Lamborn, H.I. Robins, et al. 2010. Phase II trial of pazopanib (GW786034), an oral multi-targeted angiogenesis inhibitor, for adults with recurrent glioblastoma (North American Brain Tumor Consortium Study 06-02). *Neuro-Oncology* 12: 855–861.

James, C.D., J. He, E. Carlbom, M. Nordenskjold, W.K. Cavenee, and V.P. Collins. 1991. Chromosome 9 deletion mapping reveals interferon alpha and interferon beta-1 gene deletions in human glial tumors. *Cancer Research* 51: 1684–1688.

Jaros, E., R.H. Perry, L. Adam, et al. 1992. Prognostic implications of p53 protein, epidermal growth factor receptor, and Ki-67 labelling in brain tumours. *British Journal of Cancer* 66: 373–385.

Jo, M., D.B. Stolz, J.E. Esplen, K. Dorko, G.K. Michalopoulos, and S.C. Strom. 2000. Cross-talk between epidermal growth factor receptor and c-Met signal pathways in transformed cells. *The Journal of Biological Chemistry* 275: 8806–8811.

Jue, T.R., and K.L. McDonald. 2016. The challenges associated with molecular targeted therapies for glioblastoma. *Journal of Neuro-Oncology* 127: 427–434.

Kamijo, T., F. Zindy, M.F. Roussel, et al. 1997. Tumor suppression at the mouse INK4a locus mediated by the alternative reading frame product p19ARF. *Cell* 91: 649–659.

Kamijo, T., J.D. Weber, G. Zambetti, F. Zindy, M.F. Roussel, and C.J. Sherr. 1998. Functional and physical interactions of the ARF tumor suppressor with p53 and Mdm2. *Proceedings of the National Academy of Sciences of the United States of America* 95: 8292–8297.

Karavasilis, V., V. Kotoula, G. Pentheroudakis, et al. 2013. A phase I study of temozolomide and lapatinib combination in patients with recurrent high-grade gliomas. *Journal of Neurology* 260: 1469–1480.

Kim, D.H., D.D. Sarbassov, S.M. Ali, et al. 2002. mTOR interacts with raptor to form a nutrient-sensitive complex that signals to the cell growth machinery. *Cell* 110: 163–175.

Kong, D.S., S.Y. Song, D.H. Kim, et al. 2009. Prognostic significance of c-Met expression in glioblastomas. *Cancer* 115: 140–148.

Koochekpour, S., M. Jeffers, S. Rulong, et al. 1997. Met and hepatocyte growth factor/scatter factor expression in human gliomas. *Cancer Research* 57: 5391–5398.

Koul, D. 2008. PTEN signaling pathways in glioblastoma. *Cancer Biology & Therapy* 7: 1321–1325.

Kreisl, T.N., L. Kim, K. Moore, et al. 2009a. Phase II trial of single-agent bevacizumab followed by bevacizumab plus irinotecan at tumor progression in recurrent glioblastoma. *Journal of Clinical Oncology* 27: 740–745.

Kreisl, T.N., A.B. Lassman, P.S. Mischel, et al. 2009b. A pilot study of everolimus and gefitinib in the treatment of recurrent glioblastoma (GBM). *Journal of Neuro-Oncology* 92: 99–105.

Kreisl, T.N., S. Kotliarova, J.A. Butman, et al. 2010. A phase I/II trial of enzastaurin in patients with recurrent high-grade gliomas. *Neuro-Oncology* 12: 181–189.

Kreisl, T.N., K.A. McNeill, J. Sul, F.M. Iwamoto, J. Shih, and H.A. Fine. 2012. A phase I/II trial of vandetanib for patients with recurrent malignant glioma. *Neuro-Oncology* 14: 1519–1526.

Kreisl, T.N., P. Smith, J. Sul, et al. 2013. Continuous daily sunitinib for recurrent glioblastoma. *Journal of Neuro-Oncology* 111: 41–48.

Krishnan, S., P.D. Brown, K.V. Ballman, et al. 2006. Phase I trial of erlotinib with radiation therapy in patients with glioblastoma multiforme: Results of North Central Cancer Treatment Group protocol N0177. *International Journal of Radiation Oncology, Biology, Physics* 65: 1192–1199.

Kruser, T.J., M.P. Mehta, and K.R. Kozak. 2016. Identification of patients who benefit from bevacizumab in high-grade glioma-an easy question turned difficult: Treat the scan or the patient? *Journal of Clinical Oncology* 34: 1281–1282.

Kwon, C.H., D. Zhao, J. Chen, et al. 2008. Pten haploinsufficiency accelerates formation of high-grade astrocytomas. *Cancer Research* 68: 3286–3294.

Lamszus, K., J. Laterra, M. Westphal, and E.M. Rosen. 1999. Scatter factor/hepatocyte growth factor (SF/HGF) content and function in human gliomas. *International Journal of Developmental Neuroscience* 17: 517–530.

Lassen, U., M. Sorensen, T.B. Gaziel, B. Hasselbalch, and H.S. Poulsen. 2013. Phase II study of bevacizumab and temsirolimus combination therapy for recurrent glioblastoma multiforme. *Anticancer Research* 33: 1657–1660.

Lassman, A.B., S.L. Pugh, M.R. Gilbert, et al. 2015. Phase 2 trial of dasatinib in target-selected patients with recurrent glioblastoma (RTOG 0627). *Neuro-Oncology* 17: 992–998.

Lee, E.Q., J. Kuhn, K.R. Lamborn, et al. 2012. Phase I/II study of sorafenib in combination with temsirolimus for recurrent glioblastoma or gliosarcoma: North American Brain Tumor Consortium study 05-02. *Neuro-Oncology* 14: 1511–1518.

Li, J., C. Yen, D. Liaw, et al. 1997. PTEN, a putative protein tyrosine phosphatase gene mutated in human brain, breast, and prostate cancer. *Science* 275: 1943–1947.

Li, A., J. Walling, S. Ahn, et al. 2009. Unsupervised analysis of transcriptomic profiles reveals six glioma subtypes. *Cancer Research* 69: 2091–2099.

Lin, F., M.C. de Gooijer, D. Hanekamp, D. Brandsma, J.H. Beijnen, and O. van Tellingen. 2013. Targeting core (mutated) pathways of high-grade gliomas: Challenges of intrinsic resistance and drug efflux. *CNS Oncology* 2: 271–288.

Liu, W., C.D. James, L. Frederick, B.E. Alderete, and R.B. Jenkins. 1997. PTEN/MMAC1 mutations and EGFR amplification in glioblastomas. *Cancer Research* 57: 5254–5257.

Loenarz, C., and C.J. Schofield. 2008. Expanding chemical biology of 2-oxoglutarate oxygenases. *Nature Chemical Biology* 4: 152–156.

Louis, D.N., A. Perry, G. Reifenberger, et al. 2016. The 2016 World Health Organization Classification of Tumors of the Central Nervous System: A summary. *Acta Neuropathologica* 131: 803–820.

Ma, D.J., E. Galanis, S.K. Anderson, et al. 2015. A phase II trial of everolimus, temozolomide, and radiotherapy in patients with newly diagnosed glioblastoma: NCCTG N057K. *Neuro-Oncology* 17: 1261–1269.

Mandel, J.J., D. Cachia, D. Liu, et al. 2016. Impact of IDH1 mutation status on outcome in clinical trials for recurrent glioblastoma. *Journal of Neuro-Oncology* 129: 147–154.

Mao, H., D.G. Lebrun, J. Yang, V.F. Zhu, and M. Li. 2012. Deregulated signaling pathways in glioblastoma multiforme: Molecular mechanisms and therapeutic targets. *Cancer Investigation* 30: 48–56.

Masui, K., T.F. Cloughesy, and P.S. Mischel. 2012. Review: Molecular pathology in adult high-grade gliomas: from molecular diagnostics to target therapies. *Neuropathology and Applied Neurobiology* 38: 271–291.

Matlashewski, G., P. Lamb, D. Pim, J. Peacock, L. Crawford, and S. Benchimol. 1984. Isolation and characterization of a human p53 cDNA clone: expression of the human p53 gene. *The EMBO Journal* 3: 3257–3262.

Matsui, T., M. Heidaran, T. Miki, et al. 1989. Isolation of a novel receptor cDNA establishes the existence of two PDGF receptor genes. *Science* 243: 800–804.

May, P., and E. May. 1999. Twenty years of p53 research: Structural and functional aspects of the p53 protein. *Oncogene* 18: 7621–7636.

McGillicuddy, L.T., J.A. Fromm, P.E. Hollstein, et al. 2009. Proteasomal and genetic inactivation of the NF1 tumor suppressor in gliomagenesis. *Cancer Cell* 16: 44–54.

Mellinghoff, I.K., M.Y. Wang, I. Vivanco, et al. 2005. Molecular determinants of the response of glioblastomas to EGFR kinase inhibitors. *The New England Journal of Medicine* 353: 2012–2024.

Moodie, S.A., B.M. Willumsen, M.J. Weber, and A. Wolfman. 1993. Complexes of Ras.GTP with Raf-1 and mitogen-activated protein kinase kinase. *Science* 260: 1658–1661.

Morgensztern, D., and H.L. McLeod. 2005. PI3K/Akt/mTOR pathway as a target for cancer therapy. *Anti-Cancer Drugs* 16: 797–803.

Muhic, A., H.S. Poulsen, M. Sorensen, K. Grunnet, and U. Lassen. 2013. Phase II open-label study of nintedanib in patients with recurrent glioblastoma multiforme. *Journal of Neuro-Oncology* 111: 205–212.

Mukherjee, B., N. Tomimatsu, K. Amancherla, C.V. Camacho, N. Pichamoorthy, and S. Burma. 2012. The dual PI3K/mTOR inhibitor NVP-BEZ235 is a potent inhibitor of ATM- and DNA-PKCs-mediated DNA damage responses. *Neoplasia* 14: 34–43.

Murphree, A.L., and W.F. Benedict. 1984. Retinoblastoma: Clues to human oncogenesis. *Science* 223: 1028–1033.

Neyns, B., J. Sadones, E. Joosens, et al. 2009. Stratified phase II trial of cetuximab in patients with recurrent high-grade glioma. *Annals of Oncology* 20: 1596–1603.

Neyns, B., J. Sadones, C. Chaskis, et al. 2011. Phase II study of sunitinib malate in patients with recurrent high-grade glioma. *Journal of Neuro-Oncology* 103: 491–501.

Nghiemphu, P.L., P.Y. Wen, K.R. Lamborn, et al. 2011. A phase I trial of tipifarnib with radiation therapy, with and without temozolomide, for patients with newly diagnosed glioblastoma. *International Journal of Radiation Oncology, Biology, Physics* 81: 1422–1427.

Nghiemphu, P.L., A. Lai, R.M. Green, D.A. Reardon, and T. Cloughesy. 2012. A dose escalation trial for the combination of erlotinib and sirolimus for recurrent malignant gliomas. *Journal of Neuro-Oncology* 110: 245–250.

Nigro, J.M., A. Misra, L. Zhang, et al. 2005. Integrated array-comparative genomic hybridization and expression array profiles identify clinically relevant molecular subtypes of glioblastoma. *Cancer Research* 65: 1678–1686.

Nishikawa, R., X.D. Ji, R.C. Harmon, et al. 1994. A mutant epidermal growth factor receptor common in human glioma confers enhanced tumorigenicity. *Proceedings of the National Academy of Sciences of the United States of America* 91: 7727–7731.

Nishikawa, R., T. Sugiyama, Y. Narita, F. Furnari, W.K. Cavenee, and M. Matsutani. 2004. Immunohistochemical analysis of the mutant epidermal growth factor, deltaEGFR, in glioblastoma. *Brain Tumor Pathology* 21: 53–56.

Nissan, M.H., C.A. Pratilas, A.M. Jones, et al. 2014. Loss of NF1 in cutaneous melanoma is associated with RAS activation and MEK dependence. *Cancer Research* 74: 2340–2350.

Noushmehr, H., D.J. Weisenberger, K. Diefes, et al. 2010. Identification of a CpG island methylator phenotype that defines a distinct subgroup of glioma. *Cancer Cell* 17: 510–522.

Ohgaki, H., and P. Kleihues. 2005. Population-based studies on incidence, survival rates, and genetic alterations in astrocytic and oligodendroglial gliomas. *Journal of Neuropathology and Experimental Neurology* 64: 479–489.

———. 2009. Genetic alterations and signaling pathways in the evolution of gliomas. *Cancer Science* 100: 2235–2241.

Pan, E., D. Yu, B. Yue, et al. 2012. A prospective phase II single-institution trial of sunitinib for recurrent malignant glioma. *Journal of Neuro-Oncology* 110: 111–118.

Parsons, D.W., S. Jones, X. Zhang, et al. 2008. An integrated genomic analysis of human glioblastoma multiforme. *Science* 321: 1807–1812.

Peereboom, D.M., D.R. Shepard, M.S. Ahluwalia, et al. 2010. Phase II trial of erlotinib with temozolomide and radiation in patients with newly diagnosed glioblastoma multiforme. *Journal of Neuro-Oncology* 98: 93–99.

Peereboom, D.M., M.S. Ahluwalia, X. Ye, et al. 2013. NABTT 0502: A phase II and pharmacokinetic study of erlotinib and sorafenib for patients with progressive or recurrent glioblastoma multiforme. *Neuro-Oncology* 15: 490–496.

Peraud, A., K. Watanabe, K.H. Plate, Y. Yonekawa, P. Kleihues, and H. Ohgaki. 1997. p53 mutations versus EGF receptor expression in giant cell glioblastomas. *Journal of Neuropathology and Experimental Neurology* 56: 1236–1241.

Phillips, H.S., S. Kharbanda, R. Chen, et al. 2006. Molecular subclasses of high-grade glioma predict prognosis, delineate a pattern of disease progression, and resemble stages in neurogenesis. *Cancer Cell* 9: 157–173.

Phillips, A.C., E.R. Boghaert, K.S. Vaidya, et al. 2016. ABT-414, an Antibody-Drug Conjugate Targeting a Tumor-Selective EGFR Epitope. *Molecular Cancer Therapeutics* 15: 661–669.

Porter, K.R., B.J. McCarthy, S. Freels, Y. Kim, and F.G. Davis. 2010. Prevalence estimates for primary brain tumors in the United States by age, gender, behavior, and histology. *Neuro-Oncology* 12: 520–527.

Prados, M.D., K.R. Lamborn, S. Chang, et al. 2006. Phase 1 study of erlotinib HCl alone and combined with temozolomide in patients with stable or recurrent malignant glioma. *Neuro-Oncology* 8: 67–78.

Prados, M.D., S.M. Chang, N. Butowski, et al. 2009. Phase II study of erlotinib plus temozolomide during and after radiation therapy in patients with newly diagnosed glioblastoma multiforme or gliosarcoma. *Journal of Clinical Oncology* 27: 579–584.

Prados, M.D., S.A. Byron, N.L. Tran, et al. 2015. Toward precision medicine in glioblastoma: The promise and the challenges. *Neuro-Oncology* 17: 1051–1063.

Purow, B., and D. Schiff. 2009. Advances in the genetics of glioblastoma: Are we reaching critical mass? *Nature Reviews. Neurology* 5: 419–426.

Raizer, J.J., L.E. Abrey, A.B. Lassman, et al. 2010. A phase II trial of erlotinib in patients with recurrent malignant gliomas and nonprogressive glioblastoma multiforme postradiation therapy. *Neuro-Oncology* 12: 95–103.

Razis, E., P. Selviaridis, S. Labropoulos, et al. 2009. Phase II study of neoadjuvant imatinib in glioblastoma: Evaluation of clinical and molecular effects of the treatment. *Clinical Cancer Research* 15: 6258–6266.

Reardon, D.A., M.J. Egorin, J.A. Quinn, et al. 2005. Phase II study of imatinib mesylate plus hydroxyurea in adults with recurrent glioblastoma multiforme. *Journal of Clinical Oncology* 23: 9359–9368.

Reardon, D.A., J.A. Quinn, J.J. Vredenburgh, et al. 2006. Phase 1 trial of gefitinib plus sirolimus in adults with recurrent malignant glioma. *Clinical Cancer Research* 12: 860–868.

Reardon, D.A., G. Dresemann, S. Taillibert, et al. 2009a. Multicentre phase II studies evaluating imatinib plus hydroxyurea in patients with progressive glioblastoma. *British Journal of Cancer* 101: 1995–2004.

Reardon, D.A., M.J. Egorin, A. Desjardins, et al. 2009b. Phase I pharmacokinetic study of the vascular endothelial growth factor receptor tyrosine kinase inhibitor vatalanib (PTK787) plus imatinib and hydroxyurea for malignant glioma. *Cancer* 115: 2188–2198.

Reardon, D.A., A. Desjardins, J.J. Vredenburgh, et al. 2010. Phase 2 trial of erlotinib plus sirolimus in adults with recurrent glioblastoma. *Journal of Neuro-Oncology* 96: 219–230.

Reardon, D.A., J.J. Vredenburgh, A. Desjardins, et al. 2011a. Effect of CYP3A-inducing anti-epileptics on sorafenib exposure: Results of a phase II study of sorafenib plus daily temozolomide in adults with recurrent glioblastoma. *Journal of Neuro-Oncology* 101: 57–66.

Reardon, D.A., J.J. Vredenburgh, A. Coan, et al. 2011b. Phase I study of sunitinib and irinotecan for patients with recurrent malignant glioma. *Journal of Neuro-Oncology* 105: 621–627.

Reardon, D.A., J.J. Vredenburgh, A. Desjardins, et al. 2012. Phase 1 trial of dasatinib plus erlotinib in adults with recurrent malignant glioma. *Journal of Neuro-Oncology* 108: 499–506.

Reardon, D.A., M.D. Groves, P.Y. Wen, et al. 2013. A phase I/II trial of pazopanib in combination with lapatinib in adult patients with relapsed malignant glioma. *Clinical Cancer Research* 19: 900–908.

Reardon, D.A., P.Y. Wen, and I.K. Mellinghoff. 2014. Targeted molecular therapies against epidermal growth factor receptor: Past experiences and challenges. *Neuro-Oncology* 16 Suppl 8: viii7–vii13.

Reardon, D.A., A. Desjardins, J. Schuster, et al. 2015. IMCT-08ReACT: LONG-TERM SURVIVAL FROM A RANDOMIZED PHASE II STUDY OF RINDOPEPIMUT (CDX-110) PLUS BEVACIZUMAB IN RELAPSED GLIOBLASTOMA. *Neuro-Oncology* 17: v109.

Reifenberger, G., L. Liu, K. Ichimura, E.E. Schmidt, and V.P. Collins. 1993. Amplification and overexpression of the MDM2 gene in a subset of human malignant gliomas without p53 mutations. *Cancer Research* 53: 2736–2739.

Reifenberger, G., J. Reifenberger, K. Ichimura, and V.P. Collins. 1995. Amplification at 12q13-14 in human malignant gliomas is frequently accompanied by loss of heterozygosity at loci proximal and distal to the amplification site. *Cancer Research* 55: 731–734.

Rey, J.A., M.J. Bello, J.M. de Campos, M.E. Kusak, C. Ramos, and J. Benitez. 1987. Chromosomal patterns in human malignant astrocytomas. *Cancer Genetics and Cytogenetics* 29: 201–221.

Rich, J.N., D.A. Reardon, T. Peery, et al. 2004. Phase II trial of gefitinib in recurrent glioblastoma. *Journal of Clinical Oncology* 22: 133–142.

Riemenschneider, M.J., R. Buschges, M. Wolter, et al. 1999. Amplification and overexpression of the MDM4 (MDMX) gene from 1q32 in a subset of malignant gliomas without TP53 mutation or MDM2 amplification. *Cancer Research* 59: 6091–6096.

Ruas, M., and G. Peters. 1998. The p16INK4a/CDKN2A tumor suppressor and its relatives. *Biochimica et Biophysica Acta* 1378: F115–F177.

Sami, A., and M. Karsy. 2013. Targeting the PI3K/AKT/mTOR signaling pathway in glioblastoma: Novel therapeutic agents and advances in understanding. *Tumour Biology* 34: 1991–2002.

Sandmann, T., R. Bourgon, J. Garcia, et al. 2015. Patients with proneural glioblastoma may derive overall survival benefit from the addition of bevacizumab to first-line radiotherapy and temozolomide: Retrospective analysis of the AVAglio trial. *Journal of Clinical Oncology* 33: 2735–2744.

Sanson, M., Y. Marie, S. Paris, et al. 2009. Isocitrate dehydrogenase 1 codon 132 mutation is an important prognostic biomarker in gliomas. *Journal of Clinical Oncology* 27: 4150–4154.

Sarbassov, D.D., S.M. Ali, D.H. Kim, et al. 2004. Rictor, a novel binding partner of mTOR, defines a rapamycin-insensitive and raptor-independent pathway that regulates the cytoskeleton. *Current Biology* 14: 1296–1302.

Sarbassov, D.D., D.A. Guertin, S.M. Ali, and D.M. Sabatini. 2005. Phosphorylation and regulation of Akt/PKB by the rictor-mTOR complex. *Science* 307: 1098–1101.

Sarkaria, J.N., E. Galanis, W. Wu, et al. 2010. Combination of temsirolimus (CCI-779) with chemoradiation in newly diagnosed glioblastoma multiforme (GBM) (NCCTG trial N027D) is associated with increased infectious risks. *Clinical Cancer Research* 16: 5573–5580.

Sathornsumetee, S., A. Desjardins, J.J. Vredenburgh, et al. 2010. Phase II trial of bevacizumab and erlotinib in patients with recurrent malignant glioma. *Neuro-Oncology* 12: 1300–1310.

Schlegel, J., G. Stumm, K. Brandle, et al. 1994. Amplification and differential expression of members of the erbB-gene family in human glioblastoma. *Journal of Neuro-Oncology* 22: 201–207.

Schmidt, E.E., K. Ichimura, G. Reifenberger, and V.P. Collins. 1994. CDKN2 (p16/MTS1) gene deletion or CDK4 amplification occurs in the majority of glioblastomas. *Cancer Research* 54: 6321–6324.

See, W.L., I.L. Tan, J. Mukherjee, T. Nicolaides, and R.O. Pieper. 2012. Sensitivity of glioblastomas to clinically available MEK inhibitors is defined by neurofibromin 1 deficiency. *Cancer Research* 72: 3350–3359.

Soffietti, R., E. Trevisan, L. Bertero, et al. 2014. Bevacizumab and fotemustine for recurrent glioblastoma: A phase II study of AINO (Italian Association of Neuro-Oncology). *Journal of Neuro-Oncology* 116: 533–541.

Solomon, M.T., J.C. Selva, J. Figueredo, et al. 2013. Radiotherapy plus nimotuzumab or placebo in the treatment of high grade glioma patients: Results from a randomized, double blind trial. *BMC Cancer* 13: 299.

Stambolic, V., A. Suzuki, J.L. de la Pompa, et al. 1998. Negative regulation of PKB/Akt-dependent cell survival by the tumor suppressor PTEN. *Cell* 95: 29–39.

Stenman, G., F. Rorsman, K. Huebner, and C. Betsholtz. 1992. The human platelet-derived growth factor alpha chain (PDGFA) gene maps to chromosome 7p22. *Cytogenetics and Cell Genetics* 60: 206–207.

Stommel, J.M., A.C. Kimmelman, H. Ying, et al. 2007. Coactivation of receptor tyrosine kinases affects the response of tumor cells to targeted therapies. *Science* 318: 287–290.

Stupp, R., W.P. Mason, M.J. van den Bent, et al. 2005. Radiotherapy plus concomitant and adjuvant temozolomide for glioblastoma. *The New England Journal of Medicine* 352: 987–996.

Sunayama, J., A. Sato, K. Matsuda, et al. 2010. Dual blocking of mTor and PI3K elicits a prodif-
ferentiation effect on glioblastoma stem-like cells. *Neuro-Oncology* 12: 1205–1219.

Swartz, A.M., Q.J. Li, and J.H. Sampson. 2014. Rindopepimut: A promising immunotherapeutic
for the treatment of glioblastoma multiforme. *Immunotherapy* 6: 679–690.

Taal, W., H.M. Oosterkamp, A.M. Walenkamp, et al. 2014. Single-agent bevacizumab or lomustine
versus a combination of bevacizumab plus lomustine in patients with recurrent glioblastoma
(BELOB trial): A randomised controlled phase 2 trial. *The Lancet Oncology* 15: 943–953.

Tanaka, S., D.N. Louis, W.T. Curry, T.T. Batchelor, and J. Dietrich. 2013. Diagnostic and therapeutic avenues for glioblastoma: No longer a dead end? *Nature Reviews. Clinical Oncology* 10:
14–26.

Teng, D.H., R. Hu, H. Lin, et al. 1997. MMAC1/PTEN mutations in primary tumor specimens and
tumor cell lines. *Cancer Research* 57: 5221–5225.

Thiessen, B., C. Stewart, M. Tsao, et al. 2010. A phase I/II trial of GW572016 (lapatinib) in recurrent glioblastoma multiforme: Clinical outcomes, pharmacokinetics and molecular correlation.
Cancer Chemotherapy and Pharmacology 65: 353–361.

Thomas, S.M., M. DeMarco, G. D'Arcangelo, S. Halegoua, and J.S. Brugge. 1992. Ras is essential
for nerve growth factor- and phorbol ester-induced tyrosine phosphorylation of MAP kinases.
Cell 68: 1031–1040.

Tohma, Y., C. Gratas, W. Biernat, et al. 1998. PTEN (MMAC1) mutations are frequent in primary
glioblastomas (de novo) but not in secondary glioblastomas. *Journal of Neuropathology and
Experimental Neurology* 57: 684–689.

Uhm, J.H., K.V. Ballman, W. Wu, et al. 2011. Phase II evaluation of gefitinib in patients with newly
diagnosed Grade 4 astrocytoma: Mayo/North Central Cancer Treatment Group Study N0074.
International Journal of Radiation Oncology, Biology, Physics 80: 347–353.

van den Bent, M.J., Y. Gao, M. Kerkhof, et al. 2015. Changes in the EGFR amplification and
EGFRvIII expression between paired primary and recurrent glioblastomas. *Neuro-Oncology*
17: 935–941.

Verhaak, R.G., K.A. Hoadley, E. Purdom, et al. 2010. Integrated genomic analysis identifies clinically relevant subtypes of glioblastoma characterized by abnormalities in PDGFRA, IDH1,
EGFR, and NF1. *Cancer Cell* 17: 98–110.

Vitucci, M., D.N. Hayes, and C.R. Miller. 2011. Gene expression profiling of gliomas: merging
genomic and histopathological classification for personalised therapy. *British Journal of
Cancer* 104: 545–553.

Vivanco, I., D. Rohle, M. Versele, et al. 2010. The phosphatase and tensin homolog regulates epidermal growth factor receptor (EGFR) inhibitor response by targeting EGFR for degradation.
Proceedings of the National Academy of Sciences of the United States of America 107:
6459–6464.

Wang, S.I., J. Puc, J. Li, et al. 1997. Somatic mutations of PTEN in glioblastoma multiforme.
Cancer Research 57: 4183–4186.

Wang, H., W. Zhang, H.J. Huang, W.S. Liao, and G.N. Fuller. 2004. Analysis of the activation
status of Akt, NFkappaB, and Stat3 in human diffuse gliomas. *Laboratory Investigation* 84:
941–951.

Ward, P.S., J. Patel, D.R. Wise, et al. 2010. The common feature of leukemia-associated IDH1 and
IDH2 mutations is a neomorphic enzyme activity converting alpha-ketoglutarate to
2-hydroxyglutarate. *Cancer Cell* 17: 225–234.

Watanabe, K., O. Tachibana, K. Sata, Y. Yonekawa, P. Kleihues, and H. Ohgaki. 1996.
Overexpression of the EGF receptor and p53 mutations are mutually exclusive in the evolution
of primary and secondary glioblastomas. *Brain Pathology* 6: 217–223; discussion 223–214.

Watanabe, T., S. Nobusawa, P. Kleihues, and H. Ohgaki. 2009. IDH1 mutations are early events in
the development of astrocytomas and oligodendrogliomas. *The American Journal of Pathology*
174: 1149–1153.

Weller, M., J. Felsberg, C. Hartmann, et al. 2009. Molecular predictors of progression-free and
overall survival in patients with newly diagnosed glioblastoma: A prospective translational
study of the German Glioma Network. *Journal of Clinical Oncology* 27: 5743–5750.

Wen, P.Y., W.K. Yung, K.R. Lamborn, et al. 2006. Phase I/II study of imatinib mesylate for recurrent malignant gliomas: North American Brain Tumor Consortium Study 99-08. *Clinical Cancer Research* 12: 4899–4907.

Wen, P.Y.P.M., D. Schiff, D.A. Reardon, T. Cloughesy, T. Mikkelsen, T. Batchelor, J. Drappatz, M.C. Chamberlain, and J.F. De Groot. 2010. Phase II study of XL184 (BMS 907351), an inhibitor of MET, VEGFR2, and RET, in patients (pts) with progressive glioblastoma (GB) [abstract]. *Journal of Clinical Oncology* 28: 181s.

Wick, W., V.K. Puduvalli, M.C. Chamberlain, et al. 2010. Phase III study of enzastaurin compared with lomustine in the treatment of recurrent intracranial glioblastoma. *Journal of Clinical Oncology* 28: 1168–1174.

Wick, W., J.P. Steinbach, M. Platten, et al. 2013. Enzastaurin before and concomitant with radiation therapy, followed by enzastaurin maintenance therapy, in patients with newly diagnosed glioblastoma without MGMT promoter hypermethylation. *Neuro-Oncology* 15: 1405–1412.

Wong, A.J., J.M. Ruppert, S.H. Bigner, et al. 1992. Structural alterations of the epidermal growth factor receptor gene in human gliomas. *Proceedings of the National Academy of Sciences of the United States of America* 89: 2965–2969.

Yan, H., D.W. Parsons, G. Jin, et al. 2009. IDH1 and IDH2 mutations in gliomas. *The New England Journal of Medicine* 360: 765–773.

Yung, W.K., J.J. Vredenburgh, T.F. Cloughesy, et al. 2010. Safety and efficacy of erlotinib in first-relapse glioblastoma: A phase II open-label study. *Neuro-Oncology* 12: 1061–1070.

Yust-Katz, S., D. Liu, Y. Yuan, et al. 2013. Phase 1/1b study of lonafarnib and temozolomide in patients with recurrent or temozolomide refractory glioblastoma. *Cancer* 119: 2747–2753.

Zhang, Y., Y. Xiong, and W.G. Yarbrough. 1998. ARF promotes MDM2 degradation and stabilizes p53: ARF-INK4a locus deletion impairs both the Rb and p53 tumor suppression pathways. *Cell* 92: 725–734.

Zhu, Y., F. Guignard, D. Zhao, et al. 2005. Early inactivation of p53 tumor suppressor gene cooperating with NF1 loss induces malignant astrocytoma. *Cancer Cell* 8: 119–130.

Zwick, E., J. Bange, and A. Ullrich. 2001. Receptor tyrosine kinase signalling as a target for cancer intervention strategies. *Endocrine-Related Cancer* 8: 161–173.

Chapter 5
Targeting EGFR in Glioblastoma: Molecular Biology and Current Understanding

Juan Manuel Sepúlveda, Cristina Zahonero, and Pilar Sánchez Gómez

Abstract Glioblastoma (GBM) is a heterogeneous disease comprising a multitude of genetically and epigenetically different cancers, all of them highly resistant to conventional chemo and radiotherapy. Greater characterization of GBM at the molecular level has improved its initial pathophysiological staging and classification. With this knowledge came the hope that more efficacious therapies to combat this highly lethal disease were on the horizon. One possibility for intervention was represented by the targeting of epidermal growth factor receptor (EGFR), which is amplified and/or mutated in more than 50% of patients. However, several tirosinkinase inhibitors and EGFR-directed antibodies have been tested in clinical trials and only modest results have been obtained. Here, we provide an overview of the structure and expression of EGFR and its mutant forms in GBM, describing the canonical and non-canonical downstream pathways activated by the receptor. Furthermore, we enumerate some of the most relevant therapeutic strategies that have been tested so far to inhibit EGFR, discussing the possible explanations for their failure as well as novel alternative approaches.

Keywords Glioblastoma • EGFR • EGFRvIII • Canonical signaling • Non canonical signaling • Molecular therapy • Treatment failure

J.M. Sepúlveda
Unidad Multidisciplinar de Neurooncología. Hospital Universitario 12 de Octubre, Madrid, Spain
e-mail: juanmanuel.sepulveda@salud.madrid.org

C. Zahonero
Institute for Cancer Genetics, Columbia University, New York, NY, USA
e-mail: cz2394@cumc.columbia.edu

P.S. Gómez (✉)
Neuro-oncology Unit, Instituto de Salud Carlos III-Chronic Disease Program (UFIEC), Madrid, Spain
e-mail: psanchezg@isciii.es

© Springer International Publishing AG 2017   117
K. Somasundaram (ed.), *Advances in Biology and Treatment of Glioblastoma*,
Current Cancer Research, DOI 10.1007/978-3-319-56820-1_5

5.1   Introduction

In the most recent years, the massive use of the different –omic platforms with large cohort of glioma samples (like the one from The Cancer Genome Atlas, TCGA, consortium) have allowed the identification of distinct genetic and epigenetic profiles in different types of gliomas. The new (2016) World Health Organization (WHO) classification of gliomas incorporates these new molecular biomarkers for a more accurate classification. In this new scenario, glioblastomas (GBM) (the most common and malignant type of glioma) is subdivided into two major entities, namely the common isocitrate dehydrogenase 1 and 2 (*IDH1/2*) wild-type (*IDH* wt) GBM, which accounts for more than 90% of all the tumors, and the less common *IDH* mutant GBM that is found in less than 10% of patients (Masui et al. 2016). The majority of *IDH* wt GBM correspond to primary tumors (those that occur preferentially in older patients with no evidence of a pre-existing, grade 2 or grade 3 tumor). In contrast, *IDH* mutant GBMs are typically seen in young adults and include the vast majority of secondary GBM (tumors that develop by progression from a pre-existing less malignant astrocytoma) (Ohgaki and Kleihues 2013). Moreover, patients with *IDH* mutant GBMs show a significantly longer overall survival (OS) (Weller et al. 2015).

In the *IDH* wt GBMs, the most common alterations are copy number gains on chromosome 7, loss of chromosome 10, mutations in the phosphatase and tensin homolog (*PTEN*), homozygous deletion of the cyclin-dependent kinase inhibitors 2A and 2B (*CDKN2A* and *CDKN2B*), as well as telomerase reverse transcriptase (*TERT* promoter) mutations that leads to increased expression or TERT, which promote telomere length maintenance. In addition, recurrent mutations in *TP53*, phosphatidylinositol 3-kinase, catalytic, alpha (*PIK3CA*), Phosphatidylinositol 3-kinase, regulatory subunit 1 (*PIK3R1*), and neurofibromatosis type 1 (*NF1*) (a negative modulator of Ras activation), occur in more than 10% of tumors. Moreover, adult GBMs typically carry amplifications of proto-onocogenes, affecting epidermal growth factor receptor (*EGFR*) (altered in more than 40% of IDH wt GBMs), platelet-derived growth factor receptor A (PDGFRA) (mostly in young patients), cyclin-dependent kinase genes (*CDK4* and *CDK6*) (positive modulators of the retinoblastoma, RB, activation), and murine double minute genes (*MDM2* and *MDM4*) (negative regulators of the p53 pathway) (Aldape et al. 2015; Masui et al. 2016). Among *IDH* wt GBMs, two main subgroups have been proposed. The first one is characterized by the high frequency of *NF1* and *TP53* mutations and shows a mesenchymal transcriptomic profile. The second one is characterized by a high proportion of *EGFR* amplifications and loss of the *CDKN2A* locus, and is associated with the "classical" subgroup (Brennan et al. 2013; Verhaak et al. 2010).

EGFR activation is associated with increased proliferation and migration of GBM cells (Lal et al. 2002; Talasila et al. 2013). Moreover, the extraordinary presence of *EGFR* alterations in primary GBMs suggests that this receptor participates not only in tumor growth but also during the initial steps of tumor formation. In fact, numerous investigations carried out in animal models, including transgenic mice, show that the enhanced expression of EGFRwt, and especially the vIII truncated version, in neural progenitors, can cooperate with other genetic alterations to induce primary brain cancer initiation and progression (Zahonero and Sanchez-Gomez 2014; Huse and Holland 2009). In addition, several reports suggest that EGFR participates in the well-known resistance to chemotherapy and radiotherapy in GBM (Barker et al. 2001; Leuraud et al. 2004; Munoz et al. 2014; Bouras et al. 2015). All these findings make the EGFR pathway a very attractive target for therapy. However, while EGFR kinase inhibitors have proven to be useful in treating other types of tumors, they offer poor outcomes in GBM patients, underlying the special oncogenic function of this receptor in gliomas. In this chapter we will try to summarize the molecular features of EGFR signaling in GBM, reviewing conventional pathways as well as other novel functions of EGFR that do not depend on ligand stimulation and/or kinase activity. We will also summarize past, current and future clinical trials based on an EGFR-directed rationale, trying to offer a comprehensive explanation for the lack of response of these approaches in GBM patients.

5.2 EGFR Structure and Mutations in Glioblastomas

EGFR is a transmembrane glycoprotein and the first of the 4 ErbB receptor tyrosine kinases described, together with ErbB2 (Her2/Neu), ErbB3, and ErbB4. All of them share similarities in structure and function. EGFR is classically activated through ligand binding by factors such as EGF, transforming growth factor-α (TGF-α), amphiregulin (AR), betacellulin, epiregulin, and the Heparin- binding EGF-like growth factor (HB-EGF) (Yarden 2001). EGFR consists of a 1, 186-amino acid single polypeptide chain with three main regions: an extracellular receptor domain, a transmembrane region (TM), and an intracellular domain with a tyrosine kinase (TK) and a regulatory domain (RD) (Fig. 5.1). The amino-terminal portion of the receptor has, in an alternative disposition, two ligand-binding (LB) domains and two cysteine-rich (CR) domains. Within these four segments, there are 12 asparagines that are potential N-linked glycosylation sites, required for proper configuration of the ligand binding site (Bishayee 2000). When the ligand is not around, the extracellular domain folds back on itself. In the presence of the ligand, the receptor opens up and binds to another copy of the receptor through the CR domains. This brings together two copies of the kinase domain that can now phosphorylate each other at tyrosine residues at the RD. Of the 20 tyrosines in the carboxy-terminus, a subset of seven has been reported to get phosphorylated and serve as docking sites for downstream signaling proteins (Endres et al. 2011).

Many GBMs with *EGFR* amplification also carry mutations in *EGFR* (Fig. 5.1) (Brennan et al. 2013; Frattini et al. 2013). The first identified EGFR mutant was EGFRvIII, a genomic rearrangement in the extracellular domain (present in 50% of *EGFR* amplified (*EGFR*amp) GBMs.). EGFR vIII lacks 267 amino acids of the extracelullar domain (leaving a small portion of the CR1 domain). With a fully intact intracellular domain, downstream signaling is not impeded. Hyperactivation of the

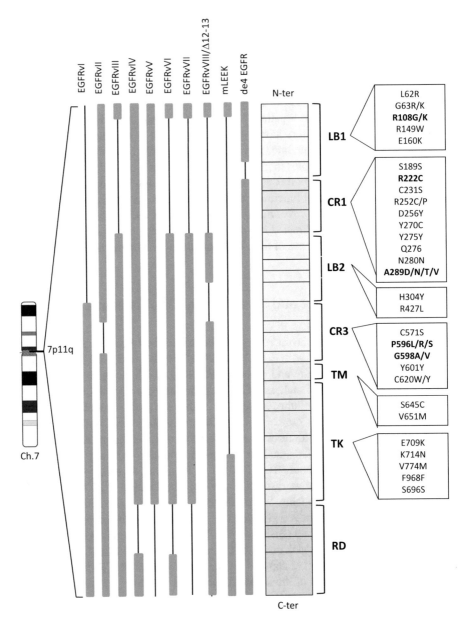

Fig. 5.1 EGFR gene structure and mutations found in GBM. EGFR gene is located in the 7p11q chromosomic region. It contains XX exons coding for the 7 protein domains of EGFR: ligand-binding 1 (LB1), cysteine-rich 1 (CR1), L2, CR2, transmembrane (TM), tyrosine kinase (TK) and regulatory domain (RD). On the right side, listed in boxes, the main point mutations found in GBM samples, with most frequent mutations in bold letters. On the left side, the EGFR mutant forms. The *black lines* represent the genetic regions deleted in the receptor aberrant isoforms

receptor is likely due to the spontaneous dimerization of the receptor and induction of the kinase domain (Batra et al. 1995; Bishayee 2000). The study of several mouse glioma models has demonstrated that the vIII variant is more tumorigenic that the wt receptor (Holland et al. 1998; Bachoo et al. 2002). Moreover, there are reports of selective and/or constitutive activation of several pathways: Phosphoinositide 3-kinase (PI3K) pathway, Ras, c-jun N-terminal kinase (JNK), Src family kinases (SFK), urokinase-type plasminogen activator receptor (uPAR) and nuclear factor kappa-light-chain-enhancer of activated B cells (NF-κB) (Zahonero and Sanchez-Gomez 2014). Moreover EGFRvIII confers drug resistance to GBM cells through the modulation of B-cell lymphoma-extralarge (Bcl-XL) and caspase 3-like proteases (Nagane et al. 1998).

Some other deletions have been described like EGFRvV, a truncation of the intracellular region at amino acid 958, which is present in 15% of *EGFR*amp GBMs. This mutant receptor is internalization-deficient and therefore, it has enhanced ligand-dependent kinase activity (Pines et al. 2010). Oncogenic missense point mutations in the extracellular domain of the receptor were also recently reported, presumably promoting receptor dimerization and enhancing EGFR activity (Lee et al. 2006). Mutations of the intracellular portion of *EGFR* are more common in other neoplasms. In fact, the tyrosine mutations in the kinase domain found in lung cancer that predict response to specific EGFR inhibition, have not been detected in GBMs (Pines et al. 2010). More recently, a genomic study has revealed the presence of recurrent in-frame fusions involving EGFR (in 7.6% of GBMs), with the most recurrent partners being septin 14 (SEPT14) and phosphoserin phosphatase (PSPH). Interestingly, the EGFR-SEPT14 fusions produce mitogen-independent growth and they constitutively activate signal transducer and activator of transcription 3 (STAT3) signaling, although they are especially sensitive to tyrosin kinase inhibitors (Frattini et al. 2013). Notably, 30% of *EGFR*amp GBMs express two or more aberrant receptor variants. Although multiple mutations can sometimes be seen in the same amplified *EGFR* gene (a finding unique to GBM), in most cases they represent different subclonal populations (Frederick et al. 2000; Francis et al. 2014).

5.3   Canonical EGFR Signaling

Classically, EGFR signalling has been broadly divided into four basic steps: ligand binding, receptor dimerization, transphosphorylation of tyrosine residues on the receptor pair, and communication with downstream effectors. There are seven tyrosine residues at the carboxy terminus of the receptor (Y992, Y1045, Y1068, Y1086, Y1114, Y1148, and Y1173) that become phosphorylated upon EGFR activation and serve as docking sites for several signaling molecules containing a Src homology domain 2 (SH2) or a phospho-tyrosine binding domain (PTB) (Endres et al. 2011). Those proteins, in turn, recruit a plethora of downstream mediators (Fig. 5.2).

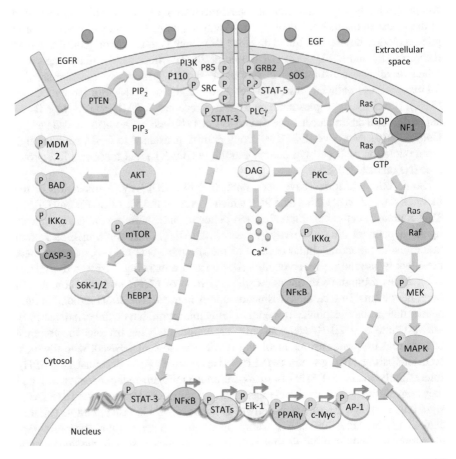

Fig. 5.2 EGFR canonical signaling pathway. After the interaction of EGFR with its ligand (EGF in this case), several effector and adaptor intracellular proteins are recruited to the phosphorylated tyrosine residues of the receptor. This triggers the activation of a variety of signaling pathways. Among other, the MAPK/ERK, PI3K, STATs and PLCγ-PKC-NFκB signal transducers are activated. These signaling events result in changes in gene expression, protein synthesis, cell growth, apoptosis, immune suppression, and cellular metabolism changes

5.3.1 MAP/ERK Pathway

One of the major pathways downstream of EGFR is the mitogen-activated protein kinase (MAPK)/extracellular signal-regulated kinase (ERK) route. EGFR recruits the upstream components Grb2 and Shc, which bind to SOS. SOS exchanges GDP for GTP and activates Ras that then binds to and allosterically activates the Raf kinase. Raf is the first member of a cascade of three kinases in the MAPK pathway, with Raf activating MEK and MEK activating ERKs. Upon activation, ERK kinases translocate to the nucleus and activate several transcription factors (TFs), including Elk-1, Elk-1 (ETS domain-containing protein), peroxisome-proliferator-activated receptor γ (PPARγ), STAT1 and STAT3, C-myc and activating protein- 1 (AP-1) (Nicholas et al. 2006; Hatanpaa et al. 2010). Although gliomas do not normally contain Ras mutations, the the GTPase-activating NF1 that inhibits Ras is inactivated in 23% of cases (Brennan et al. 2013) and high levels of active Ras-GTP are found in wild-type *NF1* tumors, probably due to upstream activation of EGFR or other receptors (Guha et al. 1997).

5.3.2 PI3K Pathway

The other main pathway activated by EGFR is the PI3K pathway. When recruited to phosphotyrosines in the activated receptor, Class I PI3K phosphorylates phosphatidylinositol 4, 5-bisphosphate (PIP2) to generate PI(3, 4, 5)P3 (also referred to as PIP3). PIP3 recruits the AKT kinase to the membrane, which phosphorylates several substrates that inhibit apoptosis. Those include BAD, caspase-9, the p53 regulator MDM2, and members of the FoxO family of transcription factors. The other major role of AKT is to activate mammalian target of rapamycin (mTOR), which regulates protein translation and cholesterol biosynthesis, thereby providing protein and lipid material to cells upon growth factor stimulation (Hatanpaa et al. 2010; Nicholas et al. 2006). Alterations of this pathway are frequent in GBM and include activating mutations and/or amplifications of the catalytic and regulatory subunit of PI3K and *PTEN* deletions or inactivating mutations (see above). Moreover, the status of AKT phosphorylation has been associated with the response to EGFR kinase inhibitors (Haas-Kogan et al. 2005).

5.3.3 PKC-NF-kB Pathway

Phospho-lipase C γ (PLC-γ) is also recruited and phosphorylated by EGFR. At the membrane, PLCγ cleaves PIP2 to inositol triphosphate (IP3) and diacylglycerol (DAG). Together with DAG, IP3-mediated induction of calcium (Ca2+) can activate protein kinase C (PKC), which in turn can phosphorylate the inhibitor of nuclear factor kappa B kinase subunit alpha (IKKα). Then, activated IKKα phosphorylates inhibitor of κB (IκB), targeting it for ubiquitination and proteosomal degradation, and provoking the activation and nuclear translocation of NF-κB (Yang et al. 2012). NF-κB can be activated by the AKT pathway as well and it plays and important role in inflammation and cancer, inducing pro-survival genes like Bcl-XL or caspase inhibitors (Bai et al. 2009). Aberrant constitutive activation of NF-κB has been observed in GBM (Nogueira et al. 2011) and it was recently demonstrated that *NFκI1A*, the gene that codes for the NF-κB inhibitor (IκBα), is often deleted in these tumors. Indeed, deletion of IκBα has a similar effect to that of EGFR amplification in the pathogenesis of GBM and it is associated with comparatively short survival (Bredel et al. 2011). These results suggest that activation of NF-κB is another fundamental pathway for glioma progression and that it can be achieved either by genetic deletion of its inhibitor, or by *EGFR* amplification.

5.3.4 STATs

Other important downstream targets of EGFR are the STAT proteins, which bind to the receptor and become phosphorylated, by EGFR itself or by non-receptor tyrosine kinases like Src. Upon phosphorylation, STATs dimerize via reciprocal SH2 domain/phosphotyrosine interactions, localize to the nucleus and induce transcription of their target genes. STAT3 is associated with cell-cycle progression, apoptosis, and immunosuppression in GBM, although there are no reports of gain-of-function mutations in these tumors (Brantley and Benveniste 2008; See et al. 2012). STAT5 is also overexpressed in GBM compared to normal tissue or lower-grade gliomas and it seems to be preferentially activated by the vIII isoform.

5.4 Non Canonical EGFR Signaling

In the traditional view, EGFR signalling was believed to occur at the plasma membrane, after ligand binding and tyrosine kinase activation. However, a more complex picture of multifaceted, spatial, and temporal regulation is emerging. We know now that EGFR can be activated by ligand-independent mechanisms as well as by multiple ligands, often with differing signalling outcomes. Moreover, EGFR-mediated signals can continue in diverse subcellular locations and these functions do not always depend on its kinase activity. Figure 5.3 resumes some of these non-canonical pathways that we describe herein.

5.4.1 EGFR Turnover

EGFR is regulated by membrane trafficking and there is a continuous movement from the cell surface to endosomes via clathrin-mediated endocytosis. In the absence of ligand, the rate of internalization is slow, and recycling of the receptor back to the membrane is rapid. Ligand binding dramatically increases the rate of receptor internalization and recycling is slowed, favouring receptor degradation at the lysosomes. Therefore, EGFR internalization works as a negative feedback loop and serves to signal attenuation. CBL is the primary E3 ubiquitin ligase that is recruited to the regulatory domain in the receptor's tail after ligand stimulation. This protein can bind directly to phospho-Y1045, or indirectly via Grb2, and it recruits E2 enzymes to its ring-finger domain to promote the ubiquitination and internalization of EGFR (Citri and Yarden 2006). There is a growing body of evidence to suggest that

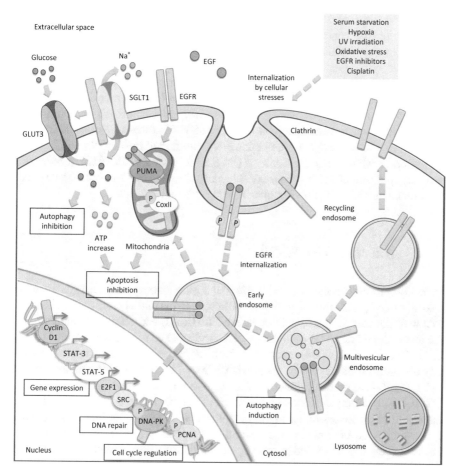

Fig. 5.3 EGFR turnover and non-canonical signaling. After ligand interaction, EGFR is internalized and mobilized to different organelles. This process can be also triggered by cellular stresses such as hypoxia, oxidative stress and EGFR inhibitors, among others. EGFR is internalized through early endosomes and then sorted to multivesicular endodomes, the mitochondria or the nucleus. At the mitochondria and the endosomes, EGFR is involved in inhibiting apoptosis and promoting cell survival. When internalized to the nucleus, EGFR interacts with some transcription factors (STATs, E2F1, SRC...) modulating gene expression and with proteins involved in DNA damage repair (DNA-PK) and cell cycle regulation (PCNA). Additionally EGFR interacts with glucose transporters, increasing glucose intracellular levels, which leads to autophagy and apoptosis inhibition of cancer cells

perturbations in EGFR trafficking play a role in the initiation and propagation of cancer (Mellman and Yarden 2013; Zahonero and Sanchez-Gomez 2014). In GBM, molecules like leucine rich repeats and immunoglobulin-like domains-1 (LRIG1) (which increases the amount of CBL recruited to EGFR (Gur et al. 2004; Laederich et al. 2004)), and mitogen-inducible gene 6 (MIG-6) (which enhances the trafficking of EGFR into late endosomes/lysosomes (Ying et al. 2010)), are downregulated in gliomas compared to normal tissue, especially in *EGFR*amp tumors. Moreover, the 19q13 allele that contains the CBL sequence is frequently lost in these tumors (Mizoguchi et al. 2004) and deletions in the 1p36 allele, where *MIG-6* gene is located, has been recently associated with overexpression of EGFR (Furgason et al. 2014). All these data reinforce the notion that stabilization of membrane EGFR is necessary for GBM growth. In fact, overexpression of LRIG1 and MIG-6 in glioma cells reduces EGFR at the cell surface and triggers cell growth inhibition and impaired invasion, enhancing apoptosis (Ye et al. 2009; Johansson et al. 2013; Ying et al. 2010). Similar results were obtained by inhibition of the dual-specificity tyrosine phosphorylation-regulated kinase (DYRK1A) (Pozo et al. 2013), a molecule that acts upstream of SPRY2 (Sprouty2), which removes CBL from activated EGFR and blocks its ubiquitination (Egan et al. 2002; Rubin et al. 2003).

5.4.2   Mitochondrial EGFR

In addition to these recycling and lysosomal sorting pathways, recent studies have also reported ligand-stimulated EGFR trafficking to the mitochondria where it interacts with the cytochrome-c oxidase subunit II (CoxII) and reduces its activity and the levels of cellular ATP, modulating cell survival (Yue et al. 2008; Demory et al. 2009; Boerner et al. 2004). Moreover, both EGFR and EGFRvIII associate with p53-upregulated modulator of apoptosis (PUMA), a pro-apoptotic member of the Bcl-2 family of proteins primarily located on the mitochondria (Zhu et al. 2010). EGFR-PUMA interaction is independent of EGF stimulation or kinase activity and induces PUMA sequestration in the cytoplasm, where it cannot initiate apoptosis. Interestingly, the amount of mitochondrial EGFR seems to be fine-tuned by the balance between autophagy and apoptosis, and inhibition of the former or induction of the latter provokes accumulation of EGFR in this organelle as a pro-survival mechanism (Yue et al. 2008). In adition, mitochondrial translocation can be enhanced by rapamycin, an mTOR inhibitor, and gefitinib, an EGFR inhibitor, (Cao et al. 2011; Yue et al. 2008) so it could be participating in the known role of EGFR in therapy-resistance.

5.4.3   Nuclear Functions of EGFR

EGFR has also been detected in the nuclei of cancer cells, where it is associated with increased proliferation and poor clinical outcome (Lin et al. 2001). In gliomas, both EGFRwt and EGFRvIII have been detected in the nucleus, where they cooperate with STAT3 (de la Iglesia et al. 2008; Lo et al. 2010; Chua et al. 2016). Regarding translocation mechanism, a nuclear localization sequence (NLS) at amino acids 645–657 has been characterized EGFR, adjacent to the TM domain, which allows nuclear translocation of members of this receptor family via binding to importin β (Hsu and Hung 2007). Moreover, receptor endocytosis has been proposed as a necessary step to transport the receptor from the cell surface to the nucleus (Lo et al. 2006). Once there, EGFR still functions as a tyrosine kinase, phosphorylating and stabilizing PCNA, and thus enhancing the proliferative potential of cancer cells (Wang et al. 2006). This could explain the strong correlation between the nuclear localization of EGFR and the highly proliferative status of tissues (Lin et al. 2001). Moreover, radiation-induced EGFR has been proposed to act as a modulator of DNA repair through interaction with DNA-dependent protein kinase (DNA-PK) (Bandyopadhyay et al. 1998; Dittmann et al. 2005). These data suggest that EGFR inhibitors may represent an effective strategy to increase radio-sensitivity of GBM tumors.

Nuclear EGFR has also been defined as a transcriptional co-factor that contains a transactivation domain in its C-terminus. As such, it would be able to modulate several transcriptional targets, mostly implicated in cell cycle progression (cyclin D1, c-Myc) and the nitric oxide pathway (iNOS). Mechanisms of EGFR-mediated gene regulation involve direct interaction of EGFR with other transcription factors like STAT3, STAT5, E2F1 or Src, in a kinase-independent manner (Han and Lo 2012).

5.4.4 Ligand-Independent EGFR Signalling

One of the mechanisms that could justify the activation of the EGFR pathway in GBM is the high expression of receptor ligands reported in certain samples (Schlegel et al. 1990; Ekstrand et al. 1991; Mishima et al. 1998). Moreover, there are evidences of *TGFα* amplification, mainly in recurrent gliomas (Yung et al. 1990). However, glioma cells grown *in vitro* in the presence of its ligand EGF, rapidly lose *EGFR* amplification, and this event leads to the loss of its tumorigenic capacity (Pandita et al. 2004; Talasila et al. 2013; Schulte et al. 2012). This emphasizes the relevance of EGFR over-expression for the progression of GBM *in vivo*. In fact, overexpression on its own could provoke a local accumulation of the kinase domain that would induce its activation in the absence of ligand (Endres et al. 2013). Apparently, this constitutive signalling still depends on EGFR kinase activity and it has been associated with the activation of the transcription factor IRF3. In fact, it seems to be mutually exclusive with the ligand-dependent signals (Chakraborty et al. 2014).

Weihua and coworkers have found that the receptor prevents autophagic cell death by maintaining intracellular glucose levels through interaction and stabilization of the sodium/glucose cotransporter 1 (SGLT1) (Weihua et al. 2008). SGLTs are capable to take up glucose into the tumor cell even against a high chemical gradient and this seems to protect the cells from apoptosis inducers (Ganapathy et al. 2009). In this case, EGFR-SGLT1 interaction does not respond to EGF stimulation or EGFR tyrosine kinase inhibition (Ren et al. 2013). Although there are no reports of SGLT1 expression in GBM, this is one of the cancers with the highest glucose consumption. Therefore, one would expect glioma cells to express significant amounts of glucose transporters, which could be modulated by the over-expression of EGFR (independent of its ligand).

Recent advances have shown that several cellular stresses (UV irradiation, aniso-mycin, cisplatin, TNFα) induce ligand-independent EGFR internalization and endosomal arrest mediated by p38MAPK activation (Tomas et al. 2015). Moreover, other stimuli like hypoxia, oxidative stress and serum starvation activate Src, which potentially stimulates caveolin-mediated internalization of EGFR. The accumula-tion of this inactive EGFR in non-degradative endosomes has been associated with a pro-survival function through the activation of the autophagy-initiating Beclin1 complex (Tan et al. 2015). In addition, many groups have found that inhibitors of EGFR tyrosin kinase activity could induce accumulation of EGFR in endosomes, activating a cytoprotective autophagy mechanism in cancer cells as an innate resis-tance mechanism (Fung et al. 2012; Han et al. 2011; Eimer et al. 2011). Moreover, autophagy inhibitors seem to cooperate with EGFR blockade in GBM (Fung et al. 2012; Han et al. 2011; Eimer et al. 2011).

5.5 Outcomes of Clinical Trials with EGFR Inhibitors in Glioblastoma

Several anti-EGFR-based therapeutic strategies have been assessed in pre-clinical and clinical trials as monotherapy, or in combination with radiotherapy and conven-tional chemotherapy (Fig. 5.4). The most advanced EGFR-based therapies currently used clinically are the small-molecule tyrosine kinase inhibitors (TKIs). Erlotinib and gefitinib are first-generation EGFR inhibitors successfully used in non-small-cell lung cancer. Both drugs are reversible TKIs and have been tested in recurrent GBMs. The EORTC 26034, a randomized phase II trial of erlotinib Vs chemother-apy, included 110 patients, 54 treated with erlotinib and 56 with temozolomide or carmustine (van den Bent et al. 2009). The progression-free survival (PFS) at 6 months was 12% for erlotinib and 24% for the control arm with similar overall sur-vival (OS) in both arms. A phase II clinical trial with 57 recurrent GBMs treated with gefitinib showed similar results: The median PFS was 8 weeks, the PFS at 6 months was 14% and the median OS was 40 weeks (Rich et al. 2004). Other studies with lapatinib (Thiessen et al. 2010) and afatinib (Reardon et al. 2015) have been also negative in in recurrent GBMs.

One of the major issues of the trials with EGFR inhibitors is the fact that these drugs have been tested without any patient selection according to EGFR status. However, the Spanish Group for Research in Neurooncology (GEINO) has evalu-ated erlotinib after selecting patients by their *EGFR* status. In this study erlotinib was tested in recurrent GBM with expression of EGFRvIII and PTEN by immunohistochemistry. The study showed no significant activity with a 20% PFS rate and only one partial response (Gallego et al. 2014). GEINO has carried out a second clinical trial assessing the efficacy and safety of dacomitinib, a second-gen-eration, oral irreversible, pan-HER TKI, in patients with recurrent GBM with *EGFR* amplification. Preclinical data suggested that dacomitinib has an effect on cell viability, self-renewal and proliferation in *EGFR*-amp GBM cells. Moreover, systematic administration of this compound strongly impaired the *in vivo* tumor growth rates in *EGFR*amp xenograft models (Zhu and Shah 2014). The tumour growth inhibition was based on the dephosphorylation of the downstream effectors of EGFR and it was also evident in the presence of EGFR-mutant isoforms (Zahonero et al. 2015). With these preclinical data and, in an attempt to improve the results with first-generation, reversible EGFR inhibitors, the GEINO11 phase II clinical trial evaluated dacomitinib in recurrent *EGFR*amp GBM. However, the 6-month progression free survival was 13% for patients without the EGFRvIII mutation (Fig. 5.5a) and 6.3% for those with the mutation (Fig. 5.5b). The median OS was 7, 3 months for the whole series (Fig. 5.5c) (2015 European Cancer Congress (ECC). Vienna, September 2015. GEINO-11: A Prospective Multicenter, Open Label, Phase II Pilot Clinical Trial To Evaluate Safety And Efficacy Of Dacomitinib, A Pan-her Irreversible Inhibitor, In Patients With Recurrent Glioblastoma With EGFR Amplification With Or Without EGFRvIII Mutation. Sepúlveda JM, et al.). Therefore, despite the preclinical facts, the observed activity with dacomitinib was comparable with that observed for reversible EGFR TKIs in non-molecularly selected recurrent GBMs.

Unconjugated antibodies targeting EGFR such as cetuximab and nimotuzumab have been tested in GBM despite the fact that these drugs do not cross very efficiently the Blood-Brain-Barrier (BBB) (Fig. 5.4). Cetuximab binds the extracellular domain of EGFR and is able to decrease proliferation in subcutaneous and intracraneal

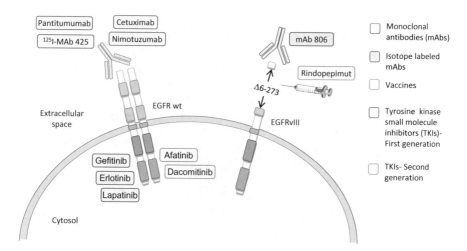

Fig. 5.4 Anti EGFR strategies for GBM therapy. The different approaches aimed at inhibiting EGFR signaling in GBM can be classified in three main groups: (i) anti-EGFR monoclonal antibodies (mAbs) that bind to the extracellular domain of either the wt receptor or the vIII mutant form; (ii) the tyrosine kinase small molecular inhibitors, able to bind the intracellular domain of wt EGFR and the mutant receptor and to block the downstream signaling in a reversible (first generation) or irreversible (second generation) way; (iii) anti-EGFRvIII vaccines designed to develop an immune response against the mutant receptor and the consequent destruction of the GBM cells

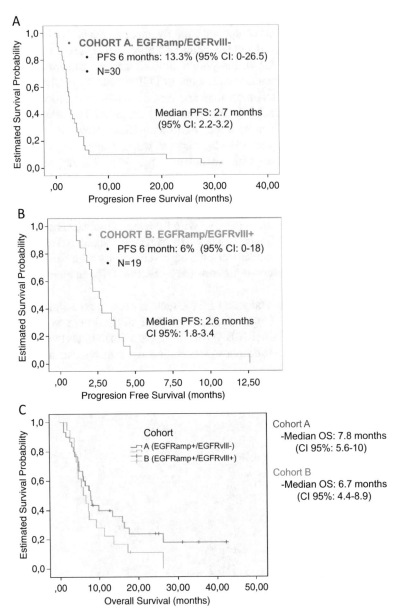

Fig. 5.5 Results of the GEINO11 clinical trial. PFS Kaplan Meier curve for patients with EGFR amplification without (**a**) or with (**b**) EGFRvIII mutation treated with dacomitinib. (**c**) OS Kaplan Meier curve for patients with EGFR amplification, with (Cohort B) or without (Cohort A) EGFRvIII mutation, treated with dacomitinib

mouse xenografts of GBM (Eller et al. 2002). However, a phase II study that tested cetuximab in recurrent GBM patients with and without *EGFR* amplification did not show significant activity since the median overall survival was 5 months (Neyns et al. 2009).

Nimotuzumab is a humanized IgG1 monoclonal antibody that also binds to the extracellular domain of EGFR. It has been approved for brainstem glioma in some countries, based on the results of a phase II clinical trial assessing nimotuzumab in recurrent progressive diffuse intrinsic pontine glioma in 44 paediatric patients. The treatment was well tolerated, with minimal cutaneous toxicity and there were 2 partial responses (PR) and 6 Stable Disease (SD). Median OS was 3, 2 months, confirming only modest activity in this group of patients (Bode et al. 2012). Nimotuzumab has also been assessed in newly diagnosed adult GBM patients in a phase III trial conducted in Germany. In this study 149 patients were randomized to receive the Stupp regimen with or without nimotuzumab, concurrent with radiotherapy. The OS was around 20 months in both arms but in a post-hoc analysis there were a benefit in OS for those patients with non-methylated *MGMT* (O6-methylguanine–DNA methyltransferase) and EGFR-positive GBMs (Westphal et al. 2015).

Despite the lack of effectiveness of anti-EGFR targeting by antibodies or TKIs, other strategies based on immune-mediated therapies are being tested in clinical trials with strong preclinical data. Rindopepimut is a peptide-based vaccine against EGFRvIII that has been assessed in several phase I, II and III clinical trials in EGFRvIII-positive glioma patients (Fig. 5.4). The in-frame deletion of *EGFRvIII* generates a novel antigen that could be exploited to generate a strong immune response against the tumour cells. However, despite promising results from the phase II trials (Gatson et al. 2016), the ACT-IV study, a phase III clinical trial in newly diagnosed GBM with EGFRvIII mutation, has not found a survival benefit in those patients treated with rindopepimut. The results has not been published yet so that it is not possible to discuss if any subgroup of patients has a benefit (http://www.celldex.com/pipeline/ rindopepimut.php).

Other strategies targeting EGFR using toxins or radioisotopes are under development in clinical trials. ^{125}I–MAb 425 is a radiolabelled conjugated antibody that has been assessed in a randomized phase II clinical trial in newly-diagnosed GBM with a median survival of 20 months for the combination arm (TMZ plus ^{125}I–MAb 425) Vs 14, 6 months for those patients treated with ^{125}I–MAb 425 in monotherapy (Li et al. 2010).

5.6 Reasons for Therapeutic Failure

TKIs are ATP competitors that have been active in non-small cell lung cancer patients carrying EGFR mutations. The high prevalence of *EGFR* amplification in GBM had made this receptor an excellent target so the failure of TKIs in these tumors was somehow unexpected. Drug-delivery limitations due to the presence of the BBB or to the use of antiepileptic drugs in most GBM clinical trials, could explain the lack of success of these compounds. Moreover, tumour heterogeneity, insufficient target inhibition and activation of resistance mechanisms have been argued by several authors (Reardon et al. 2014; Hegi et al. 2012; Karpel-Massler et al. 2009). On top of that, it has been suggested that the point mutations present in lung, but not in brain tumors, could render the first ones more sensitive to TKIs (Vivanco et al. 2012; Barkovich et al. 2012).

Based on the non-canonical mechanisms of EGFR function (Fig. 5.3), other possible explanation for the lack of TKI effectiveness would be the relevance of kinase-independent functions of the receptor. In fact, Hegi et al. analysed 22 GBM patients operated after treatment failure with gefinib. Resected tumours exhibited high concentrations of the drug and showed that EGFR was dephosphorylated. However, no effect on the EGFR downstream pathway was found. This study showed that EGFR pathway in GBM seems to be dominated by regulatory circuits independent of EGFR phosphorylation (Hegi et al. 2011). As we have reviewed here, EGFR can promote transcriptional activation of genes associated with cell growth in a kinase-independent manner. Moreover, many of the survival and antiapoptotic functions of endosomal and mitochondrial EGFR do not require kinase activity. Therefore, targeting EGFR stability could be an attractive alternative to EGFR inhibitors, either by direct downregulation with siRNA strategies (Kang et al. 2006; Mazzoleni et al. 2010; Verreault et al. 2013), or by targeting one of the modulators of EGFR turnover (Zahonero and Sanchez-Gomez 2014). Moreover, the constitutive presence of EGFR in the nuclei may be beneficial to the tumors that encounter EGFR-targeted antibodies and TKIs. In fact, cancer cells that have acquired resistance to cetuximab (Li et al. 2009) or gefitinib (Huang et al. 2011) accumulate more nuclear EGFR. These observations provide a rationale for the combined use of inhibitors of this receptor with molecules that could block EGFR nuclear translocation or for the use of inhibitors that affect both processes.

Regarding heterogeneity, recent technological innovations have allowed the analysis of cancer genetics to be conducted on the single-cell level. In fact, Patel et al. profiled 430 cells from 5 GBMs and found that individual cells could be classified as different types of GBM according to the TCGA classification scheme (Patel et al. 2014). Tumor heterogeneity may be the reason of the lack of efficacy of targeted therapies in GBM as the treatment would be only active in a group of the tumour cells. Additionally, other studies have confirmed the observation of heterogeneous amplification EGFR and other receptors with tyrosin kinase activity in GBM, hindering the efficacy of these targeted therapies (Snuderl et al. 2011; Szerlip et al. 2012; Chakravarti et al. 2002). Activation of resistance could be derived from the expansion of clones without *EGFR* amplification but also to a redundancy in activation of PI3K/AKT due to the stimulation of tyrosine kinases upstream such as MET, PDGFR (Platelet Derived Growth Factor Receptor), or IGFR (Insulin Growth Factor Receptor) (Chakravarti et al. 2002; Stommel et al. 2007). Additionally, the loss of PTEN, with or without the activation of other ErbB receptors, could make EGFR signaling dispensable for tumour growth and proliferation (Mellinghoff et al. 2005).

Although EGFR inhibition for NSCLC has been active, EGFR point mutations have been found as drivers of treatment resistance. These mutations are detected in relapse tumour tissue and also in circulating DNA (Piotrowska et al. 2015). TKI point mutations following EGFR therapy have not been found in GBM patients, but it can be theorized that a selective pressure from anti-EGFR drugs may produce the growth and expansion of EGFR-resistance clones.

5.7 Future Direction in Clinical Research: Ongoing Clinical Trials Targeting EGFR in GBM

Amplification of *EGFR* and expression of EGFRvIII could be utilized for immunotherapies. As it was reviewed above, rindopepimut, an EGFRvIII-specific peptide conjugated with immunogenic proteins, has been the first drug with promising results in phase II trials. However, it has not been confirmed in phase III studies. Another strategy with an immune-mediated therapy is production of chimeric antigen receptor T cells (CART), which are T lymphocytes genetically modified to recognize and bind cells expressing EGFRvIII. Clinical trials with CART have shown positive results in leukemia and lymphoma and they are now being assessed in other malignancies, including GBM (Ramos et al. 2016).

Other strategies targeting EGFR include conjugate antibodies that combine an anti-EGFR antibody with cytotoxins enabling tumour cell injury. Their objective is not to inhibit EGFR signaling, but to use EGFR as a target for toxin release. ABT414 is an antibody-directed against EGFR combined with a cytotoxic agent (MMAF, Monomethyl Auristatin F) with encouraging preclinical results. Nowadays it is being investigated in large randomized clinical trials both in newly diagnosed and recurrent GBM (Phillips et al. 2016). AMG595 and MR1–1 are other conjugates targeting EGFRvIII that are under investigation in early clinical trials.

There are also therapies targeting EGFR under preclinical investigation such as gene silencing by RNA interference, drugs conjugates with diphtheria toxin and oncolytic viruses that use EGFR as the binding protein on the target malignant cells. Very promising is the use of bivalent recombinant immunotoxins such as mAb806 that combines a high specific antibody against EGFR and EGFRvIII with a diphtheria toxin fragment (Fig. 5.4). The first preclinical studies have shown a significant efficacy of the drug in tumour xenografts (Meng et al. 2015).

5.8 Concluding Remarks

The inhibition of EGFR-driven signalling network is a treatment strategy with strong rationale in GBM. However, this approach has been ineffective to date and tumour heterogeneity has been proposed as the main reason for the failure of EGFR targeted therapies. Resistance to EGFR inhibitors is caused by complex mechanisms that could trigger compensatory pathways such as PDGFR/mTOR/AKT. Those molecules could be also pharmacologically hindered, although combination of TKIs has not been properly explored yet in GBM. Moreover, compelling evidence links EGFR with the regulation of cell cycle and survival by non-canonical signaling at different cellular locations. Therefore, targeting receptor stability and/or translocation could be more effective than the use of kinase inhibitors. Furthermore, EGFR and its mutants could be used not just as targets to be inhibited but as markers for activated immune cells or antibodies linked to toxins or viruses. Hopefully, these new approaches will reach satisfactory clinical results, at least for a subset of patients with this terrible disease.

References

Aldape, K., G. Zadeh, S. Mansouri, G. Reifenberger, and A. von Deimling. 2015. Glioblastoma: Pathology, molecular mechanisms and markers. *Acta Neuropathologica* 129: 829–848.

Bachoo, R.M., E.A. Maher, K.L. Ligon, N.E. Sharpless, S.S. Chan, M.J. You, Y. Tang, J. DeFrances, E. Stover, R. Weissleder, D.H. Rowitch, D.N. Louis, and R.A. DePinho. 2002. Epidermal growth factor receptor and Ink4a/Arf: Convergent mechanisms governing terminal differentiation and transformation along the neural stem cell to astrocyte axis. *Cancer Cell* 1: 269–277.

Bai, D., L. Ueno, and P.K. Vogt. 2009. Akt-mediated regulation of NFkappaB and the essentialness of NFkappaB for the oncogenicity of PI3K and Akt. *International Journal of Cancer* 125: 2863–2870.

Bandyopadhyay, D., M. Mandal, L. Adam, J. Mendelsohn, and R. Kumar. 1998. Physical interaction between epidermal growth factor receptor and DNA-dependent protein kinase in mammalian cells. *The Journal of Biological Chemistry* 273: 1568–1573.

Barker, F.G., M.L. Simmons, S.M. Chang, M.D. Prados, D.A. Larson, P.K. Sneed, W.M. Wara, M.S. Berger, P. Chen, M.A. Israel, and K.D. Aldape. 2001. EGFR overexpression and radiation response in glioblastoma multiforme. *International Journal of Radiation Oncology, Biology, Physics* 51: 410–418.

Batra, S.K., S. Castelino-Prabhu, C.J. Wikstrand, X. Zhu, P.A. Humphrey, H.S. Friedman, and D.D. Bigner. 1995. Epidermal growth factor ligand-independent, unregulated, cell-transforming potential of a naturally occurring human mutant EGFRvIII gene. *Cell Growth & Differentiation* 6: 1251–1259.

Barkovich, K.J., S. Hariono, A.L. Garske, J. Zhang, J.A. Blair, Q.W. Fan, K.M. Shokat, T. Nicolaides, and W.A. Weiss. 2012. Kinetics of inhibitor cycling underlie therapeutic disparities between EGFR-driven lung and brain cancers. *Cancer Discovery* 2 (5): 450–457.

Bishayee, S. 2000. Role of conformational alteration in the epidermal growth factor receptor (EGFR) function. *Biochemical Pharmacology* 60: 1217–1223.

Bode, U., M. Massimino, F. Bach, M. Zimmermann, E. Khuhlaeva, M. Westphal, and G. Fleischhack. 2012. Nimotuzumab treatment of malignant gliomas. *Expert Opinion on Biological Therapy* 12: 1649–1659.

Boerner, J.L., M.L. Demory, C. Silva, and S.J. Parsons. 2004. Phosphorylation of Y845 on the epidermal growth factor receptor mediates binding to the mitochondrial protein cytochrome c oxidase subunit II. *Molecular and Cellular Biology* 24: 7059–7071.

Bouras, A., M. Kaluzova, and C.G. Hadjipanayis. 2015. Radiosensitivity enhancement of radioresistant glioblastoma by epidermal growth factor receptor antibody-conjugated iron-oxide nanoparticles. *Journal of Neuro-Oncology* 124: 13–22.

Brantley, E.C., and E.N. Benveniste. 2008. Signal transducer and activator of transcription-3: A molecular hub for signaling pathways in gliomas. Mol. *Cancer Research* 6: 675–684.

Bredel, M., D.M. Scholtens, A.K. Yadav, A.A. Alvarez, J.J. Renfrow, J.P. Chandler, I.L. Yu, M.S. Carro, F. Dai, M.J. Tagge, R. Ferrarese, C. Bredel, H.S. Phillips, P.J. Lukac, P.A. Robe, A. Weyerbrock, H. Vogel, S. Dubner, B. Mobley, X. He, A.C. Scheck, B.I. Sikic, K.D. Aldape, A. Chakravarti, and G.R. Harsh. 2011. NFKBIA deletion in glioblastomas. *The New England Journal of Medicine* 364: 627–637.

Brennan, C.W., R.G. Verhaak, A. McKenna, B. Campos, H. Noushmehr, S.R. Salama, S. Zheng, D. Chakravarty, J.Z. Sanborn, S.H. Berman, R. Beroukhim, B. Bernard, C.J. Wu, G. Genovese, I. Shmulevich, J. Barnholtz-Sloan, L. Zou, R. Vegesna, S.A. Shukla, G. Ciriello, W.K. Yung, W. Zhang, C. Sougnez, T. Mikkelsen, K. Aldape, D.D. Bigner, E.G. Van Meir, M. Prados, A. Sloan, K.L. Black, J. Eschbacher, G. Finocchiaro, W. Friedman, D.W. Andrews, A. Guha, M. Iacocca, B.P. O'Neill, G. Foltz, J. Myers, D.J. Weisenberger, R. Penny, R. Kucherlapati, C.M. Perou, D.N. Hayes, R. Gibbs, M. Marra, G.B. Mills, E. Lander, P. Spellman, R. Wilson, C. Sander, J. Weinstein, M. Meyerson, S. Gabriel, P.W. Laird, D. Haussler, G. Getz, and L. Chin. 2013. The somatic genomic landscape of glioblastoma. *Cell* 155: 462–477.

Cao, X., H. Zhu, F. Ali-Osman, and H.W. Lo. 2011. EGFR and EGFRvIII undergo stress- and EGFR kinase inhibitor-induced mitochondrial translocalization: A potential mechanism of EGFR-driven antagonism of apoptosis. *Molecular Cancer* 10: 26.

Chakraborty, S., L. Li, V.T. Puliyappadamba, G. Guo, K.J. Hatanpaa, B. Mickey, R.F. Souza, P. Vo, J. Herz, M.R. Chen, D.A. Boothman, T.K. Pandita, D.H. Wang, G.C. Sen, and A.A. Habib. 2014. Constitutive and ligand-induced EGFR signalling triggers distinct and mutually exclusive downstream signalling networks. *Nature Communications* 5: 5811.

Chakravarti, A., J.S. Loeffler, and N.J. Dyson. 2002. Insulin-like growth factor receptor I mediates resistance to anti-epidermal growth factor receptor therapy in primary human glioblastoma cells through continued activation of phosphoinositide 3-kinase signaling. *Cancer Research* 62: 200–207.

Chua, C.Y., Y. Li, K.J. Granberg, L. Hu, H. Haapasalo, M.J. Annala, D.E. Cogdell, M. Verploegen, L.M. Moore, G.N. Fuller, M. Nykter, W.K. Cavenee, and W. Zhang. 2016. IGFBP2 potentiates nuclear EGFR-STAT3 signaling. *Oncogene* 35: 738–747.

Citri, A., and Y. Yarden. 2006. EGF-ERBB signalling: Towards the systems level. *Nature Reviews. Molecular Cell Biology* 7: 505–516.

de la Iglesia, N., G. Konopka, S.V. Puram, J.A. Chan, R.M. Bachoo, M.J. You, D.E. Levy, R.A. DePinho, and A. Bonni. 2008. Identification of a PTEN-regulated STAT3 brain tumor suppressor pathway. *Genes & Development* 22: 449–462.

Demory, M.L., J.L. Boerner, R. Davidson, W. Faust, T. Miyake, I. Lee, M. Huttemann, R. Douglas, G. Haddad, and S.J. Parsons. 2009. Epidermal growth factor receptor translocation to the mitochondria: Regulation and effect. *The Journal of Biological Chemistry* 284: 36592–36604.

Dittmann, K., C. Mayer, B. Fehrenbacher, M. Schaller, U. Raju, L. Milas, D.J. Chen, R. Kehlbach, and H.P. Rodemann. 2005. Radiation-induced epidermal growth factor receptor nuclear import is linked to activation of DNA-dependent protein kinase. *The Journal of Biological Chemistry* 280: 31182–31189.

Egan, J.E., A.B. Hall, B.A. Yatsula, and D. Bar-Sagi. 2002. The bimodal regulation of epidermal growth factor signaling by human Sprouty proteins. *Proceedings of the National Academy of Sciences of the United States of America* 99: 6041–6046.

Eimer, S., M.A. Belaud-Rotureau, K. Airiau, M. Jeanneteau, E. Laharanne, N. Veron, A. Vital, H. Loiseau, J.P. Merlio, and F. Belloc. 2011. Autophagy inhibition cooperates with erlotinib to induce glioblastoma cell death. *Cancer Biology & Therapy* 11: 1017–1027.

Ekstrand, A.J., C.D. James, W.K. Cavenee, B. Seliger, R.F. Pettersson, and V.P. Collins. 1991. Genes for epidermal growth factor receptor, transforming growth factor alpha, and epidermal growth factor and their expression in human gliomas in vivo. *Cancer Research* 51: 2164–2172.

Eller, J.L., S.L. Longo, D.J. Hicklin, and G.W. Canute. 2002. Activity of anti-epidermal growth factor receptor monoclonal antibody C225 against glioblastoma multiforme. *Neurosurgery* 51: 1005–1013.

Endres, N.F., K. Engel, R. Das, E. Kovacs, and J. Kuriyan. 2011. Regulation of the catalytic activity of the EGF receptor. *Current Opinion in Structural Biology* 21: 777–784.

Endres, N.F., R. Das, A.W. Smith, A. Arkhipov, E. Kovacs, Y. Huang, J.G. Pelton, Y. Shan, D.E. Shaw, D.E. Wemmer, J.T. Groves, and J. Kuriyan. 2013. Conformational coupling across the plasma membrane in activation of the EGF receptor. *Cell* 152: 543–556.

Francis, J.M., C.Z. Zhang, C.L. Maire, J. Jung, V.E. Manzo, V.A. Adalsteinsson, H. Homer, S. Haidar, B. Blumenstiel, C.S. Pedamallu, A.H. Ligon, J.C. Love, M. Meyerson, and K.L. Ligon. 2014. EGFR variant heterogeneity in glioblastoma resolved through single-nucleus sequencing. *Cancer Discovery* 4: 956–971.

Frattini, V., V. Trifonov, J.M. Chan, A. Castano, M. Lia, F. Abate, S.T. Keir, A.X. Ji, P. Zoppoli, F. Niola, C. Danussi, I. Dolgalev, P. Porrati, S. Pellegatta, A. Heguy, G. Gupta, D.J. Pisapia, P. Canoll, J.N. Bruce, R.E. McLendon, H. Yan, K. Aldape, G. Finocchiaro, T. Mikkelsen, G.G. Prive, D.D. Bigner, A. Lasorella, R. Rabadan, and A. Iavarone. 2013. The integrated landscape of driver genomic alterations in glioblastoma. *Nature Genetics* 45: 1141–1149.

Frederick, L., X.Y. Wang, G. Eley, and C.D. James. 2000. Diversity and frequency of epidermal growth factor receptor mutations in human glioblastomas. *Cancer Research* 60: 1383–1387.

Fung, C., X. Chen, J.R. Grandis, and U. Duvvuri. 2012. EGFR tyrosine kinase inhibition induces autophagy in cancer cells. *Cancer Biology & Therapy* 13: 1417–1424.

Furgason, J.M., W. Li, B. Milholland, E. Cross, Y. Li, C.M. McPherson, R.E. Warnick, O. Rixe, P.J. Stambrook, J. Vijg, and E.M. Bahassi. 2014. Whole genome sequencing of glioblastoma multiforme identifies multiple structural variations involved in EGFR activation. *Mutagenesis* 29: 341–350.

Gallego, O., M. Cuatrecasas, M. Benavides, P.P. Segura, A. Berrocal, N. Erill, A. Colomer, M.J. Quintana, C. Balana, M. Gil, A. Gallardo, P. Murata, and A. Barnadas. 2014. Efficacy of erlotinib in patients with relapsed gliobastoma multiforme who expressed EGFRVIII and PTEN determined by immunohistochemistry. *Journal of Neuro-Oncology* 116: 413–419.

Ganapathy, V., M. Thangaraju, and P.D. Prasad. 2009. Nutrient transporters in cancer: Relevance to Warburg hypothesis and beyond. *Pharmacology & Therapeutics* 121: 29–40.

Gatson, N.T., S.P. Weathers, and J.F. de Groot. 2016. ReACT Phase II trial: a critical evaluation of the use of rindopepimut plus bevacizumab to treat EGFRvIII-positive recurrent glioblastoma. *CNS Oncology* 5: 11–26.

Guha, A., M.M. Feldkamp, N. Lau, G. Boss, and A. Pawson. 1997. Proliferation of human malignant astrocytomas is dependent on Ras activation. *Oncogene* 15: 2755–2765.

Gur, G., C. Rubin, M. Katz, I. Amit, A. Citri, J. Nilsson, N. Amariglio, R. Henriksson, G. Rechavi, H. Hedman, R. Wides, and Y. Yarden. 2004. LRIG1 restricts growth factor signaling by enhancing receptor ubiquitylation and degradation. *The EMBO Journal* 23: 3270–3281.

Haas-Kogan, D.A., M.D. Prados, T. Tihan, D.A. Eberhard, N. Jelluma, N.D. Arvold, R. Baumber, K.R. Lamborn, A. Kapadia, M. Malec, M.S. Berger, and D. Stokoe. 2005. Epidermal growth factor receptor, protein kinase B/Akt, and glioma response to erlotinib. *Journal of the National Cancer Institute* 97: 880–887.

Han, W., and H.W. Lo. 2012. Landscape of EGFR signaling network in human cancers: Biology and therapeutic response in relation to receptor subcellular locations. *Cancer Letters* 318 (2): 124–134.

Han, W., H. Pan, Y. Chen, J. Sun, Y. Wang, J. Li, W. Ge, L. Feng, X. Lin, X. Wang, X. Wang, and H. Jin. 2011. EGFR tyrosine kinase inhibitors activate autophagy as a cytoprotective response in human lung cancer cells. *PLoS One* 6: e18691.

Hatanpaa, K.J., S. Burma, D. Zhao, and A.A. Habib. 2010. Epidermal growth factor receptor in glioma: Signal transduction, neuropathology, imaging, and radioresistance. *Neoplasia* 12: 675–684.

Hegi, M.E., A.C. Diserens, P. Bady, Y. Kamoshima, M.C. Kouwenhoven, M. Delorenzi, W.L. Lambiv, M.F. Hamou, M.S. Matter, A. Koch, F.L. Heppner, Y. Yonekawa, A. Merlo, K. Frei, L. Mariani, and S. Hofer. 2011. Pathway analysis of glioblastoma tissue after preoperative treatment with the EGFR tyrosine kinase inhibitor gefitinib – A phase II trial. *Molecular Cancer Therapeutics* 10: 1102–1112.

Hegi, M.E., P. Rajakannu, and M. Weller. 2012. Epidermal growth factor receptor: A re-emerging target in glioblastoma. *Current Opinion in Neurology* 25: 774–779.

Holland, E.C., W.P. Hively, V. Gallo, and H.E. Varmus. 1998. Modeling mutations in the G1 arrest pathway in human gliomas: Overexpression of CDK4 but not loss of INK4a-ARF induces hyperploidy in cultured mouse astrocytes. *Genes & Development* 12: 3644–3649.

Hsu, S.C., and M.C. Hung. 2007. Characterization of a novel tripartite nuclear localization sequence in the EGFR family. *The Journal of Biological Chemistry* 282: 10432–10440.

Huang, W.C., Y.J. Chen, L.Y. Li, Y.L. Wei, S.C. Hsu, S.L. Tsai, P.C. Chiu, W.P. Huang, Y.N. Wang, C.H. Chen, W.C. Chang, W.C. Chang, A.J. Chen, C.H. Tsai, and M.C. Hung. 2011. Nuclear translocation of epidermal growth factor receptor by Akt-dependent phosphorylation enhances breast cancer-resistant protein expression in gefitinib-resistant cells. *The Journal of Biological Chemistry* 286: 20558–20568.

Huse, J.T., and E.C. Holland. 2009. Genetically engineered mouse models of brain cancer and the promise of preclinical testing. *Brain Pathology* 19: 132–143.

Johansson, M., A. Oudin, K. Tiemann, A. Bernard, A. Golebiewska, O. Keunen, F. Fack, D. Stieber, B. Wang, H. Hedman, and S.P. Niclou. 2013. The soluble form of the tumor suppressor Lrig1 potently inhibits in vivo glioma growth irrespective of EGF receptor status. *Neuro-Oncology* 15: 1200–1211.

Kang, C.S., Z.Y. Zhang, Z.F. Jia, G.X. Wang, M.Z. Qiu, H.X. Zhou, S.Z. Yu, J. Chang, H. Jiang, and P.Y. Pu. 2006. Suppression of EGFR expression by antisense or small interference RNA inhibits U251 glioma cell growth in vitro and in vivo. *Cancer Gene Therapy* 13: 530–538.

Karpel-Massler, G., U. Schmidt, A. Unterberg, and M.E. Halatsch. 2009. Therapeutic inhibition of the epidermal growth factor receptor in high-grade gliomas: Where do we stand? Mol. *Cancer Research* 7: 1000–1012.

Laederich, M.B., M. Funes-Duran, L. Yen, E. Ingalla, X. Wu, K.L. Carraway III, and C. Sweeney. 2004. The leucine-rich repeat protein LRIG1 is a negative regulator of ErbB family receptor tyrosine kinases. *The Journal of Biological Chemistry* 279: 47050–47056.

Lal, A., C.A. Glazer, H.M. Martinson, H.S. Friedman, G.E. Archer, J.H. Sampson, and G.J. Riggins. 2002. Mutant epidermal growth factor receptor up-regulates molecular effectors of tumor invasion. *Cancer Research* 62: 3335–3339.

Lee, J.C., I. Vivanco, R. Beroukhim, J.H. Huang, W.L. Feng, R.M. DeBiasi, K. Yoshimoto, J.C. King, P. Nghiemphu, Y. Yuza, Q. Xu, H. Greulich, R.K. Thomas, J.G. Paez, T.C. Peck, D.J. Linhart, K.A. Glatt, G. Getz, R. Onofrio, L. Ziaugra, R.L. Levine, S. Gabriel, T. Kawaguchi, K. O'Neill, H. Khan, L.M. Liau, S.F. Nelson, P.N. Rao, P. Mischel, R.O. Pieper, T. Cloughesy, D.J. Leahy, W.R. Sellers, C.L. Sawyers, M. Meyerson, and I.K. Mellinghoff. 2006. Epidermal growth factor receptor activation in glioblastoma through novel missense mutations in the extracellular domain. *PLoS Medicine* 3: e485.

Leuraud, P., L. Taillandier, J. Medioni, L. Aguirre-Cruz, E. Criniere, Y. Marie, M. Kujas, J.L. Golmard, A. Duprez, J.Y. Delattre, M. Sanson, and M.F. Poupon. 2004. Distinct responses of xenografted gliomas to different alkylating agents are related to histology and genetic alterations. *Cancer Research* 64: 4648–4653.

Li, C., M. Iida, E.F. Dunn, A.J. Ghia, and D.L. Wheeler. 2009. Nuclear EGFR contributes to acquired resistance to cetuximab. *Oncogene* 28: 3801–3813.

Li, L., T.S. Quang, E.J. Gracely, J.H. Kim, J.G. Emrich, T.E. Yaeger, J.M. Jenrette, S.C. Cohen, P. Black, and L.W. Brady. 2010. A Phase II study of anti-epidermal growth factor receptor radioimmunotherapy in the treatment of glioblastoma multiforme. *Journal of Neurosurgery* 113: 192–198.

Lin, S.Y., K. Makino, W. Xia, A. Matin, Y. Wen, K.Y. Kwong, L. Bourguignon, and M.C. Hung. 2001. Nuclear localization of EGF receptor and its potential new role as a transcription factor. *Nature Cell Biology* 3: 802–808.

Lo, H.W., M. Ali-Seyed, Y. Wu, G. Bartholomeusz, S.C. Hsu, and M.C. Hung. 2006. Nuclear-cytoplasmic transport of EGFR involves receptor endocytosis, importin beta1 and CRM1. *Journal of Cellular Biochemistry* 98: 1570–1583.

Lo, H.W., X. Cao, H. Zhu, and F. Ali-Osman. 2010. Cyclooxygenase-2 is a novel transcriptional target of the nuclear EGFR-STAT3 and EGFRvIII-STAT3 signaling axes. Mol. *Cancer Research* 8: 232–245.

Masui, K., P.S. Mischel, and G. Reifenberger. 2016. Molecular classification of gliomas. *Handbook of Clinical Neurology* 134: 97–120.

Mazzoleni, S., L.S. Politi, M. Pala, M. Cominelli, A. Franzin, S.L. Sergi, A. Falini, M. De Palma, A. Bulfone, P.L. Poliani, and R. Galli. 2010. Epidermal growth factor receptor expression identifies functionally and molecularly distinct tumor-initiating cells in human glioblastoma multiforme and is required for gliomagenesis. *Cancer Research* 70: 7500–7513.

Mellinghoff, I.K., M.Y. Wang, I. Vivanco, D.A. Haas-Kogan, S. Zhu, E.Q. Dia, K.V. Lu, K. Yoshimoto, J.H. Huang, D.J. Chute, B.L. Riggs, S. Horvath, L.M. Liau, W.K. Cavenee, P.N. Rao, R. Beroukhim, T.C. Peck, J.C. Lee, W.R. Sellers, D. Stokoe, M. Prados, T.F. Cloughesy, C.L. Sawyers, and P.S. Mischel. 2005. Molecular determinants of the response of glioblastomas to EGFR kinase inhibitors. *The New England Journal of Medicine* 353: 2012–2024.

Mellman, I., and Y. Yarden. 2013. Endocytosis and cancer. *Cold Spring Harbor Perspectives in Biology* 5: a016949.

Meng, J., Y. Liu, S. Gao, S. Lin, X. Gu, M.G. Pomper, P.C. Wang, and L. Shan. 2015. A bivalent recombinant immunotoxin with high potency against tumors with EGFR and EGFRvIII expression. *Cancer Biology & Therapy* 16: 1764–1774.

Mishima, K., S. Higashiyama, A. Asai, K. Yamaoka, Y. Nagashima, N. Taniguchi, C. Kitanaka, T. Kirino, and Y. Kuchino. 1998. Heparin-binding epidermal growth factor-like growth factor stimulates mitogenic signaling and is highly expressed in human malignant gliomas. *Acta Neuropathologica* 96: 322–328.

Mizoguchi, M., C.L. Nutt, and D.N. Louis. 2004. Mutation analysis of CBL-C and SPRED3 on 19q in human glioblastoma. *Neurogenetics* 5: 81–82.

Munoz, J.L., V. Rodriguez-Cruz, S.J. Greco, V. Nagula, K.W. Scotto, and P. Rameshwar. 2014. Temozolomide induces the production of epidermal growth factor to regulate MDR1 expression in glioblastoma cells. *Molecular Cancer Therapeutics* 13: 2399–2411.

Nagane, M., A. Levitzki, A. Gazit, W.K. Cavenee, and H.J. Huang. 1998. Drug resistance of human glioblastoma cells conferred by a tumor-specific mutant epidermal growth factor receptor through modulation of Bcl-XL and caspase-3-like proteases. *Proceedings of the National Academy of Sciences of the United States of America* 95: 5724–5729.

Neyns, B., J. Sadones, E. Joosens, F. Bouttens, L. Verbeke, J.F. Baurain, L. D'Hondt, T. Strauven, C. Chaskis, V.P. In't, A. Michotte, and J. De Greve. 2009. Stratified phase II trial of cetuximab in patients with recurrent high-grade glioma. *Annals of Oncology* 20: 1596–1603.

Nicholas, M.K., R.V. Lukas, N.F. Jafri, L. Faoro, and R. Salgia. 2006. Epidermal growth factor receptor – Mediated signal transduction in the development and therapy of gliomas. *Clinical Cancer Research* 12: 7261–7270.

Nogueira, L., P. Ruiz-Ontanon, A. Vazquez-Barquero, F. Moris, and J.L. Fernandez-Luna. 2011. The NFkappaB pathway: A therapeutic target in glioblastoma. *Oncotarget* 2: 646–653.

Ohgaki, H., and P. Kleihues. 2013. The definition of primary and secondary glioblastoma. *Clinical Cancer Research* 19: 764–772.

Pandita, A., K.D. Aldape, G. Zadeh, A. Guha, and C.D. James. 2004. Contrasting in vivo and in vitro fates of glioblastoma cell subpopulations with amplified EGFR. *Genes, Chromosomes & Cancer* 39: 29–36.

Patel, A.P., I. Tirosh, J.J. Trombetta, A.K. Shalek, S.M. Gillespie, H. Wakimoto, D.P. Cahill, B.V. Nahed, W.T. Curry, R.L. Martuza, D.N. Louis, O. Rozenblatt-Rosen, M.L. Suva, A. Regev, and B.E. Bernstein. 2014. Single-cell RNA-seq highlights intratumoral heterogeneity in primary glioblastoma. *Science* 344: 1396–1401.

Phillips, A.C., E.R. Boghaert, K.S. Vaidya, M.J. Mitten, S. Norvell, H.D. Falls, P.J. DeVries, D. Cheng, J.A. Meulbroek, F.G. Buchanan, L.M. McKay, N.C. Goodwin, and E.B. Reilly. 2016. ABT-414, an antibody-drug conjugate targeting a tumor-selective EGFR epitope. *Molecular Cancer Therapeutics* 15: 661–669.

Pines, G., W.J. Kostler, and Y. Yarden. 2010. Oncogenic mutant forms of EGFR: Lessons in signal transduction and targets for cancer therapy. *FEBS Letters* 584: 2699–2706.

Piotrowska, Z., M.J. Niederst, C.A. Karlovich, H.A. Wakelee, J.W. Neal, M. Mino-Kenudson, L. Fulton, A.N. Hata, E.L. Lockerman, A. Kalsy, S. Digumarthy, A. Muzikansky, M. Raponi,

A.R. Garcia, H.E. Mulvey, M.K. Parks, R.H. DiCecca, D. Dias-Santagata, A.J. Iafrate, A.T. Shaw, A.R. Allen, J.A. Engelman, and L.V. Sequist. 2015. Heterogeneity underlies the emergence of EGFRT790 wild-type clones following treatment of T790M-positive cancers with a third-generation EGFR inhibitor. *Cancer Discovery* 5: 713–722.

Pozo, N., C. Zahonero, P. Fernandez, J.M. Linares, A. Ayuso, M. Hagiwara, A. Perez, J.R. Ricoy, A. Hernandez-Lain, J.M. Sepulveda, and P. Sanchez-Gomez. 2013. Inhibition of DYRK1A destabilizes EGFR and reduces EGFR-dependent glioblastoma growth. *The Journal of Clinical Investigation* 123: 2475–2487.

Ramos, C.A., B. Savoldo, V. Torrano, B. Ballard, H. Zhang, O. Dakhova, E. Liu, G. Carrum, R.T. Kamble, A.P. Gee, Z. Mei, M.F. Wu, H. Liu, B. Grilley, C.M. Rooney, M.K. Brenner, H.E. Heslop, and G. Dotti. 2016. Clinical responses with T lymphocytes targeting malignancy-associated kappa light chains. *The Journal of Clinical Investigation* 126: 2588–2596.

Reardon, D.A., P.Y. Wen, and I.K. Mellinghoff. 2014. Targeted molecular therapies against epidermal growth factor receptor: Past experiences and challenges. *Neuro-Oncology* 16 Suppl 8: viii7–vii13.

Reardon, D.A., L.B. Nabors, W.P. Mason, J.R. Perry, W. Shapiro, P. Kavan, D. Mathieu, S. Phuphanich, A. Cseh, Y. Fu, J. Cong, S. Wind, and D.D. Eisenstat. 2015. Phase I/randomized phase II study of afatinib, an irreversible ErbB family blocker, with or without protracted temozolomide in adults with recurrent glioblastoma. *Neuro-Oncology* 17: 430–439.

Ren, J., L.R. Bollu, F. Su, G. Gao, L. Xu, W.C. Huang, M.C. Hung, and Z. Weihua. 2013. EGFR-SGLT1 interaction does not respond to EGFR modulators, but inhibition of SGLT1 sensitizes prostate cancer cells to EGFR tyrosine kinase inhibitors. *Prostate* 73: 1453–1461.

Rich, J.N., D.A. Reardon, T. Peery, J.M. Dowell, J.A. Quinn, K.L. Penne, C.J. Wikstrand, L.B. Van Duyn, J.E. Dancey, R.E. McLendon, J.C. Kao, T.T. Stenzel, B.K. Ahmed Rasheed, S.E. Tourt-Uhlig, J.E. Herndon, J.J. Vredenburgh, J.H. Sampson, A.H. Friedman, D.D. Bigner, and H.S. Friedman. 2004. Phase II trial of gefitinib in recurrent glioblastoma. *Journal of Clinical Oncology* 22: 133–142.

Rubin, C., V. Litvak, H. Medvedovsky, Y. Zwang, S. Lev, and Y. Yarden. 2003. Sprouty fine-tunes EGF signaling through interlinked positive and negative feedback loops. *Current Biology* 13: 297–307.

Schlegel, U., P.L. Moots, M.K. Rosenblum, H.T. Thaler, and H.M. Furneaux. 1990. Expression of transforming growth factor alpha in human gliomas. *Oncogene* 5: 1839–1842.

Schulte, A., H.S. Gunther, T. Martens, S. Zapf, S. Riethdorf, C. Wulfing, M. Stoupiec, M. Westphal, and K. Lamszus. 2012. Glioblastoma stem-like cell lines with either maintenance or loss of high-level EGFR amplification, generated via modulation of ligand concentration. *Clinical Cancer Research* 18: 1901–1913.

See, A.P., J.E. Han, J. Phallen, Z. Binder, G. Gallia, F. Pan, D. Jinasena, C. Jackson, Z. Belcaid, S.J. Jeong, C. Gottschalk, J. Zeng, J. Ruzevick, S. Nicholas, Y. Kim, E. Albesiano, D.M. Pardoll, and M. Lim. 2012. The role of STAT3 activation in modulating the immune microenvironment of GBM. *Journal of Neuro-Oncology* 110: 359–368.

Snuderl, M., L. Fazlollahi, L.P. Le, M. Nitta, B.H. Zhelyazkova, C.J. Davidson, S. Akhavanfard, D.P. Cahill, K.D. Aldape, R.A. Betensky, D.N. Louis, and A.J. Iafrate. 2011. Mosaic amplification of multiple receptor tyrosine kinase genes in glioblastoma. *Cancer Cell* 20: 810–817.

Stommel, J.M., A.C. Kimmelman, H. Ying, R. Nabioullin, A.H. Ponugoti, R. Wiedemeyer, A.H. Stegh, J.E. Bradner, K.L. Ligon, C. Brennan, L. Chin, and R.A. DePinho. 2007. Coactivation of receptor tyrosine kinases affects the response of tumor cells to targeted therapies. *Science* 318: 287–290.

Szerlip, N.J., A. Pedraza, D. Chakravarty, M. Azim, J. McGuire, Y. Fang, T. Ozawa, E.C. Holland, J.T. Huse, S. Jhanwar, M.A. Leversha, T. Mikkelsen, and C.W. Brennan. 2012. Intratumoral heterogeneity of receptor tyrosine kinases EGFR and PDGFRA amplification in glioblastoma defines subpopulations with distinct growth factor response. *Proceedings of the National Academy of Sciences of the United States of America* 109: 3041–3046.

Talasila, K.M., A. Soentgerath, P. Euskirchen, G.V. Rosland, J. Wang, P.C. Huszthy, L. Prestegarden, K.O. Skaftnesmo, P.O. Sakariassen, E. Eskilsson, D. Stieber, O. Keunen, N. Brekka, I. Moen,

J.M. Nigro, O.K. Vintermyr, M. Lund-Johansen, S. Niclou, S.J. Mork, P.O. Enger, R. Bjerkvig, and H. Miletic. 2013. EGFR wild-type amplification and activation promote invasion and development of glioblastoma independent of angiogenesis. *Acta Neuropathologica* 125: 683–698.

Tan, X., N. Thapa, Y. Sun, and R.A. Anderson. 2015. A kinase-independent role for EGF receptor in autophagy initiation. *Cell* 160: 145–160.

Thiessen, B., C. Stewart, M. Tsao, S. Kamel-Reid, P. Schaiquevich, W. Mason, J. Easaw, K. Belanger, P. Forsyth, L. McIntosh, and E. Eisenhauer. 2010. A phase I/II trial of GW572016 (lapatinib) in recurrent glioblastoma multiforme: Clinical outcomes, pharmacokinetics and molecular correlation. *Cancer Chemotherapy and Pharmacology* 65: 353–361.

Tomas, A., S.O. Vaughan, T. Burgoyne, A. Sorkin, J.A. Hartley, D. Hochhauser, and C.E. Futter. 2015. WASH and Tsg101/ALIX-dependent diversion of stress-internalized EGFR from the canonical endocytic pathway. *Nature Communications* 6: 7324.

van den Bent, M.J., A.A. Brandes, R. Rampling, M.C. Kouwenhoven, J.M. Kros, A.F. Carpentier, P.M. Clement, M. Frenay, M. Campone, J.F. Baurain, J.P. Armand, M.J. Taphoorn, A. Tosoni, H. Kletzl, B. Klughammer, D. Lacombe, and T. Gorlia. 2009. Randomized phase II trial of erlotinib versus temozolomide or carmustine in recurrent glioblastoma: EORTC brain tumor group study 26034. *Journal of Clinical Oncology* 27: 1268–1274.

Verhaak, R.G., K.A. Hoadley, E. Purdom, V. Wang, Y. Qi, M.D. Wilkerson, C.R. Miller, L. Ding, T. Golub, J.P. Mesirov, G. Alexe, M. Lawrence, M. O'Kelly, P. Tamayo, B.A. Weir, S. Gabriel, W. Winckler, S. Gupta, L. Jakkula, H.S. Feiler, J.G. Hodgson, C.D. James, J.N. Sarkaria, C. Brennan, A. Kahn, P.T. Spellman, R.K. Wilson, T.P. Speed, J.W. Gray, M. Meyerson, G. Getz, C.M. Perou, and D.N. Hayes. 2010. Integrated genomic analysis identifies clinically relevant subtypes of glioblastoma characterized by abnormalities in PDGFRA, IDH1, EGFR, and NF1. *Cancer Cell* 17: 98–110.

Verreault, M., S.A. Weppler, A. Stegeman, C. Warburton, D. Strutt, D. Masin, and M.B. Bally. 2013. Combined RNAi-mediated suppression of Rictor and EGFR resulted in complete tumor regression in an orthotopic glioblastoma tumor model. *PLoS One* 8: e59597.

Vivanco, I., H.I. Robins, D. Rohle, C. Campos, C. Grommes, P.L. Nghiemphu, S. Kubek, B. Oldrini, M.G. Chheda, N. Yannuzzi, H. Tao, S. Zhu, A. Iwanami, D. Kuga, J. Dang, A. Pedraza, C.W. Brennan, A. Heguy, L.M. Liau, F. Lieberman, W.K. Yung, M.R. Gilbert, D.A. Reardon, J. Drappatz, P.Y. Wen, K.R. Lamborn, S.M. Chang, M.D. Prados, H.A. Fine, S. Horvath, N. Wu, A.B. Lassman, L.M. DeAngelis, W.H. Yong, J.G. Kuhn, P.S. Mischel, M.P. Mehta, T.F. Cloughesy, and I.K. Mellinghoff. 2012. Differential sensitivity of glioma- versus lung cancer-specific EGFR mutations to EGFR kinase inhibitors. *Cancer Discovery* 2(5): 458-471.

Wang, S.C., Y. Nakajima, Y.L. Yu, W. Xia, C.T. Chen, C.C. Yang, E.W. McIntush, L.Y. Li, D.H. Hawke, R. Kobayashi, and M.C. Hung. 2006. Tyrosine phosphorylation controls PCNA function through protein stability. *Nature Cell Biology* 8: 1359–1368.

Weihua, Z., R. Tsan, W.C. Huang, Q. Wu, C.H. Chiu, I.J. Fidler, and M.C. Hung. 2008. Survival of cancer cells is maintained by EGFR independent of its kinase activity. *Cancer Cell* 13: 385–393.

Weller, M., R.G. Weber, E. Willscher, V. Riehmer, B. Hentschel, M. Kreuz, J. Felsberg, U. Beyer, H. Loffler-Wirth, K. Kaulich, J.P. Steinbach, C. Hartmann, D. Gramatzki, J. Schramm, M. Westphal, G. Schackert, M. Simon, T. Martens, J. Bostrom, C. Hagel, M. Sabel, D. Krex, J.C. Tonn, W. Wick, S. Noell, U. Schlegel, B. Radlwimmer, T. Pietsch, M. Loeffler, A. von Deimling, H. Binder, and G. Reifenberger. 2015. Molecular classification of diffuse cerebral WHO grade II/III gliomas using genome- and transcriptome-wide profiling improves stratification of prognostically distinct patient groups. *Acta Neuropathologica* 129: 679–693.

Westphal, M., O. Heese, J.P. Steinbach, O. Schnell, G. Schackert, M. Mehdorn, D. Schulz, M. Simon, U. Schlegel, C. Senft, K. Geletneky, C. Braun, J.G. Hartung, D. Reuter, M.W. Metz, F. Bach, and T. Pietsch. 2015. A randomised, open label phase III trial with nimotuzumab, an anti-epidermal growth factor receptor monoclonal antibody in the treatment of newly diagnosed adult glioblastoma. *European Journal of Cancer* 51: 522–532.

Yang, W., Y. Xia, Y. Cao, Y. Zheng, W. Bu, L. Zhang, M.J. You, M.Y. Koh, G. Cote, K. Aldape, Y. Li, I.M. Verma, P.J. Chiao, and Z. Lu. 2012. EGFR-induced and PKCepsilon monoubiquitylation-dependent NF-kappaB activation upregulates PKM2 expression and promotes tumorigenesis. *Molecular Cell* 48: 771–784.

Yarden, Y. 2001. The EGFR family and its ligands in human cancer. Signalling mechanisms and therapeutic opportunities. *European Journal of Cancer* 37 Suppl 4: S3–S8.

Ye, F., Q. Gao, T. Xu, L. Zeng, Y. Ou, F. Mao, H. Wang, Y. He, B. Wang, Z. Yang, D. Guo, and T. Lei. 2009. Upregulation of LRIG1 suppresses malignant glioma cell growth by attenuating EGFR activity. *Journal of Neuro-Oncology* 94: 183–194.

Ying, H., H. Zheng, K. Scott, R. Wiedemeyer, H. Yan, C. Lim, J. Huang, S. Dhakal, E. Ivanova, Y. Xiao, H. Zhang, J. Hu, J.M. Stommel, M.A. Lee, A.J. Chen, J.H. Paik, O. Segatto, C. Brennan, L.A. Elferink, Y.A. Wang, L. Chin, and R.A. DePinho. 2010. Mig-6 controls EGFR trafficking and suppresses gliomagenesis. *Proceedings of the National Academy of Sciences of the United States of America* 107: 6912–6917.

Yue, X., W. Song, W. Zhang, L. Chen, Z. Xi, Z. Xin, and X. Jiang. 2008. Mitochondrially localized EGFR is subjected to autophagic regulation and implicated in cell survival. *Autophagy* 4: 641–649.

Yung, W.K., X. Zhang, P.A. Steck, and M.C. Hung. 1990. Differential amplification of the TGF-alpha gene in human gliomas. *Cancer Communications* 2: 201–205.

Zahonero, C., and P. Sanchez-Gomez. 2014. EGFR-dependent mechanisms in glioblastoma: Towards a better therapeutic strategy. *Cellular and Molecular Life Sciences* 71 (18): 3465–3488.

Zahonero, C., P. Aguilera, C. Ramirez-Castillejo, M. Pajares, M.V. Bolos, D. Cantero, A. Perez-Nunez, A. Hernandez-Lain, P. Sanchez-Gomez, and J.M. Sepulveda. 2015. Preclinical test of dacomitinib, an irreversible EGFR inhibitor, confirms its effectiveness for glioblastoma. *Molecular Cancer Therapeutics* 14 (7): 1548–1558.

Zhu, Y., and K. Shah. 2014. Multiple lesions in receptor tyrosine kinase pathway determine glioblastoma response to pan-ERBB inhibitor PF-00299804 and PI3K/mTOR dual inhibitor PF-05212384. *Cancer Biology & Therapy* 15: 815–822.

Zhu, H., X. Cao, F. Ali-Osman, S. Keir, and H.W. Lo. 2010. EGFR and EGFRvIII interact with PUMA to inhibit mitochondrial translocation of PUMA and PUMA-mediated apoptosis independent of EGFR kinase activity. *Cancer Letters* 294: 101–110.

Chapter 6
Radiogenomics and Histomics in Glioblastoma: The Promise of Linking Image-Derived Phenotype with Genomic Information

Michael Lehrer, Reid T. Powell, Souptik Barua, Donnie Kim, Shivali Narang, and Arvind Rao

Abstract Intra-tumor heterogeneity is the fundamental challenge in finding a cure for late-stage cancers. Physical biopsies do not sufficiently cover the diversity of molecular phenotypes within the tumor. Treatments are only effective on a subset of vulnerable tumor cells due to the prevalence of tumor stem-like cells. GBM tumors exemplify these general properties of late-stage cancers, with heterogeneous molecular profiles, histology, and radiology. Radiomics aims to characterize disease phenotypes from radiology scans in order to provide an alternative view of tumor heterogeneity, enabling models built from retrospective analysis of radiology scan data, and their integration with clinical data and molecular profiles. Computational histology (histomics) follows a workflow analogous to that of radiomics, with preprocessing, segmentation, feature extraction and analytics. The goal of histomics is to compute cellular morphometry and heterogeneity features from histology datasets. Genomic traits can potentially be inferred from histologic features by analysis of large, linked pathology-genomic data sets. There is also an active investigation of computer vision and machine learning applications to classify gliomas using radiology and histology images. The potential of radiomics, radiogenomics and histomics

M. Lehrer • D. Kim • S. Narang
Department of Bioinformatics and Computational Biology, University of Texas MD Anderson Cancer Center, Houston, TX, USA

R.T. Powell
Institute of Biosciences and Technology, Texas A&M University Health Science Center, Houston, TX, USA

S. Barua
Department of Electrical and Computer Engineering, Rice University, Houston, TX, USA

A. Rao, PhD (✉)
Department of Bioinformatics and Computational Biology, Unit 1410, The University of Texas MD Anderson Cancer Center, 1515 Holcombe Blvd, Houston, TX 77030, USA
e-mail: aruppore@mdanderson.org

© Springer International Publishing AG 2017
K. Somasundaram (ed.), *Advances in Biology and Treatment of Glioblastoma*,
Current Cancer Research, DOI 10.1007/978-3-319-56820-1_6

studies is to advance personalized cancer treatment by enabling interpretation of biological mechanisms underlying imaging phenotypes. These efforts aim to make personalized therapies more accessible. Results from preliminary imaging could direct administration of precision assays to guide treatment, measure treatment response and identify targetable genetic alterations from image-derived phenotype data, across biological scale. Radiomics and histomics promises to revolutionize the practice of personalized medicine, by providing an important complement to molecular strategies.

Keywords Radiomics • Radiogenomics • Histomics • Glioma • Glioblastoma • Magnetic Resonance Imaging • Computed Tomography • Positron Emission Tomography

6.1 Introduction

Intra-tumor heterogeneity is the fundamental challenge in characterizing therapy-induced treatment changes and resistance mechanisms. Physical biopsies do not provide sufficient coverage of molecular phenotypes within the tumor. Treatments for late stage tumors are only effective on a subset of vulnerable tumor cells. Due to the prevalence of tumor stem-like cells expressing the stem cell surface protein marker CD133, resistant tumor cells survive and continue to proliferate (Liu et al. 2006; Yuan et al. 2004). Glioblastoma (GBM) tumors exemplify these general properties of late-stage cancers, with varying molecular profiles, histology, and radiology (Verhaak et al. 2010). The field of radiomics aims to meet these challenges through comprehensive analysis of tumor radiology data, as a way to complement the tumor genomic characteristics with image-derived tumor characteristics, to provide some insight into the molecular and phenotypic heterogeneity of the tumor. Radiomic data obtains hundreds or thousands of measurements describing the shape, morphology, and distribution of gray-level pixel intensity values in the radiology scans. Through these measurements, radiomics aim to gain additional insight from image analysis (Lambin et al. 2012). Statistical models built from retrospective analysis of radiology data with matched clinical and molecular profiles integrate these disparate data sets to better predict disease and patient outcomes. Radiogenomics takes the radiomics approach further to discern the correlations between the molecular features of GBM, clinical outcomes and radiological phenotypes.

Through recent efforts by The Cancer Genome Atlas (TCGA) to comprehensively describe brain tumors at the genomic and molecular level, a complex picture of GBM molecular and cell biology has emerged. GBM tumors are driven by altered p53, Rb, and PI3K signaling, sustaining uncontrolled cellular growth and proliferation (Chin et al. 2008). These redundant growth mechanisms are responsible for the recalcitrance of GBM tumors (Brennan et al. 2013). GBM manifests as multiple subtypes: classical, mesenchymal, and proneural, each with distinct histological, genomic and gene expression phenotypes (Verhaak et al. 2010). For instance, proneural GBM tumors feature increased activation of PI3K signaling compared to mesenchymal tumors (Brennan et al. 2013). Overactive PI3K signaling is due to the most common mutations, deletions and rearrangements residing in the receptor tyrosine kinase (RTK) *EGFR* (Brennan et al. 2013). Other RTKs less often found to be mutated were *PDFGRA, FGFR,* and *MET* (Brennan et al. 2013). In addition to the deregulated canonical signaling pathways and cell surface receptor molecules, microRNAs including miR-141, 200c (Guo et al. 2016), and 204 (Song et al. 2016) have been described as tumor suppressors in GBM are mutated as well. MicroRNAs (miRs) regulate translation of messenger RNA by binding mRNA target sequences, facilitating formation of the RISC silencing enzymatic complex, and degrading the targeted transcript. There is crosstalk between miRs and regulatory networks in GBM, as miR-422a interacts with PI3K signaling through suppression of *PIK3CA* transcript (Liang et al. 2016). These mechanisms and interactions are responsible for the aggressiveness of GBM tumors. Radiomics and Radiogenomics provides the computational tools to determine how this pathobiology manifests in radiological data. Radiogenomics asks the question: what, if any, effect does a genetic mutation (or some such alteration) have on the phenotypes apparent in radiological data?

6.2 Radiomics (Extracting Information from Radiology Data)

Radiomics is the process of extracting features from radiological acquisitions. The radiomics workflow compasses data acquisition, image pre-processing, feature extraction, and data analysis (Fig. 6.1). Magnetic resonance imaging (MRI), computed tomography (CT), and positron emission tomography (PET) provide the core data for radiomics analysis. Pre-processing of this data prior to feature computation ensures the integrity and reproducibility of the results. Feature extraction is the core of the radiomics approach. Finally, radiomics feature statistics are compared with matched clinical and genomic data, drawing associations and correlations with survival, mutational status, and other molecular information. This approach has been possible through the large-scale efforts of the TCGA, which has made large data sets of matched radiology, genomics, transcript, and expression data publicly available. Radiomics studies the entire tumor, in contrast to current genetic profiling, in which coverage is limited to the number of biopsies taken. This process aims to parse out the variation in gray-level intensities with underlying genomic or transcriptomic causes.

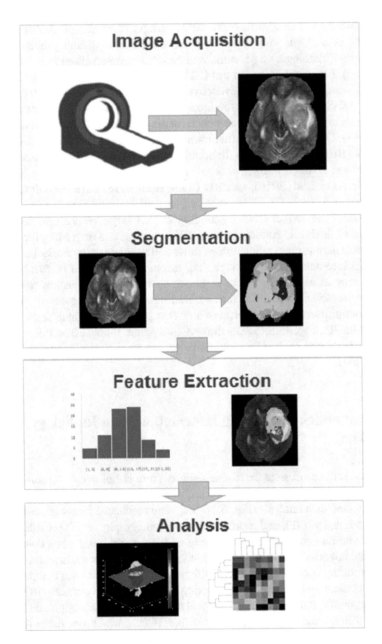

Fig. 6.1 The radiomics analytical pipeline. Radiological scans data acquired by CT, PET, or MR are pre-processed and segmented. Features are extracted and analysis performed using clinical data

6.2.1   Data Acquisition

MRI is the standard technique for GBM diagnostics, as PET scans suffer from comparatively lower sensitivity and specificity (la Fougère et al. 2011). MR imaging is acquired using multiple modalities, with distinct parameters for phenotype characterization. These include T1-weighted, T2-weighted, diffusion-weighted, perfusion, and fluid attenuated inversion recovery (FLAIR). Gadolinium contrast enhanced MRI is used to diagnose gliomas and GBM, and FDG-PET has been evaluated as well (Nihashi et al. 2013; Pötzi et al. 2007). Contrast agents such as gadolinium with MR, or fluoro-deoxyglucose (FDG) or FDOPA with PET, allow metabolic and other data to be derived (Karunanithi et al. 2013). FDOPA-PET imaging of lower grade gliomas has shown the ability to predict recurrence (Harris et al. 2012). With so many imaging modalities and variants, considerable care must be taken to ensure consistent acquisition parameters are used so that quantitative downstream analyses remain valid. This ensures the reproducibility of radiomics studies.

6.2.2   Image Pre-processing

In radiomics studies, acquired radiological datasets undergo extensive pre-processing to ensure accuracy and reproducibility. Registration, inhomogeneity correction, intensity normalization, and voxel re-slicing ensure radiomic feature robustness and make the data more interpretable. Image registration ensures consistency in the segmentation results. Inhomogeneity correction and intensity normalization aim to mitigate acquisition-associated artifacts ensuring that quantitative features are computed accurately and with consistency. Voxel re-slicing matches image resolution across multiple acquisitions and data collection sites, correcting inconsistent acquisition parameters. Segmentation using manual software, semi-automatic software such as 3D Slicer (Parmar et al. 2014) or fully-automated software such as BraTumIA (Rios Velazquez et al. 2015), delineates the region-of-interest (ROI) defining the tumor. Automated segmentation of GBM tumors using BraTumIA software compares favorably with manual segmentation by trained radiologists (Porz et al. 2014). Further, radiomic features are extracted from the segmented ROI, i.e. the tumor portion. These quantitative radiomics features are computed from the morphological characteristics and distribution of gray-level intensities within and across the radiograph.

6.2.3   Feature Extraction

Radiomics analyses extract either semantic or computational features from radiology images. Semantic features, such as the Visually Accessible REMBRANDT Images (VASARI) for GBM, are scored manually by the radiologists based on visual appearance of tumor characteristics. The twenty-six VASARI features scored from T1-weighted and T2-weighted FLAIR acquisitions predict GBM patient survival and are shown to demonstrate associations with genetic alterations (Gutman et al. 2013). In computational radiomics analysis, volumetric, habitat and heterogeneity (first or second-order texture) features are computed from radiological images.

Texture features include first-order (histogram) statistics, second-order statistics (or Haralick features such as energy, entropy, etc.) (Haralick et al. 1973), and spectral features (Kassner and Thornhill 2010). These features describe the arrangement and patterns of gray-level intensities within a two-dimensional or three-dimensional image. First-order texture features are computed on subsets or "neighborhoods" of adjacent pixels, and are mathematically defined as mean gray level (MGL), variance of gray levels (VGL), absolute gradient value, mean gradient (MGR) and variance gradient (VGR) (Kassner and Thornhill 2010). Second-order texture features are computed from gray level co-occurrence matrices (GLCM) or run-length matrices (RLM). The GLCM of an image defines the distribution of intensities of adjacent pixels over a specified distance (Haralick et al. 1973). The RLM of an image tabulates the number of runs of a given length of a certain gray level intensity within the image (Galloway 1975). Spectral features are mathematical transformations applied to the images and include Fourier transform (Zhu et al. 2003), wavelet transform (Mallat 1989) and Stockwell transform (Kassner and Thornhill 2010).

Imaging habitats are computed from multi-modal MR imaging and represent unique combinations of relative high- and low-intensity pixel values across the various MR acquisitions (Lee et al. 2015). Pixels in each MR acquisition are dichotomized as either high or low intensity by k-means clustering. Each pixel in the tumor volume therefore has a binary designation for each modality. For example, a particular imaging habitat might be defined as having relatively low pixel intensities in the T1-weighted acquisition, high intensity pixels in the T1-contrast enhanced images, and low intensity in both the FLAIR and T2-weighted acquisitions. There are therefore sixteen possible combinations of pixel intensity designations and sixteen possible habitats.

Segmentation is typically performed prior to feature extraction to delineate the tumor region, but the segmentation process itself can define radiomic volumetric features. Volumetric features can be defined to describe total tumor volume and other tumor dimensions (Coroller et al. 2015). These volumetrics can include edema, tumor enhancing region, non-enhancing region, and necrosis (Gutman et al. 2015). One study calculated the T2/FLAIR hyperintense volume ratio to contrast enhancing volume and necrotic volume in their radiomics feature set (Naeini et al. 2013). Segmentation can also be used to derive shape features which can predict GBM tissue phenotypes (Chaddad et al. 2016).

6.2.4   Data Analysis

A variety of statistical methods are employed in the correlation of extracted radiomic features with clinical or molecular parameters. Benjamini-Hochberg correction (Benjamini and Hochberg 1995) and bootstrap-based correction of p-values (Efron 1979) associated with correlation coefficients describing the relationship between features and other parameters remove spurious correlations and minimize false-detection results (Kim et al. 2002). Cox proportional hazards regression models are used to screen potential traditional molecular and histological biomarkers, and have been used to interrogate radiomic features for their ability to predict GBM patient outcomes, such as survival (Wangaryattawanich et al. 2015). More recently, machine learning algorithms such as neural networks, support vector machines, decision trees, k-nearest neighbor, and logistic regression have been applied to predict survival of GBM patients based on radiomics features (Kim et al. 2002). Regression models, classification models and other statistical methods relating radiomics features with molecular and clinical parameters are necessarily high-dimensional and could suffer from model overfitting. This can be ameliorated by dimension reduction techniques such as principal components analysis (PCA) (Mishra et al. 2011), sparse PCA (sPCA), non-linear PCA (Kramer 1991), partial least squares regression (PLS) (Wold et al. 1984), and auto-encoders (Kumar et al. 2015). Supervised PCA isolated eleven radiomic features which predicted survival more accurately than existing risk models (Kickingereder et al. 2016). Calculation of the area under the receiver operating characteristic curve (AUC) analysis is often used to gauge the predictive power of radiomic features. This technique was used in a study of volumetric radiomic features and their correlation with mutations in TP53, RB1, NF1, EGFR, and PDGFRA (Gutman et al. 2015). Cross validation of radiomics findings shows correlations are not spurious or artifacts of the analytic pipeline (Kassner and Thornhill 2010).

6.3 Radiogenomics

Radiogenomics (also termed "imaging-genomics") correlates imaging features with genomics data (Lambin et al. 2012; Kumar et al. 2012; Pope et al. 2005; Kuo et al. 2007; Ellingson 2015) and *de novo* mutations that exist in the tumor or may emerge in response to radiation therapy (Rosenstein et al. 2014; Kerns et al. 2014; Best et al. 2011; Lambin et al. 2013). A number of studies have studied radiogenomics in GBM. MRI contrast and mass effect features have been shown to predict EGFR mutation status (Diehn et al. 2008). MRI FLAIR features associated with disease infiltration were correlated with Periostin expression and survival (Zinn et al. 2011). The volume of enhancing tumor in MR imaging was correlated with the proneural GBM molecular subtype, with proneural tumors having relatively low levels of enhancement (Gutman et al. 2013). Gene-set enrichment analysis (GSEA) found contrast-necrosis ratio to be significantly associated with mutations in genes such as KLK3, FOXP1, and PIK3IP1 (Jamshidi et al. 2014). Hierarchical clustering of imaging data from a cohort of 55 GBM patients revealed enhancement features associated with survival and molecular sub-type (Gevaert et al. 2014). Analysis of MR texture features computed from multiple modalities predicted survival and molecular sub-types (Yang et al. 2015). MR enhancement, cerebral blood volume and apparent diffusion coefficients were correlated with histopathologic classifications and differential RNA expression patterns (Barajas et al. 2010). *MGMT* promoter methylation, an epigenetic trait of tumor associated with survival, was stratified by the level of intra-tumoral edema (Carrillo et al. 2012). Contrast enhancing tumor was inversely correlated with *IDH1* mutations (Carrillo et al. 2012). This was further borne out in another study which showed a strong negative correlation between ring enhancement and *MGMT* promoter methylation, but using texture features to classify *MGMT* status based on T2 images had poor accuracy (Drabycz et al. 2010). Several volumetric features including volume of contrast enhancement, volume of central necrosis, combined volume of contrast enhancement and central necrosis, and the ratio of T2/FLAIR to contrast enhancement and necrosis differentiated mesenchymal GBM from the classical, neural and proneural subtypes (Naeini et al. 2013).

These reports highlight the numerous associations between MR features and genomic profiles through state-of-the-art of radiogenomics. Current challenges in the field of radiogenomics include consistency of radiological data acquisition, sample size, feature robustness, and the reproducibility of correlations (through validation). An ideal radiogenomics study would ensure identical radiological acquisition parameters and a large study population, with access to a validation cohort. However, often acquisition parameters vary due to radiologist or institutional preference and practice. In many cases, the size of the eligible population is limited, and the cohort must be constructed from a multi-center study, leading to challenges ensuring consistent modalities and acquisitions are used. This challenge is particularly acute in GBM, which is one of the rarer tumor types, with relatively fewer eligible study participants. The multi-institutional TCGA effort has in part ameliorated this difficulty by compiling extensive data sets from multiple studies and institutions. Even so, a suitable validation cohort may not be available to assess correctness and reproducibility. Despite these issues, radiogenomics shows exciting promise to overcome the many logistical and computational challenges it faces, obtaining novel insights into tumor biology and the nature of phenotype-genomic relationships.

6.4   Radioproteomics

Radioproteomics (or "imaging-proteomics") correlates protein expression with imaging features. This extension of radiogenomics describes the relationship between translation products and radiomics features. Expression of many proteins is not directly proportional to mRNA transcript levels, and thus modeling correlations between genomic alterations and imaging features may not fully capture the entire landscape of molecular-phenotypic interactions within the tumor. The proteomic context can be explored by using protein expression data derived from high-throughput proteomics technologies such as reverse-phase protein arrays and mass spectrometry which allows the molecular status of the tumor to be comprehensively determined. These techniques also assay post-translational modifications, such as phosphorylation, indicating signaling pathway activation. Such data provides a unique opportunity to discern the correlation between intra/intercellular signaling and imaging phenotypes.

6.5   Computational Pathology and Histomics

At a different scale of biology, i.e. tissue, histological evaluation of tumors has long been an important tool in the classification and grading of gliomas. More recently, molecular analysis has shown that molecular sub-classes (i.e. mesenchymal, neural, proneural, classical) can be defined and have prognostic value (Cancer Genome Atlas Research Network et al. 2015; Eckel-Passow et al. 2015). Computational histology (or "histomics") follows a workflow analogous to that of radiomics, with pre-processing, segmentation, feature extraction and analytics. The goal of histomics is to compute morphology and texture features from histology correlated with molecular characteristics. Genomic traits can be inferred from histologic features (semantic or computational) by high-throughput analysis of large pathology data sets. This has led to a revolution in how gliomas are classified which now include both histological classifications in addition to molecular features (Louis et al. 2016). Despite utilizing a more integrative classification in the diagnosis and prognosis of a patient, there is still the recognized variability in histological classifications amongst diagnostic centers and pathologists. To help minimize inter-user variability and standardize histological classification, multiple quantitative analysis pipelines have been proposed. These range from relatively low-complexity approaches which quantify morphometric features of nuclei, commonly termed as histomorphometry, to much more complex machine learning approaches which learn to discriminate morphology-based features between glioma subtypes. Analysis of histological sections can be applied to many different tissue types including those in cancer using both pre-configured software from vendors such as Aperio (Lieca Biosystems) and Vectra (PerkinElmer). Other 3rd party software developers provide quantitative services and offer development of highly customizable scripts in multiple proprietary or open source languages.

In glioma, evaluation of the composition and orientation of nuclei are used to infer cellular origin and levels of differentiation are used to classify glioma (Louis et al. 2007, 2016). It therefore stands to reason that spatial organization of nuclei in addition to the morphometric properties can be used to quantify these changes between histological classifications. To this end, pipelines have been developed using open source software such as ImageJ (NIH) to segment and extract morphological features from regions of interest defined by a pathologist (Surowka et al. 2014; Nafe and Schlote 2004). Collectively, these results showed that morphological features of nuclei could be associated with malignancy grade and histological classifications. In addition to quantifying morphological features of nuclei, the spatial distributions of nuclei has also been considered as a quantitative feature associated with malignancy status (Nafe and Schlote 2004; Jiao et al. 2011). These results show the density of nuclei can distinguish normal from high grade tissue and provide evidence that the tumor microenvironment is not spatially random in its organization. Other techniques have been developed to identify higher order tissue structures that are associated with malignancy status including pseudo - palisading necrosis and microvascular proliferation (MVP) which delineate a high grade glioma from lower grades (Mousavi et al. 2015).

In addition to methods which provide direct morphological and spatial readouts, there is active investigation of computer vision and machine learning applications to classify gliomas. Examples of this include single cell classifiers which provide a feature rich machine-learned ranking of individual cells. This pipeline method classifies individual nuclei into oligodendroglioma or astrocytoma-like and stratifies risk on the basis of the oligodendroglioma component (Kong et al. 2013). Many of the discussed methods heavily rely on the ability to segment individual nuclei, however, techniques which do not require segmentation have also been developed. In general, many of these techniques partition an image into multiple smaller patches from which features are extracted. Identification of discriminant patches which best represent the conceptual class of the larger tissue can then be identified using multiple supervised and unsupervised machine learning techniques. These include but are not limited to convolutional neural networks (Ertosun and Rubin 2015; Xu et al. 2015), decision tree models (Mousavi et al. 2015), convolutional sparse coding (Zhou et al. 2014) and restricted Boltzmann machines (Nayak et al. 2013). These techniques are also not mutually-exclusive and can be combined. Examples of this include feature extraction followed by data reduction (i.e. principal component analysis and/or clustering) and subsequent implementation of a supervised learning technique (Barker et al. 2016). An additional example includes utilization of modular supervised learning where discrimination of higher grade from lower grade gliomas is achieved using one model and then further those determined to belong to the lower grade gliomas are sub-classified using a different model (Ertosun and Rubin 2015), i.e. through classifier cascading. Many of the methods to discriminate GBM from LGG do so through the identification of disease associated phenotypes such as necrosis and MVP, demonstrating that these techniques are identifying relevant visually interpretable phenotypes (Mousavi et al. 2015; Zhou et al. 2014; Vu et al. 2015).

As previously stated, there is an overwhelming trend of classifying gliomas using histology and molecular profiling. Likewise, researchers have begun to explore how quantitative imaging of histological sections can be combined with molecular information, however, there is still much to be explored in this field. At this point correlative studies are typically utilized which attempt to understand the molecular etiology of visual features (Kong et al. 2013). While these types of studies can help validate the relevance of machine learned visual features, the ultimate goal is to create an integrated molecular and machine learned visual dictionary used to interpret gliomas. Towards widespread adoption, some key challenges pertain to the use of harmonization and data standardization techniques for the development of standard H&E/IHC datasets for image mining.

6.6   The Future of Imaging Genomics

The potential of radiomics, radiogenomics and histomics studies is to advance personalized cancer treatment by enabling interpretation of biological mechanisms jointly with imaging-derived phenotypes (Fig. 6.2). Through these efforts, the goal has been

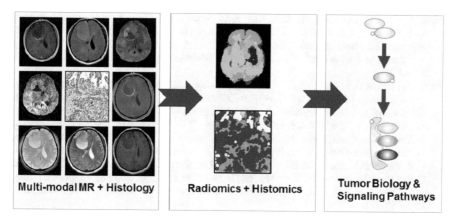

Fig. 6.2 Radiomics, radiogenomics and histomics interrogate the biology of tumor regions from radiology (MR modalities) and pathology images through integrated analysis pipelines. Describing tumor regions with integrated radiomics and histomics can discern underlying tumor signaling and biological functions

to make personalized therapies more economically viable and to facilitate the integrated biological interpretation of radiological and histological phenotypes. Personalized treatment has created additional challenges in data management and treatment cost. Improvements in the reproducibility, precision and economics of genetics have made possible the detailed characterization of the mutational status of individual patients' tumors. As this personalized approach becomes widespread, additional logistics, clinical, and informatics challenges such as image characterization, image management, and clinical decision support systems arise (Hsu et al. 2013; Williams et al. 2015). Radiogenomics addresses many of these challenges by reducing the need for biopsy in preliminary patient screening procedures. Rendering initial genetic testing unnecessary in certain cases, radiogenomics would help prioritize data from next-generation sequencing (Noor et al. 2015; O'Driscoll et al. 2013). Results from preliminary imaging, already in widespread use, would be able to direct administration of precision assays to guide treatment and identify targetable genetic alterations. Phenotype-genomic correlation thus promises to revolutionize personalized medicine and cancer care.

References

Barajas, R.F., J.G. Hodgson, J.S. Chang, S.R. Vandenberg, R.F. Yeh, A.T. Parsa, M.W. McDermott, M.S. Berger, W.P. Dillon, and S. Cha. 2010. Glioblastoma multiforme regional genetic and cellular expression patterns: Influence on anatomic and physiologic MR imaging. *Radiology* 254: 564–576.

Barker, J., A. Hoogi, A. Depeursinge, and D.L. Rubin. 2016. Automated classification of brain tumor type in whole-slide digital pathology images using local representative tiles. *Medical image analysis* 30: 60–71.

Benjamini, Y., and Y. Hochberg. 1995. Controlling the false discovery rate – A practical and powerful approach to multiple testing. *Journal of the Royal Statistical Society Series B-Methodological* 57: 289–300.

Best, T., D. Li, A.D. Skol, T. Kirchhoff, S.A. Jackson, Y. Yasui, S. Bhatia, L.C. Strong, S.M. Domchek, K.L. Nathanson, O.I. Olopade, R.S. Huang, T.M. Mack, D.V. Conti, K. Offit, W. Cozen, L.L. Robison, and K. Onel. 2011. Variants at 6q21 implicate PRDM1 in the etiology of therapy-induced second malignancies after Hodgkin's lymphoma. *Nature Medicine* 17: 941–943.

Brennan, C.W., R.G.W. Verhaak, A. McKenna, B. Campos, H. Noushmehr, S.R. Salama, S. Zheng, D. Chakravarty, J.Z. Sanborn, S.H. Berman, R. Beroukhim, B. Bernard, C.-J. Wu, G. Genovese, I. Shmulevich, J. Barnholtz-Sloan, L. Zou, R. Vegesna, S.A. Shukla, G. Ciriello, W.K. Yung, W. Zhang, C. Sougnez, T. Mikkelsen, K. Aldape, D.D. Bigner, E.G. Van Meir, M. Prados, A. Sloan, K.L. Black, J. Eschbacher, G. Finocchiaro, W. Friedman, D.W. Andrews, A. Guha, M. Iacocca, B.P. O'Neill, G. Foltz, J. Myers, D.J. Weisenberger, R. Penny, R. Kucherlapati, C.M. Perou, D.N. Hayes, R. Gibbs, M. Marra, G.B. Mills, E. Lander, P. Spellman, R. Wilson, C. Sander, J. Weinstein, M. Meyerson, S. Gabriel, P.W. Laird, D. Haussler, G. Getz, L. Chin, and TCGA Research Network. 2013. The somatic genomic landscape of glioblastoma. *Cell* 155: 462–477.

Cancer Genome Atlas Research Network, D.J. Brat, R.G. Verhaak, K.D. Aldape, W.K. Yung, S.R. Salama, L.A. Cooper, E. Rheinbay, C.R. Miller, M. Vitucci, O. Morozova, A.G. Robertson, H. Noushmehr, P.W. Laird, A.D. Cherniack, R. Akbani, J.T. Huse, G. Ciriello, L.M. Poisson, J.S. Barnholtz-Sloan, M.S. Berger, C. Brennan, R.R. Colen, H. Colman, A.E. Flanders, C. Giannini, M. Grifford, A. Iavarone, R. Jain, I. Joseph, J. Kim, K. Kasaian, T. Mikkelsen, B.A. Murray, B.P. O'Neill, L. Pachter, D.W. Parsons, C. Sougnez, E.P. Sulman, S.R. Vandenberg, E.G. Van Meir, A. von Deimling, H. Zhang, D. Crain, K. Lau, D. Mallery, S. Morris, J. Paulauskis, R. Penny, T. Shelton, M. Sherman, P. Yena, A. Black, J. Bowen, K. Dicostanzo, J. Gastier-Foster, K.M. Leraas, T.M. Lichtenberg, C.R. Pierson, N.C. Ramirez, C. Taylor, S. Weaver, L. Wise, E. Zmuda, T. Davidsen, J.A. Demchok, G. Eley, M.L. Ferguson, C.M. Hutter, K.R. Mills Shaw, B.A. Ozenberger, M. Sheth, H.J. Sofia, R. Tarnuzzer, Z. Wang, L. Yang, J.C. Zenklusen, B. Ayala, J. Baboud, S. Chudamani, M.A. Jensen, J. Liu, T. Pihl, R. Raman, Y. Wan, Y. Wu, A. Ally, J.T. Auman, M. Balasundaram, S. Balu, S.B. Baylin, R. Beroukhim, M.S. Bootwalla, R. Bowlby, C.A. Bristow, D. Brooks, Y. Butterfield, R. Carlsen, S. Carter, L. Chin, A. Chu, E. Chuah, K. Cibulskis, A. Clarke, S.G. Coetzee, N. Dhalla, T. Fennell, S. Fisher, S. Gabriel, G. Getz, R. Gibbs, R. Guin, A. Hadjipanayis, D.N. Hayes, T. Hinoue, K. Hoadley, R.A. Holt, A.P. Hoyle, S.R. Jefferys, S. Jones, C.D. Jones, R. Kucherlapati, P.H. Lai, E. Lander, S. Lee, L. Lichtenstein, Y. Ma, D.T. Maglinte, H.S. Mahadeshwar, M.A. Marra, M. Mayo, S. Meng, M.L. Meyerson, P.A. Mieczkowski, R.A. Moore, L.E. Mose, A.J. Mungall, A. Pantazi, M. Parfenov, P.J. Park, J.S. Parker, C.M. Perou, A. Protopopov, X. Ren, J. Roach, T.S. Sabedot, J. Schein, S.E. Schumacher, J.G. Seidman, S. Seth, H. Shen, J.V. Simons, P. Sipahimalani, M.G. Soloway, X. Song, H. Sun, B. Tabak, A. Tam, D. Tan, J. Tang, N. Thiessen, T. Triche Jr., D.J. Van Den Berg, U. Veluvolu, S. Waring, D.J. Weisenberger, M.D. Wilkerson, T. Wong, J. Wu, L. Xi, A.W. Xu, L. Yang, T.I. Zack, J. Zhang, B.A. Aksoy, H. Arachchi, C. Benz, B. Bernard, D. Carlin, J. Cho, D. DiCara, S. Frazer, G.N. Fuller, J. Gao, N. Gehlenborg, D. Haussler, D.I. Heiman, L. Iype, A. Jacobsen, Z. Ju, S. Katzman, H. Kim, T. Knijnenburg, R.B. Kreisberg, M.S. Lawrence, W. Lee, K. Leinonen, P. Lin, S. Ling, W. Liu, Y. Liu, Y. Liu, Y. Lu, G. Mills, S. Ng, M.S. Noble, E. Paull, A. Rao, S. Reynolds, G. Saksena, Z. Sanborn, C. Sander, N. Schultz, Y. Senbabaoglu, R. Shen, I. Shmulevich, R. Sinha, J. Stuart, S.O. Sumer, Y. Sun, N. Tasman, B.S. Taylor, D. Voet, N. Weinhold, J.N. Weinstein, D. Yang, K. Yoshihara, S. Zheng, W. Zhang, L. Zou, T. Abel, S. Sadeghi, M.L. Cohen, J. Eschbacher, E.M. Hattab, A. Raghunathan, M.J. Schniederjan, D. Aziz, G. Barnett, W. Barrett, D.D. Bigner, L. Boice, C. Brewer, C. Calatozzolo, B. Campos, C.G. Carlotti Jr., T.A. Chan, L. Cuppini, E. Curley, S. Cuzzubbo, K. Devine, F. DiMeco, R. Duell, J.B. Elder, A. Fehrenbach, G. Finocchiaro, W. Friedman, J. Fulop, J. Gardner, B. Hermes, C. Herold-Mende, A. Jungk, A. Kendler, N.L. Lehman, E. Lipp, O. Liu, R. Mandt, M. McGraw, R. McLendon, C. McPherson, L. Neder, P. Nguyen, A. Noss, R. Nunziata, Q.T. Ostrom, C. Palmer, A. Perin, B. Pollo, A. Potapov, O. Potapova,

W.K. Rathmell, D. Rotin, L. Scarpace, C. Schilero, K. Senecal, K. Shimmel, V. Shurkhay, S. Sifri, R. Singh, A.E. Sloan, K. Smolenski, S.M. Staugaitis, R. Steele, L. Thorne, D.P. Tirapelli, A. Unterberg, M. Vallurupalli, Y. Wang, R. Warnick, F. Williams, Y. Wolinsky, S. Bell, M. Rosenberg, C. Stewart, F. Huang, J.L. Grimsby, A.J. Radenbaugh, and J. Zhang. 2015. Comprehensive, integrative genomic analysis of diffuse lower-grade gliomas. *N Engl J Med* 372: 2481–2498.

Carrillo, J.A., A. Lai, P.L. Nghiemphu, H.J. Kim, H.S. Phillips, S. Kharbanda, P. Moftakhar, S. Lalaezari, W. Yong, B.M. Ellingson, T.F. Cloughesy, and W.B. Pope. 2012. Relationship between tumor enhancement, edema, IDH1 mutational status, MGMT promoter methylation, and survival in glioblastoma. *AJNR Am J Neuroradiol* 33: 1349–1355.

Chaddad, A., C. Desrosiers, and M. Toews. 2016. Phenotypic characterization of glioblastoma identified through shape descriptors, Proc. SPIE 9785, Medical Imaging 2016: Computer-Aided Diagnosis, 97852M, 2016.

Chin, L., M. Meyerson, K. Aldape, D. Bigner, T. Mikkelsen, S. VandenBerg, A. Kahn, R. Penny, M.L. Ferguson, D.S. Gerhard, G. Getz, C. Brennan, B.S. Taylor, W. Winckler, P. Park, M. Ladanyi, K.A. Hoadley, R.G.W. Verhaak, D.N. Hayes, P.T. Spellman, D. Absher, B.A. Weir, L. Ding, D. Wheeler, M.S. Lawrence, K. Cibulskis, E. Mardis, J. Zhang, R.K. Wilson, L. Donehower, D.A. Wheeler, E. Purdom, J. Wallis, P.W. Laird, J.G. Herman, K.E. Schuebel, D.J. Weisenberger, S.B. Baylin, N. Schultz, J. Yao, R. Wiedemeyer, J. Weinstein, C. Sander, R.A. Gibbs, J. Gray, R. Kucherlapati, E.S. Lander, R.M. Myers, C.M. Perou, R. McLendon, A. Friedman, E.G. Van Meir, D.J. Brat, G.M. Mastrogianakis, J.J. Olson, N. Lehman, W.K.A. Yung, O. Bogler, M. Berger, M. Prados, D. Muzny, M. Morgan, S. Scherer, A. Sabo, L. Nazareth, L. Lewis, O. Hall, Y. Zhu, Y. Ren, O. Alvi, J. Yao, A. Hawes, S. Jhangiani, G. Fowler, A. San Lucas, C. Kovar, A. Cree, H. Dinh, J. Santibanez, V. Joshi, M.L. Gonzalez-Garay, C.A. Miller, A. Milosavljevic, C. Sougnez, T. Fennell, S. Mahan, J. Wilkinson, L. Ziaugra, R. Onofrio, T. Bloom, R. Nicol, K. Ardlie, J. Baldwin, S. Gabriel, R.S. Fulton, M.D. McLellan, D.E. Larson, X. Shi, R. Abbott, L. Fulton, K. Chen, D.C. Koboldt, M.C. Wendl, R. Meyer, Y. Tang, L. Lin, J.R. Osborne, B.H. Dunford-Shore, T.L. Miner, K. Delehaunty, C. Markovic, G. Swift, W. Courtney, C. Pohl, S. Abbott, A. Hawkins, S. Leong, C. Haipek, H. Schmidt, M. Wiechert, T. Vickery, S. Scott, D.J. Dooling, A. Chinwalla, G.M. Weinstock, M. O'Kelly, J. Robinson, G. Alexe, R. Beroukhim, S. Carter, D. Chiang, J. Gould, S. Gupta, J. Korn, C. Mermel, J. Mesirov, S. Monti, H. Nguyen, M. Parkin, M. Reich, N. Stransky, L. Garraway, T. Golub, A. Protopopov, I. Perna, S. Aronson, N. Sathiamoorthy, G. Ren, H. Kim, S.W. Kong, Y. Xiao, I.S. Kohane, J. Seidman, L. Cope, F. Pan, D. Van Den Berg, L. Van Neste, J.M. Yi, J.Z. Li, A. Southwick, S. Brady, A. Aggarwal, T. Chung, G. Sherlock, J.D. Brooks, L.R. Jakkula, A.V. Lapuk, H. Marr, S. Dorton, Y.G. Choi, J. Han, A. Ray, V. Wang, S. Durinck, M. Robinson, N.J. Wang, K. Vranizan, V. Peng, E. Van Name, G.V. Fontenay, J. Ngai, J.G. Conboy, B. Parvin, H.S. Feiler, T.P. Speed, N.D. Socci, A. Olshen, A. Lash, B. Reva, Y. Antipin, A. Stukalov, B. Gross, E. Cerami, W.Q. Wang, L.-X. Qin, V.E. Seshan, L. Villafania, M. Cavatore, L. Borsu, A. Viale, W. Gerald, M.D. Topal, Y. Qi, S. Balu, Y. Shi, G. Wu, M. Bittner, T. Shelton, E. Lenkiewicz, S. Morris, D. Beasley, S. Sanders, R. Sfeir, J. Chen, D. Nassau, L. Feng, E. Hickey, C. Schaefer, S. Madhavan, K. Buetow, A. Barker, J. Vockley, C. Compton, J. Vaught, P. Fielding, F. Collins, P. Good, M. Guyer, B. Ozenberger, J. Peterson, E. Thomson, Cancer Genome Atlas Research Network, Tissue Source Sites, Genome Sequencing Centers, Cancer Genome Characterization Centers, and Project Teams. 2008. Comprehensive genomic characterization defines human glioblastoma genes and core pathways. *Nature* 455: 1061–1068.

Coroller, T., P. Grossmann, Y. Hou, S. Lee, R. Mak, and H. Aerts. 2015. CT-Based Volumetric Features Are Associated with Somatic Mutations in Lung Cancer. *Medical Physics* 42: 3322.

Diehn, M., C. Nardini, D.S. Wang, S. McGovern, M. Jayaraman, Y. Liang, K. Alclape, S. Cha, and M.D. Kuo. 2008. Identification of noninvasive imaging surrogates for brain tumor gene-expression modules. *Proceedings of the National Academy of Sciences of the United States of America* 105: 5213–5218.

Drabycz, S., G. Roldán, P. de Robles, D. Adler, J.B. McIntyre, A.M. Magliocco, J.G. Cairncross, and J.R. Mitchell. 2010. An analysis of image texture, tumor location, and MGMT promoter methylation in glioblastoma using magnetic resonance imaging. *Neuroimage* 49: 1398–1405.

Eckel-Passow, J.E., D.H. Lachance, A.M. Molinaro, K.M. Walsh, P.A. Decker, H. Sicotte, M. Pekmezci, T. Rice, M.L. Kosel, I.V. Smirnov, G. Sarkar, A.A. Caron, T.M. Kollmeyer, C.E. Praska, A.R. Chada, C. Halder, H.M. Hansen, L.S. McCoy, P.M. Bracci, R. Marshall, S. Zheng, G.F. Reis, A.R. Pico, B.P. O'Neill, J.C. Buckner, C. Giannini, J.T. Huse, A. Perry, T. Tihan, M.S. Berger, S.M. Chang, M.D. Prados, J. Wiemels, J.K. Wiencke, M.R. Wrensch, and R.B. Jenkins. 2015. Glioma groups based on 1p/19q, IDH, and TERT promoter mutations in tumors. *N Engl J Med* 372: 2499–2508.

Efron, B. 1979. 1977 Rietz Lecture – Bootstrap methods – Another look at the jackknife. *Annals of Statistics* 7: 1–26.

Ellingson, B.M. 2015. Radiogenomics and imaging phenotypes in glioblastoma: Novel observations and correlation with molecular characteristics. *Curr Neurol Neurosci Rep* 15: 506.

Ertosun, M.G., D.L. Rubin. 2015. Automated grading of gliomas using deep learning in digital pathology images: A modular approach with ensemble of convolutional neural networks, AMIA Annual Symposium Proceedings, American Medical Informatics Association, 1899.

Galloway, M. 1975. Texture analysis using gray level run lengths. *Computer Graphics and Image Processing* 4: 172–179.

Gevaert, O., L.A. Mitchell, A.S. Achrol, J. Xu, S. Echegaray, G.K. Steinberg, S.H. Cheshier, S. Napel, G. Zaharchuk, and S.K. Plevritis. 2014. Glioblastoma multiforme: Exploratory radiogenomic analysis by using quantitative image features. *Radiology* 273: 168–174.

Guo, E., Z. Wang, and S. Wang. 2016. MiR-200c and miR-141 inhibit ZEB1 synergistically and suppress glioma cell growth and migration. *Eur Rev Med Pharmacol Sci* 20: 3385–3391.

Gutman, D.A., L.A.D. Cooper, S.N. Hwang, C.A. Holder, J. Gao, T.D. Aurora, W.D. Dunn Jr., L. Scarpace, T. Mikkelsen, R. Jain, M. Wintermark, M. Jilwan, P. Raghavan, E. Huang, R.J. Clifford, P. Mongkolwat, V. Kleper, J. Freymann, J. Kirby, P.O. Zinn, C.S. Moreno, C. Jaffe, R. Colen, D.L. Rubin, J. Saltz, A. Flanders, and D.J. Brat. 2013. MR imaging predictors of molecular profile and survival: Multi-institutional study of the TCGA glioblastoma data set. *Radiology* 267: 560–569.

Gutman, D.A., W.D. Dunn, P. Grossmann, L.A. Cooper, C.A. Holder, K.L. Ligon, B.M. Alexander, and H.J. Aerts. 2015. Somatic mutations associated with MRI-derived volumetric features in glioblastoma. *Neuroradiology* 57: 1227–1237.

Haralick, R.M., K. Shanmuga, and I. Dinstein. 1973. Textural features for Image Classification. *IEEE Transactions on Systems Man and Cybernetics* SMC3: 610–621.

Harris, R.J., T.F. Cloughesy, W.B. Pope, P.L. Nghiemphu, A. Lai, T. Zaw, J. Czernin, M.E. Phelps, W. Chen, and B.M. Ellingson. 2012. 18F-FDOPA and 18F-FLT positron emission tomography parametric response maps predict response in recurrent malignant gliomas treated with bevacizumab. *Neuro Oncol* 14: 1079–1089.

Hsu, W., M.K. Markey, and M.D. Wang. 2013. Biomedical imaging informatics in the era of precision medicine: Progress, challenges, and opportunities. *Journal of the American Medical Informatics Association* 20: 1010–1013.

Jamshidi, N., M. Diehn, M. Bredel, and M.D. Kuo. 2014. Illuminating radiogenomic characteristics of glioblastoma multiforme through integration of MR imaging, messenger RNA expression, and DNA copy number variation. *Radiology* 270: 1–2.

Jiao, Y., H. Berman, T.-R. Kiehl, and S. Torquato. 2011. Spatial organization and correlations of cell nuclei in brain tumors. *PLoS ONE* 6: e27323.

Karunanithi, S., P. Sharma, A. Kumar, B.C. Khangembam, G.P. Bandopadhyaya, R. Kumar, D.K. Gupta, A. Malhotra, and C. Bal. 2013. 18F-FDOPA PET/CT for detection of recurrence in patients with glioma: Prospective comparison with 18F-FDG PET/CT. *Eur J Nucl Med Mol Imaging* 40: 1025–1035.

Kassner, A., and R.E. Thornhill. 2010. Texture analysis: A review of neurologic MR imaging applications. *AJNR Am J Neuroradiol* 31: 809–816.

Kerns, S.L., H. Ostrer, and B.S. Rosenstein. 2014. Radiogenomics : Using genetics to identify cancer patients at risk for development of adverse effects following radiotherapy. *Cancer Discovery* 4: 155–165.

Kickingereder, P., S. Burth, A. Wick, M. Götz, O. Eidel, H.P. Schlemmer, K.H. Maier-Hein, W. Wick, M. Bendszus, A. Radbruch, and D. Bonekamp. 2016. Radiomic profiling of glioblastoma: Identifying an imaging predictor of patient survival with improved performance over established clinical and radiologic risk models. *Radiology* 280: 880–889.

Kim, S., E. Dougherty, J. Barrera, Y. Chen, M. Bittner, and J. Trent. 2002. Strong feature sets from small samples. *Journal of Computational Biology* 9: 127–146.

Kong, J., L.A. Cooper, F. Wang, J. Gao, G. Teodoro, L. Scarpace, T. Mikkelsen, M.J. Schniederjan, C.S. Moreno, and J.H. Saltz. 2013. Machine-based morphologic analysis of glioblastoma using whole-slide pathology images uncovers clinically relevant molecular correlates. *PloS one* 8: e81049.

Kramer, M.A. 1991. Nonlinear principal component analysis using autoassociative neural networks. *Aiche Journal* 37: 233–243.

Kumar, V., Y. Gu, S. Basu, A. Berglund, S.A. Eschrich, M.B. Schabath, K. Forster, H.J.W.L. Aerts, A. Dekker, D. Fenstermacher, D.B. Goldgof, L.O. Hall, P. Lambin, Y. Balagurunathan, R.A. Gatenby, and R.J. Gillies. 2012. Radiomics: The process and the challenges. *Magnetic Resonance Imaging* 30: 1234–1248.

Kumar, D., A. Wong, and D. Clausi. 2015. Lung nodule classification using deep features in CT Images, IEEE, Computer and Robot Vision (CRV), 2015 12th Conference on, 2015.

Kuo, M.D., J. Gollub, C.B. Sirlin, C. Ooi, and X. Chen. 2007. Radiogenomic analysis to identify imaging phenotypes associated with drug response gene expression programs in hepatocellular carcinoma. *Journal of Vascular and Interventional Radiology* 18: 821–831.

la Fougère, C., B. Suchorska, P. Bartenstein, F.-W. Kreth, and J.-C. Tonn. 2011. Molecular imaging of gliomas with PET: Opportunities and limitations. *Neuro Oncology* 13 (8): 806–819. nor054.

Lambin, P., E. Rios-Velazquez, R. Leijenaar, S. Carvalho, R.G.P.M. van Stiphout, P. Granton, C.M.L. Zegers, R. Gillies, R. Boellard, A. Dekker, H.J.W.L. Aerts, and I.C.C.C. Qu. 2012. Radiomics: Extracting more information from medical images using advanced feature analysis. *European Journal of Cancer* 48: 441–446.

Lambin, P., E. Roelofs, B. Reymen, E.R. Velazquez, J. Buijsen, C.M.L. Zegers, S. Carvalho, R.T.H. Leijenaar, G. Nalbantov, C. Oberije, M.S. Marshall, F. Hoebers, E.G.C. Troost, R.G.P.M. van Stiphout, W. van Elmpt, T. van der Weijden, L. Boersma, V. Valentini, and A. Dekker. 2013. Rapid Learning health care in oncology' – An approach towards decision support systems enabling customised radiotherapy. *Radiotherapy and Oncology* 109: 159–164.

Lee, J., S. Narang, J.J. Martinez, G. Rao, and A. Rao. 2015. Associating spatial diversity features of radiologically defined tumor habitats with epidermal growth factor receptor driver status and 12-month survival in glioblastoma: Methods and preliminary investigation. *J Med Imaging (Bellingham)* 2: 041006.

Liang, H., R. Wang, Y. Jin, J. Li, and S. Zhang. 2016. MiR-422a acts as a tumor suppressor in glioblastoma by targeting PIK3CA. *Am J Cancer Res* 6: 1695–1707.

Liu, G., X. Yuan, Z. Zeng, P. Tunici, H. Ng, I.R. Abdulkadir, L. Lu, D. Irvin, K.L. Black, and J.S. Yu. 2006. Analysis of gene expression and chemoresistance of CDI33(+) cancer stem cells in glioblastoma. *Molecular Cancer* 5: 67.

Louis, D.N., H. Ohgaki, O.D. Wiestler, W.K. Cavenee, P.C. Burger, A. Jouvet, B.W. Scheithauer, and P. Kleihues. 2007. The 2007 WHO classification of tumours of the central nervous system. *Acta neuropathologica* 114: 97–109.

Louis, D.N., A. Perry, G. Reifenberger, A. von Deimling, D. Figarella-Branger, W.K. Cavenee, H. Ohgaki, O.D. Wiestler, P. Kleihues, and D.W. Ellison. 2016. The 2016 World Health Organization classification of tumors of the Central Nervous System: A summary. *Acta Neuropathologica* 131: 803–820.

Mallat, S. 1989. A theory for multiresolution signal decomposition: The wavelet representation. *IEEE Transactions on Pattern Analysis and Machine Intelligence* 11: 674–693.

Mishra, D., R. Dash, A.K. Rath, and M. Acharya. 2011. Feature selection in gene expression data using principal component analysis and rough set theory. *Software Tools and Algorithms for Biological Systems* 696: 91–100.

Mousavi, H.S., V. Monga, G. Rao, and A.U. Rao. 2015. Automated discrimination of lower and higher grade gliomas based on histopathological image analysis. *Journal of pathology informatics* 6: 15.

Naeini, K.M., W.B. Pope, T.F. Cloughesy, R.J. Harris, A. Lai, A. Eskin, R. Chowdhury, H.S. Phillips, P.L. Nghiemphu, Y. Behbahanian, and B.M. Ellingson. 2013. Identifying the mesenchymal molecular subtype of glioblastoma using quantitative volumetric analysis of anatomic magnetic resonance images. *Neuro Oncol* 15: 626–634.

Nafe, R., and W. Schlote. 2004. Histomorphometry of brain tumours. *Neuropathology and applied neurobiology* 30: 315–328.

Nayak, N., H. Chang, A. Borowsky, and P. Spellman, B. Parvin. 2013. Classification of tumor histopathology via sparse feature learning, 2013 IEEE 10th International Symposium on Biomedical Imaging, IEEE, 410–413.

Nihashi, T., I.J. Dahabreh, and T. Terasawa. 2013. Diagnostic accuracy of PET for recurrent glioma diagnosis: A meta-analysis. *AJNR Am J Neuroradiol* 34: 944–950. S941-911.

Noor, A.M., L. Holmberg, C. Gillett, and A. Grigoriadis. 2015. Big data: The challenge for small research groups in the era of cancer genomics. *British Journal of Cancer* 113: 1405–1412.

O'Driscoll, A., J. Daugelaite, and R.D. Sleator. 2013. 'Big data', Hadoop and cloud computing in genomics. *Journal of Biomedical Informatics* 46: 774–781.

Parmar, C., E. Rios Velazquez, R. Leijenaar, M. Jermoumi, S. Carvalho, R.H. Mak, S. Mitra, B.U. Shankar, R. Kikinis, B. Haibe-Kains, P. Lambin, and H.J. Aerts. 2014. Robust Radiomics feature quantification using semiautomatic volumetric segmentation. *PLoS One* 9: e102107.

Pope, W.B., J. Sayre, A. Perlina, J.P. Villablanca, P.S. Mischel, and T.F. Cloughesy. 2005. MR imaging correlates of survival in patients with high-grade gliomas. *AJNR Am J Neuroradiol* 26: 2466–2474.

Porz, N., S. Bauer, A. Pica, P. Schucht, J. Beck, R.K. Verma, J. Slotboom, M. Reyes, and R. Wiest. 2014. Multi-modal glioblastoma segmentation: Man versus machine. *Plos One* 9: e96873.

Pötzi, C., A. Becherer, C. Marosi, G. Karanikas, M. Szabo, R. Dudczak, K. Kletter, and S. Asenbaum. 2007. [11C] methionine and [18F] fluorodeoxyglucose PET in the follow-up of glioblastoma multiforme. *J Neurooncol* 84: 305–314.

Rios Velazquez, E., R. Meier, W.D. Dunn, B. Alexander, R. Wiest, S. Bauer, D.A. Gutman, M. Reyes, and H.J. Aerts. 2015. Fully automatic GBM segmentation in the TCGA-GBM dataset: Prognosis and correlation with VASARI features. *Sci Rep* 5: 16822.

Rosenstein, B.S., C.M. West, S.M. Bentzen, J. Alsner, C.N. Andreassen, D. Azria, G.C. Barnett, M. Baumann, N. Burnet, J. Chang-Claude, E.Y. Chuang, C.E. Coles, A. Dekker, K. De Ruyck, D. De Ruysscher, K. Drumea, A.M. Dunning, D. Easton, R. Eeles, L. Fachal, S. Gutiérrez-Enríquez, K. Haustermans, L.A. Henríquez-Hernández, T. Imai, G.D. Jones, S.L. Kerns, Z. Liao, K. Onel, H. Ostrer, M. Parliament, P.D. Pharoah, T.R. Rebbeck, C.J. Talbot, H. Thierens, A. Vega, J.S. Witte, P. Wong, F. Zenhausern, and R. Consortium. 2014. Radiogenomics: Radiobiology enters the era of big data and team science. *Int J Radiat Oncol Biol Phys* 89: 709–713.

Song, S., A. Fajol, X. Tu, B. Ren, and S. Shi. 2016. miR-204 suppresses the development and progression of human glioblastoma by targeting ATF2. *Oncotarget* 7 (43): 70058–70065.

Surowka, A.D., D. Adamek, E. Radwanska, M. Lankosz, and M. Szczerbowska-Boruchowska. 2014. A methodological approach to the characterization of brain gliomas, by means of semiautomatic morphometric analysis. *Image Analysis and Stereolog* 33 (2014): 18.

Verhaak, R.G.W., K.A. Hoadley, E. Purdom, V. Wang, Y. Qi, M.D. Wilkerson, C.R. Miller, L. Ding, T. Golub, J.P. Mesirov, G. Alexe, M. Lawrence, M. O'Kelly, P. Tamayo, B.A. Weir, S. Gabriel, W. Winckler, S. Gupta, L. Jakkula, H.S. Feiler, J.G. Hodgson, C.D. James, J.N. Sarkaria, C. Brennan, A. Kahn, P.T. Spellman, R.K. Wilson, T.P. Speed, J.W. Gray, M. Meyerson, G. Getz, C.M. Perou, D.N. Hayes, and The Cancer Genome Atlas Research Network. 2010. Integrated genomic analysis identifies clinically relevant subtypes of glioblastoma characterized by abnormalities in PDGFRA, IDH1, EGFR, and NF1. *Cancer Cell* 17: 98–110.

Vu, T.H., H.S. Mousavi, V. Monga, U.A. Rao, and G. Rao. 2015. DFDL: Discriminative feature-oriented dictionary learning for histopathological image classification, 2015 IEEE 12th International Symposium on Biomedical Imaging (ISBI), IEEE, 990–994.

Wangaryattawanich, P., M. Hatami, J. Wang, G. Thomas, A. Flanders, J. Kirby, M. Wintermark, E.S. Huang, A.S. Bakhtiari, M.M. Luedi, S.S. Hashmi, D.L. Rubin, J.Y. Chen, S.N. Hwang, J. Freymann, C.A. Holder, P.O. Zinn, and R.R. Colen. 2015. Multicenter imaging outcomes study of The Cancer Genome Atlas glioblastoma patient cohort: Imaging predictors of overall and progression-free survival. *Neuro Oncol* 17: 1525–1537.

Williams, M.S., M.D. Ritchie, and P.R.O. Payne. 2015. Interdisciplinary training to build an informatics workforce for precision medicine. *Applied and Translational Genomics* 6: 28–30.

Wold, S., A. Ruhe, H. Wold, and W.J. Dunn. 1984. The collinearity problem in linear-regression – The Partial least-squares (Pls) approach to generalized inverses. *Siam Journal on Scientific and Statistical Computing* 5: 735–743.

Xu, Y., Z. Jia, Y. Ai, F. Zhang, M. Lai, I. Eric, and C. Chang. 2015. Deep convolutional activation features for large scale brain tumor histopathology image classification and segmentation, 2015 IEEE International Conference on Acoustics, Speech and Signal Processing (ICASSP), IEEE., 947–951.

Yang, D., G. Rao, J. Martinez, A. Veeraraghavan, and A. Rao. 2015. Evaluation of tumor-derived MRI-texture features for discrimination of molecular subtypes and prediction of 12-month survival status in glioblastoma. *Medical Physics* 42: 6725–6735.

Yuan, X.P., J. Curtin, Y.Z. Xiong, G.T. Liu, S. Waschsmann-Hogiu, D.L. Farkas, K.L. Black, and J.S. Yu. 2004. Isolation of cancer stem cells from adult glioblastoma multiforme. *Oncogene* 23: 9392–9400.

Zhou, Y., H. Chang, K. Barner, P. Spellman, and B. Parvin. 2014. Classification of histology sections via multispectral convolutional sparse coding, 2014. *IEEE Conference on Computer Vision and Pattern Recognition, IEEE* 2014: 3081–3088.

Zhu, H., B.G. Goodyear, M.L. Lauzon, R.A. Brown, G.S. Mayer, A.G. Law, L. Mansinha, and J.R. Mitchell. 2003. A new local multiscale Fourier analysis for medical imaging. *Medical Physics* 30: 1134–1141.

Zinn, P.O., B. Majadan, P. Sathyan, S.K. Singh, S. Majumder, F.A. Jolesz, and R.R. Colen. 2011. Radiogenomic Mapping of Edema/Cellular Invasion MRI-Phenotypes in Glioblastoma Multiforme. *Plos One* 6: e25451.

Chapter 7
Next-Generation Sequencing in Glioblastoma Personalized Therapy

Jagriti Pal, Vikas Patil, and Kumaravel Somasundaram

Abstract The most common and aggressive form of intracranial tumors is glioblastoma (GBM). These tumors show significant amount of proliferation, invasion, angiogenesis and necrosis. The current treatment modality that includes surgery, radiotherapy and temozolomide chemotherapy fails to provide great benefit with the median survival remaining at a dismal 15–17 months. The response to standard therapy is highly variable which is primarily determined by the differences in the genetic makeup of the tumor. Hence, it is required that clinicians stratify the patients based on prognostic features such that appropriate therapy can be given as per aggressiveness of the tumor. However, it has been observed that almost all GBM tumors recur. This demands the necessity of alternative therapeutic options for the treatment of GBM. In recent times, Next Generation Sequencing (NGS) based techniques help us to interrogate the genome of cells in a comprehensive manner. Intensive studies have revealed various genetic alterations typical to GBM, e.g., TP53 mutation and loss, EGFR amplification and mutation, INK4a/ARF mutation, MDM2/4 amplification or overexpression, PTEN mutation and loss of heterozygosity (LOH) in chromosome 10p and 10q. Through the past few decades, many studies have been carried out to identify small molecule inhibitors and antibodies against various molecules deregulated in different cancers such that they can be used for targeted therapy. Moreover, each tumor harbors a spectrum of genetic alterations that are different from another tumor. Hence, personalized therapy, tailored to target tumor-specific alterations is the approach to be developed for improvement of survival of GBM patients. For identification of genetic alterations in each tumor, sequencing of the tumor DNA has to be carried out. For that purpose, NGS-based targeted sequencing of all known GBM-specific driver alterations is a lucrative option. In this chapter, we have discussed about how targeted sequencing can be used for identifying all driver genetic alterations in each GBM tumor such that those molecules can be targeted using small molecule inhibitors and antibodies against them.

J. Pal • V. Patil • K. Somasundaram (✉)
Department of Microbiology and Cell Biology, Indian Institute of Science,
Bangalore 560012, India
e-mail: skumar@mcbl.iisc.ernet.in; ksomasundaram1@gmail.com

© Springer International Publishing AG 2017
K. Somasundaram (ed.), *Advances in Biology and Treatment of Glioblastoma*,
Current Cancer Research, DOI 10.1007/978-3-319-56820-1_7

Keywords Personalized therapy • Driver genetic alterations • Patient stratification • Next generation sequencing • Targeted sequencing • Targeted therapy

Abbreviations

CNA	Copy Number Alteration
CNS	Central Nervous System
GBM	Glioblastoma
Indel	Insertion/deletion
NGS	Next Generation Sequencing
SNV	Single Nucleotide Variation
TCGA	The Cancer Genome Atlas
WHO	World Health Organization

7.1 Introduction

Glial cells, the supporting cells for the neurons, comprise of approximately 50% of the nervous system with its percentage varying from 10 to 90% depending on the portion of the brain (Herculano-Houzel 2014). Malignancy of glial cells is termed as glioma. Gliomas comprise of 30% of all tumors of the central nervous system (CNS) and 80% of malignant brain tumors (ABTA 2014). The most common and lethal type of intracranial tumors include the astrocytomas which arise from particular type of glial cells called astrocytes. It is divided into four groups according to World Health organization (WHO) classification based on histopathology (Louis et al. 2007). Grade I or pilocytic astrocytoma is benign in nature. However, the other three grades are progressively more malignant, from grade II (diffused astrocytoma) to grade III (anaplastic astrocytoma) to grade IV or glioblastoma (GBM). GBM is the most common, highly aggressive tumor that arises in the brain and accounts for 12–15% of all brain tumors and 60–75% of all astrocytic tumors (D. Doyle et al. 2005). GBMs are fast growing tumors that are highly infiltrative and treatment refractory. Without treatment, a GBM patient survives only ~3 months (Schapira 2007); and even after surgical resection, chemotherapy and radiotherapy, the median survival for GBM patients is only 15–17 months (Arvold and Reardon 2014; Stupp et al. 2009). It is more prevalent among older patients in the age group of 45–70 years although it is also observed among children and young adults (Mechtler 2009). GBMs are divided into two categories on the basis of their origin - primary GBMs account for 90% of GBM cases and manifest *de novo* without prior evidence of a pre-existing tumor of lower grade; while secondary GBMs develop through malignant progression of lower grade astrocytomas (Furnari et al. 2007). Primary GBM is more common in older patients, >60 years of age, and is more aggressive in nature, while secondary GBM is more prevalent in younger adults of ~45 years of age and have a better survival rate possibly due to mutation in Isocitrate Dehydrogenase (IDH) genes. Hence, primary GBMs are referred to as IDH wild-type class while secondary GBMs are referred to as IDH mutant class as per 2016 classification scheme (Louis et al. 2016). The cellular make up comprises of poorly differentiated, fusiform, round, or pleomorphic cells and hyper chromatic nuclei. The presence of multinucleated giant cells is typical but it is associated with a more malignant clinical course. Mitotic activity is usually high (denoted by MIB-1 immunohistochemistry), the growth fraction being in the range of 5–25% (Ohgaki and Kleihues 2013). The characteristic of GBM which distinguishes it from other astrocytomas is the presence of microvascular proliferation and necrosis. Necrosis is caused by depletion in blood supply in parts of the tumor and this may comprise more than 80% of the total tumor mass. Particularly typical to GBM are foci of necrosis surrounded by radially oriented pseudopalisading tumor cell nuclei which often show a high degree of proliferative activity (Burger 1995).

7.2 Conventional Therapy for the Treatment of GBM

Traditional therapy, often referred to as conventional therapy, comprises of methods by which bulk tumor cells are surgically removed to the greatest extent possible followed by radiation therapy and chemotherapy. The combination of above three methods of treatment and their dosage depends on the type of cancer, location of the tumor and how advanced it is (Rizzo and Rhonda 2002). For GBM, this kind of therapy has been developed and applied for years. The current conventional treatment method includes maximal surgical resection followed by radiotherapy and temozolomide chemotherapy (Sathornsumetee et al. 2007). Survival of GBM patients receiving adjuvant temozolomide along with radiotherapy was found to be longer compared to those receiving radiotherapy alone (Stupp et al. 2005). Both radiotherapy and chemotherapy target rapidly dividing cancer cells by invoking DNA damage response and apoptosis. This works for cancer cells because the characteristic of enhanced cell division leads to DNA being exposed in open chromatin form and thus these cells are more susceptible to damage by agents like radiation and DNA alkylating chemicals. However, this also results in the damage and death of normal cells which are highly proliferative such as, the epithelium and lymphocytes (Mitchison 2012).

7.3 Personalized Therapy: Patient Stratification and Targeted Therapy

The response to conventional treatment is variable between different patients and this makes it difficult for oncologists in tailoring the treatment options as per the needs of patients. Moreover, treatment options should be explored such that it causes lesser health hazard to the individual patient. For example, for patients older than 70 years, less aggressive therapy is the usual course of action and this is achieved by using radiation or temozolomide alone (Glantz et al. 2003; Keime-Guibert et al. 2007). Apart from age being a reason behind differential therapeutic response, the various genetic and epigenetic changes present in tumor cells that vary between individuals are major factors in differential responses to conventional therapy. This is referred to as *inter-tumoral heterogeneity* (Almendro et al. 2013). Hence, a new approach undertaken for tailor-made or personalized treatment is *patient stratification*. Stratification of patients basically involves assessment of the clinical outcome of patients including survival and therapeutic outcome based on molecular signatures. For instance, if patients by virtue of the molecular changes present can be predicted to be better survivors, they need not be subjected to aggressive treatment as more aggressive the therapy, the suffering and health hazards for the patient is more. Few such molecular markers have been identified through the years. For example, patients harboring mutation in IDH genes have better survival and show improved outcomes with radiotherapy and temozolomide chemotherapy (Vigneswaran et al. 2015). It has been observed that O6 -methylguanine DNA methyltransferase (MGMT) promoter methylation in GBM tumor leads to better response to temozolomide and improved median survival (> 3 years); while patients with unmethylated MGMT promoter show resistance to temozolomide and hence may be subjected to alternative therapies (Martinez and Esteller 2010; Thon et al. 2013). With advances in the understanding of molecular aspects of GBM pathology, information regarding accurate risk stratification of GBM patients through prognostic signatures has been identified by various groups e.g., a 9-gene methylation signature developed by our group divides GBM patients into high risk and low risk groups with significant difference in survival (Shukla et al. 2013). There are multiple other signatures which can be used for patient stratification, such as, gene expression subtypes (Verhaak et al. 2010), G-CIMP classification (Noushmehr et al. 2010), 9 gene mRNA signature (Colman et al. 2010), 10 miRNA signature (Srinivasan et al. 2011) add 14 gene mRNA signature (Arimappamagan et al. 2013) etc. A more detailed overview of various prognostic markers/signatures identified for the stratification of GBM patients have been discussed by Shukla et al. 2014.

Due to the high infiltrative nature and aggressiveness, GBM tumor mass cannot be resected completely and they recur (Wen and Kesari 2008); the median time of recurrence after conventional/standard therapy is 6.9 months (Stupp et al. 2009). These recurrent tumors are resistant to the standard radio- and chemo-therapeutic regimes (Nakano and Mangum 2011). Also, a small percentage of GBM tumor cells are less differentiated, stem-like and quiescent in nature. They have the capacity of self-renewal and can differentiate and give rise to bulk tumor cells. The quiescent nature of these cells gives them a survival advantage because their DNA is more protected in heterochromatin form and do not undergo damage during radiotherapy and chemotherapy. Also, by lieu of over-expression of transporters, they can rapidly expel out chemotherapeutic drugs. These cells thrive even after therapy and have been shown to be responsible for tumor recurrence (Lathia et al. 2015). Further, it has been observed that tumor cells from different sections of the same tumor have different genetic alterations and this phenomenon is known as *intra-tumoral heterogeneity* (Almendro et al. 2013). This happens due to the fact that tumor cells being rapidly dividing; they keep on accumulating numerous genetic changes. Hence, two different cells of the same tumor may acquire different mutations, and the proliferation of these cells to form daughter cells creates sub-populations of tumor cells with different genetic make-ups. All these factors highlight the importance of the development and application of an alternative therapeutic option i.e., targeted therapy (Wang et al. 2015).

Targeted therapy is a new trend in cancer therapeutics in which drugs that target particular molecules that are altered in a particular tumor are used to obliterate only cancer cells with little or no damage to the normal cells (Baudino 2015). Through the last few decades, various targetable molecules altered in different types of cancer and targeted therapeutic regimes have been identified and tested of which some have been approved by Food and Drug Administration (FDA) for use while some are in clinical trials (http://www.cancer.gov/about-cancer/treatment/drugs). Of note, Herceptin (Trastuzumab) is a humanized monoclonal antibody against receptor tyrosine kinase HER2 which is an approved targeted therapy used in metastatic breast carcinoma where this receptor has been found to be frequently over-expressed (Balduzzi et al. 2014). Gleevec or Imatinib is another example of a highly popular cancer targeted therapy; it is a tyrosine kinase inhibitor which particularly targets BCR-ABL fusion protein, a fusion event found in >95% of patients having chronic myelogenous leukemia (Goldman and Melo 2003).

Development of targeted therapeutic regime is of utmost importance in GBM as conventional therapies fail to eliminate the tumor completely leading to a poor median survival in patients and recurrence occurs in almost all cases. Enormous efforts have been undertaken through decades to understand the molecular pathogenesis of GBM and there have been several attempts at developing targeted therapies. For example, GBM is characterized by extensive and sustained angiogenesis which is primarily regulated by vascular endothelial growth factor (VEGF). Bevacizumab (Avastin), a humanized monoclonal antibody against VEGF had been taken forward for clinical trial (Gilbert et al. 2014). Inhibitors of EGFR, erlotinib, lapatinib and nimotuzumab have also been put to clinical trial as well as in experimental therapies (Padfield et al. 2015). From this, we understand that although advancement have been made in understanding GBM pathogenesis, ample effort has to be put in identification of targetable molecules in each tumor and formulating effective therapeutic options for individual GBM patients.

7.4 Identification of Driver Genetic alterations for Targeted Therapy

Changes in the DNA sequence is referred to as genetic alteration. A cancer genome harbors thousands of genetic alterations of which only a small percentage of changes is responsible for attributing a survival advantage to the cancer cells. These changes are also referred to as *driver genetic alterations*. However, due to the increased cell division and failing cell cycle checkpoints caused by these driver changes, the genome of a cancer cell acquires a large number of genetic aberrations that are of no consequence to the cancer cell's survival capabilities. These are termed as *passenger genetic alterations* or *hitchhikers* (Stratton et al. 2009).

Depending on the location of the alteration in the gene, the phenotype will be perceived by the cell. For example, alteration in the amino acid sequence of the protein may lead to activation or inactivation of the protein, alteration in the promoter region of the gene may lead to over- or under-expression of the gene product, mutation in the 3'UTR region of the gene may lead to differential miRNA binding thus leading to alteration in mRNA stability etc. Genetic changes include single nucleotide variations (SNVs), insertions/deletions (indels), copy number alterations (CNAs) and gene fusions.

SNVs or point mutations are alteration in a single nucleotide/base in the DNA sequence which arises due to either error in replication or chemical modification of bases by carcinogens. Essentially, SNVs present in the protein coding region of a gene can be of various types – 1) *silent mutation* - does not lead to any change in the amino acid of the protein due to degeneracy of codons i.e., different codons can code for same amino acid, 2) *missense mutation* - leads to a change in the amino acid sequence of proteins, 3) *non-sense mutation* - introduces a premature stop codon in the protein, thus giving rise to a truncated protein product and 4) *non-stop mutation* - leads to a loss of stop codon thus creating a longer protein product. An *indel* is an insertion or deletion of 1 or more bases (<1000 bases) in the DNA sequence of an organism. Indels present in the protein coding region of the genes can be classified into two types – 1) *frameshift indel* – leads to a change in the reading frame of the protein because they do not occur in multiples of three bases and this gives rise to a new protein sequence after the insertion or deletion of bases and 2) *in-frame indel* –occurs in multiples of three bases and hence do not change the reading frame of the protein. Duplication or deletion of large segments of DNA, ranging in size from thousands to millions of DNA bases, is referred to as copy number alteration (CNA). Such CNAs can encompass genes leading to dosage imbalances. Phenotypic effects of CNAs are brought about by changes in expression levels. *Gene fusion* is a genetic aberration where a hybrid gene is created from two previously separate genes giving rise to a fused protein product. This happens as a result of translocation or interstitial deletion or chromosomal inversion. The above four types of genetic alterations can lead to formation of driver oncogenes or inactivation of important tumor suppressor genes.

There are various traditional methods that can be employed to identify important driver genetic alterations in cancer patients. For example, SNVs and indels can be identified either by Sanger sequencing or by single strand conformation polymorphism (SSCP) (Rohlin et al. 2009). Additionally, mutant protein specific antibodies can be used to detect the presence of certain mutations, e.g., mutation in TP53 leads to accumulation of the protein in the cell which can be detected by immunohistochemistry (IHC) (Wang et al. 1995); mutation in IDH1 gene occurs only in a particular nucleotide in the gene sequence and hence can be detected by an antibody which can specifically identify the mutant protein (Cai et al. 2016). Over expression of oncoproteins and down regulation of tumor suppressor proteins in tumor tissues can be detected by IHC. Also, RNA level detection of genes can be carried out by semi quantitative PCR or real time qPCR techniques (Logan et al. 2009). CNAs and gene fusion events can be detected by fluorescent *in situ* hybridization techniques (Levsky and Singer 2003).

The traditional methods of identification of genetic alterations are cumbersome, time consuming and often expensive. Moreover, each genetic alteration requires to be queried individually. As mentioned before, due to intra-tumoral heterogeneity, sub-populations of tumor cells will contain different driver gene alterations. Hence, targeting one altered molecule will not obliterate those cells which depend on a different altered molecule for their survival. This is one of the reasons why targeted therapy against one molecule alone often fails in eradicating aggressive tumors such as GBM. Also, the traditional methods for detection of genetic aberrations are not sensitive enough to detect alterations in a small percentage of cancer cells. Any remaining tumor cells that survive therapy can later give rise to a recurrent tumor. Hence, comprehensive identification of the entire in-depth picture of genetic alterations of individual GBM patients will pave the path to formulation of tailor-made therapeutic regime for each patient.

Targeted sequencing makes it possible for evaluation of the alteration status of multiple genes in one go. This technique is both cost and time effective. It is a next-generation sequencing (NGS) based technique where selected driver genes are sequenced to determine mutations, indels, CNAs and gene fusions (Meldrum et al. 2011). Another type of targeted sequencing is *deep sequencing* where sequencing is carried out at a very high depth of coverage (> 500 X) and this allows us to look at alterations that are present in a small percentage of cancer cells (Mirebrahim et al. 2015). Hence, by this method, multiple driver genes can be identified and targeted; possibly resulting in decrease in total tumor burden.

There has been an explosion of data on understanding the genetic alteration spectrum of GBM and many targeted therapies have been identified and are under clinical trials (Bastien et al. 2015). While many companies and scientific groups are working towards development of comprehensive gene panels for identifying mutations in genes frequently altered in different cancers; very minimal efforts have been put towards developing and implementing in clinics an agglomerated genetic alteration panel to identify known driver genetic alterations particular to GBM. A targeted sequencing panel called GlioSeq has been formulated for all central nervous system (CNS) tumors and it consists of 30 genes covering more than 1360 CNS tumor-related hotspots (Nikiforova et al. 2016). However, this does not cover many of the driver genes known to be altered in GBM (Brennan et al. 2013; Frattini et al. 2013). Hence, to formulate a targeted sequencing panel for GBM, a thorough understanding of the genetic alteration landscape is of utmost necessity.

7.5 Recent Advances in the Understanding of the Genetic Alteration Landscape of GBM

The first comprehensive study on GBM samples was carried out by The Cancer Genome Atlas (TCGA) in 2008. They carried out investigations on copy number alterations (CNA), gene expression and DNA methylation aberrations in 206 GBM samples. Additionally, mutation status of ~220 genes was determined in 91 of 206 GBM samples using Sanger sequencing (Cancer Genome Atlas Research 2008). This study revealed three important signaling pathways which are significantly altered in GBM by multiple mechanisms – 1) RTK/Ras/PI3K pathway, 2) TP53 pathway and, 3) Rb pathway. Subsequently in 2013, two groups independently carried out comprehensive genomic characterization of GBM samples from TCGA using high throughput sequencing and microarray data, to find out genes undergoing genetic and epigenetic alterations in GBM scenario (Brennan et al. 2013; Frattini et al. 2013). The major findings in these two studies include top mutated genes in GBM patients such as, PIK3R1, PIK3CA, TP53, EGFR, RB1, NF1 and PTEN; frequent CNA alterations like, amplification of EGFR, PDGFRA, MDM2, CDK4, CDK6 etc. and deletion of PTEN, CDKN2A/B, TP53, NF1 etc.; and frequent gene fusions in EGFR and FGFR genes. Their studies have also validated previous findings that, the three most deregulated signaling pathways in GBM are TP53, RB and RTK/Ras/PI3K pathways (Brennan et al. 2013). In the same year, three groups also identified the importance of hTERT promoter mutation in GBM pathogenesis and found that 55% of GBM patients harbor these changes in their tumor cells (Arita et al. 2013; Killela et al. 2013; Nonoguchi et al. 2013).

7.5.1 Pathways Altered in GBM

The genetic alterations in GBM mainly target pathways involved in cell proliferation, cell survival (apoptosis and necrosis), invasion, and angiogenesis. Molecular players of three main pathways are involved in the above biological processes and they acquire specific genetic aberrations which primarily lead to gliomagenesis (Brennan et al. 2013).

A. RTK/Ras/PI3K pathway: Mitogenic pathways play a major role in cell proliferation and survival (Zhang and Liu 2002). Receptor-driven mitogenic pathways get activated in GBM by different mechanisms, e.g., genomic amplification, and/or mutation of the receptor leading to its constitutive activation, overexpression of ligands and receptors etc. The epidermal growth factor (EGF) and platelet-derived growth factor (PDGF) pathways have important roles in both CNS development and gliomagenesis. EGF receptor (EGFR) is altered in >50% of GBM patients where mutation and/or amplification in the gene is observed and the amplified genes have been found to be frequently rearranged (Brennan et al. 2013). An EGFR variant called EGFRvIII (deletion of exons 2–7) is present in 20–30% of patients which is a constitutively active variant of EGFR capable of increasing proliferation of GBM cells (Holland et al. 1998). Hence, EGFR has been a prime target for targeted therapy using kinase inhibitors and immunotherapy. Another RTK, PDGF receptor (PDGFRA) gets frequently altered in ~10% of GBM patients. PDGFR and its ligands are often over-expressed suggesting an autocrine loop for this pathway (Hermanson et al. 1992).

Phosphatidylinositol-3-kinases (PI3Ks), when stimulated by mitogenic signals, catalyze phosphorylation of phosphatidylinositol-4,5-bisphosphate [PtdIns(4,5) P2] to produce phosphatidylinositol-3-4,5-trisphosphate [PtdIns(3,4,5)P3]. This creates docking sites for a various signaling proteins containing domains capable of binding to PtdIns(3,4,5)P3 and thus activates downstream pro-proliferative and pro-survival pathways (Nieto-Sampedro et al. 2011). PI3Ks comprise of catalytic subunits encoded by PIK3CA, PIK3CB and PIK3CD genes and regulatory subunits encoded by PIK3R1, PIK3R2 and PIK3R3 genes. Genetic alterations in the above genes occur in 25% of GBM patients with changes in PIK3CA gene occurring in ~15% of patients (Knobbe and Reifenberger 2003). The action of PI3Ks is antagonized by phosphatase, PTEN, which again undergoes alterations by mutation or deletion in 41% of GBM patients (Choe et al. 2003). Downstream to RTK signaling pathway, activation of small GTP-bound protein RAS leads to stimulation of downstream pro-proliferative signals like MAPK or PI3K pathways. Although RAS gets altered genetically in only 1% of GBM patients, it remains active in the cancer cells by activation of upstream signaling molecules (Guha et al. 1997). Additionally, a negative regulator of RAS is NF1 gene which gets inactivated by mutation or deletion in 10% of GBM patients (Brennan et al. 2013). Mutations in RTKs like EGFR and PDGFR or downstream molecules RAS, RAF and negative regulator of RAS i.e. NF1, results in activation of MAPK signaling cascade leading to phosphorylation of effector molecules such as MEK and ERK. In fact, it was observed that NF1-deficient GBM cells are sensitive to MEK inhibitors (See et al. 2012).

B. TP53 pathway: TP53 is a tumor suppressor that inhibits cycling of cell with unstable genomes. It achieves this function by either halting the cell cycle in the G1 phase or prompting programmed cell death. TP53 is a transcription factor, and post-translational modifications caused by various genotoxic and cytotoxic stress-sensing agents leads to its stabilization (Lavin and Gueven 2006). Consequently, it binds and transcriptionally regulates the promoters of >2500 potential effector genes. The best characterized of these effectors is CDK2 inhibitor, p21 encoded by CDKN1A gene (Lavin and Gueven 2006). TP53 itself gets altered by mutation or deletion in 28% of GBM patients. However, regulators of this pathway undergo genetic aberrations in GBM scenario, rendering this pathway to be altered in greater than 80% of GBM patients.TP53 function is regulated by a number of proteins of which the ubiquitin ligase, MDM2, and its homologue, MDM4, are prominent negative regulators. They bind to TP53 and ubiquitilate it, ultimately leading to its degradation through the proteasomal pathway. It has been observed that both MDM2 and MDM4 get altered through gene duplication and such phenomenon is seen in 7.6% and 7.2% of GBM patients respectively (Brennan et al. 2013).

C. RB pathway: In the hypo-phosphorylated state, RB blocks progression through cell cycle by sequestration of the E2F family of transcription factors, which in turn prevents the transactivation of genes essential for progression through the cell cycle. Mitogenic signal stimulation leads to the induction of cyclin D1 and its association with the cyclin-dependent kinases, CDK4 and CDK6. The activated CDK complexes then phosphorylate RB which leads to separation of RB from E2F, transactivation of direct transcriptional targets of E2F, and entry and progression through cell cycle (Giacinti and Giordano 2006). GBM tumor cells circumvent RB-mediated cell cycle inhibition via several genetic alterations. The RB1 gene is mutated/deleted in 7.6% of GBM patients. Regulators of cell cycle like CDKN2A/CDKN2B/CDKN2C function by negatively regulating MDM2 as well as cyclins/CDKs and hence they regulate both TP53 and RB pathways. These molecules have been found to be altered in GBM by mutation or deletion in >61% of patients. Positive regulators of cell cycle progression like cyclins, CDK4 and CDK6 get activated by mutations and more commonly by amplification in 2%, 14% and 1.6% of GBM patients respectively (Brennan et al. 2013).

7.6 Next Generation Sequencing: Principle and Methodology

7.6.1 Next Generation Sequencing Platforms

Development of first generation sequencing methods started in the late 1970s. In 1977, Maxam and Gilbert published their DNA sequencing method which involved nucleotide specific chemical modification followed by cleavage (Maxam and Gilbert 1977). In the same year, Sanger published the chain termination method of DNA sequencing which evolved later on to give rise to the automated capillary sequencers (Luckey et al. 1990; Sanger et al. 1977). However, it is a colossal task to sequence an entire genome using capillary sequencing. The whole process involves shearing the genomic DNA into large fragments (100–500 Kb) followed by cloning of each fragment into a bacterial artificial chromosome (BAC) cloning system. Subsequently, each larger fragment is sheared into smaller fragments and sequenced individually by Sanger sequencing method. The shorter fragment sequences are first arranged to obtain the larger contigs cloned into the BACs and finally the BAC-cloned larger fragments are assembled to get the sequence of the whole genome (Lander et al. 2001; Osoegawa et al. 2001; Venter et al. 2001). Hence, it is evident that these methods are immensely time consuming and requires tremendous man power resulting in increased cost. NGS technique, which is actually a second generation sequencing method, involves parallel sequencing of thousands to millions of DNA fragments and it represents an effective way of capturing huge amounts of genomic information at a low cost (Tucker et al. 2009). It is used for various applications such as genome sequencing, transcriptome or RNA sequencing, sequencing of exome, sequencing of immunoprecipitated chromatin-bound DNA/RNA, micro RNA sequencing etc. (Morozova and Marra 2008). Since early 1990s, many NGS platforms emerged and they differ in engineering configurations and sequencing chemistry. Each sequencing platform has different sequencing output capacity, run time, library preparation method, library fragment length and principle of sequencing (Table 7.1). Polymerase-dependent sequencing approach is referred to as sequencing by synthesis (SBS); while sequencing by ligation technique involves the enzyme DNA ligase to identify the nucleotide present at a given position in a DNA sequence (Chen 2014; Mardis 2008). Most NGS platforms use sequencing by synthesis technique. The NGS technique, irrespective of the platform, comprises of three steps – DNA/cDNA library preparation, sequencing and data analysis (Mardis 2008).

Illumina's Solexa sequencing deserves a notable mention due to its enormous technological advances with nine different sequencers developed through a span of 8 years (Goodwin et al. 2016). It utilizes SBS technology using nucleotides modified by reversible dye terminators. The library preparation involves fragmentation of the DNA followed by ligation of short stretches of double-stranded DNA of known sequence called *adapters*. During sequencing, primers complementary to these adapter sequences are used for extension. Additionally, another feature of the adapters is a short stretch (6 bp) of sequence called an *index* which varies between two different adapters and this is used for *multiplexing* different samples in the same sequencing reaction, i.e., adapter sequences containing different indices can be ligated to different DNA samples and these samples can be pooled together in the same sequencing reaction. After sequencing, the sequences from the different samples can be differentiated by virtue of the differences in their index sequences, a process in data analysis referred to as *de-multiplexing*. The double-stranded DNA library is denatured and put on a flow-cell containing covalently attached lawn of primers complementary to a portion of the adapter sequence. These fragments are amplified using a method called *bridge amplification* to produce ~1000 of similar fragments and this is referred to as a *cluster* (cluster generation). Each cluster forms a 'spot' on the flow cell. In each cycle of sequencing, all four dNTPs conjugated with a fluorophore dye and a reversible terminator modification is added. The complementary base in each fragment is added in that cycle, the image is captured and then the dye and the terminator are removed to move to the next cycle. Images for each cycle are compiled and the final sequence for each read is obtained (http://www.illumina.com/documents/products/techspotlights/techspotlight_sequencing.pdf).

Although improvements in the second generation sequencing techniques continue to be impressive, a more recent development in sequencing is a number of third generation sequencing techniques. Third-generation platforms have several characteristics over its predecessor technologies such as single-molecule templates, lower cost, easy sample preparation, faster run times and simplified data analysis. An initial DNA amplification step is necessary in second generation sequencers which produce multiple copies of the same DNA fragment and this step has been eliminated in the

Table 7.1 Next generation sequencing platforms

Company	Platforms	Output range (Gb)	Run time	Maximum read length	Library amplification	Sequencing principle
Second generation						
Illumina	MiniSeq	0.6–7.5	4–24 hrs	2 × 150 bp	Bridge-PCR on flow cell surface	Reversible terminator sequencing by synthesis
	MiSeq	0.3–15	5–55 hrs	2 × 300 bp		
	NextSeq 500	30–120	12–30 hrs	2 × 150 bp		
	HiSeq 2500	50–1000	<1–6 days	2 × 125 bp		
	HiSeq 3000	125–750	<1–3.5 days	2 × 150 bp		
	HiSeq 4000	125–1500	<1–3.5 days	2 × 150 bp		
	HiSeq X Five	900–1800	<3 days	2 × 150 bp		
	HiSeq X Ten	900–1800	<3 days	2 × 150 bp		
Roche	GS Junior+	~0.07	18 hrs	~700 bases	Emulsion PCR on microbeads	Pyro sequencing
	GS FLX Titanium XL+	~0.7	23 hrs	Up to 1000 bp		
	GS FLX Titanium XLR70	0.450	10 hrs	Up to 600 bp		
Life Technologies (SoLiD)	5500 W System	~ 80–160	8 days	1 × 75 bp, 2 × 50 mate-pair, 50 × 50 Paired-End	PCR on FlowChip surface	Sequencing by ligation
	5500xl W System	~160–320	8 days	1 × 75 bp, 2 × 50 mate-pair, 50 × 50 Paired-End		
Life Technologies (Ion Torrent)	Ion PGM	~0.03–2	2–7 hrs	200 bp, 400 bp	Emulsion PCR on microbeads	Semiconductor based sequencing by synthesis
	Ion S5	~0.6–15	2.5–4 hrs	200 bp, 400 bp		
	Ion S5 XL	~0.6–15	24 hrs	200 bp, 400 bp		
Third generation						
Pacific Bioscience	PACBIO RS II	~0.5–1	0.5–4 hrs	> 20 kb	NA	Single-molecule, real-time DNA sequencing by synthesis
	SEQUEL SYSTEM	0.75–1.25	0.5–6 hrs	> 20 kb		
Oxford nanopore	MinION	21–42	1 min–48 hrs	230–300 kb	NA	Nanopore sequencing
	Single PromethION Flow Cell	128–256	1 min–48 hrs	230–300 kb		
	PromethION (48 Flow Cells)	6000–12,000	1 min–48 hrs	230–300 kb		
Helicos	HelicosBiotechnologies	~28	>1 Gb/hr	25–30 bp	NA	Reversible terminator chemistry

hrs hours, *bp* base pair, *kb* kilo bases, *NA* not applicable third generation technologies. The sample DNA strands are subjected to sequencing directly at the single-molecule level using engineered protein polymerases. By this method, PCR amplification bias can be avoided. Additionally, longer DNA strands can be sequenced by third generation sequencers which help in easy alignment of reads to the reference genome (Schadt et al. 2010). However, it is important to note that none of the third generation technologies are currently in mass use for sequencing purposes. The three significant platforms developed include Pacific Biosciences single molecule real time sequencing, Helicos molecule fluorescence sequencing, and Oxford's nanopore sequencing (Table 7.1) (Schadt et al. 2010).

7.6.2 Whole Genome, Whole Exome and Targeted Sequencing

The entire genome of an organism can be sequenced in one go using NGS and this is referred to as *whole genome sequencing (WGS)*. This entails sequencing of the entire chromosomal DNA and mitochondrial DNA of an organism, and in case of plants it includes DNA from the chloroplasts. The isolated DNA from the cells of normal or diseased tissue is fragmented and adapter ligated to give rise to DNA library which is then subjected to sequencing. The output fragment sequences are then aligned to a previously constructed reference genome. Subsequently, the aligned sequences can be used to find out SNVs, indels, CNAs, gene fusions etc. (Ng and Kirkness 2010). The whole human genome is approximately 3.3 GB in size (Venter et al. 2001). Functionally important short stretches of the human genome that are translated into proteins are termed as exons. The human genome comprises of about 180,000 exons constituting about 1% of the entire genome and this translates to around 30 megabases in length (Ng et al. 2009). About 85% of disease causing mutations is found in these protein coding regions of the human genome (Choi et al. 2009). *Whole exome sequencing (WES)* is carried out to selectively sequence the exonic part of the human genome. The advantage of this method over WGS is its cost-effectiveness and the possibility of sequencing more number of samples at a time. The principle behind the library preparation for WES is basically pull-down of only the exonic regions of the genome. For this purpose, a pool of highly optimized probe set that delivers comprehensive coverage of exonic regions are used (Warr et al. 2015).

For targeted therapy of any diseased condition including cancer, the first step is to identify driver genetic alterations which can be targeted. Instead of sequencing the entire genome or exome of an organism, we can sequence particular genes of interest and this is referred to as *targeted sequencing*. Targeted sequencing enables in conserving resources (*increased productivity*) and generating a smaller, more easy-to-handle data set thus reducing analysis burden (*stream-lined workflow*) (Meldrum et al. 2011). This approach additionally delivers much higher coverage levels (500 – 1000X or higher) enabling identification of rare variants with high degree of confidence (*accurate results*) (Mirebrahim et al. 2015). Two methods can be employed for fishing out regions of interest for targeted sequencing – 1) custom amplicon and 2) custom enrichment (Fig. 7.1). In *custom amplicon* method, the regions of interest are amplified from the genomic DNA using primers and the amplified fragments are ligated

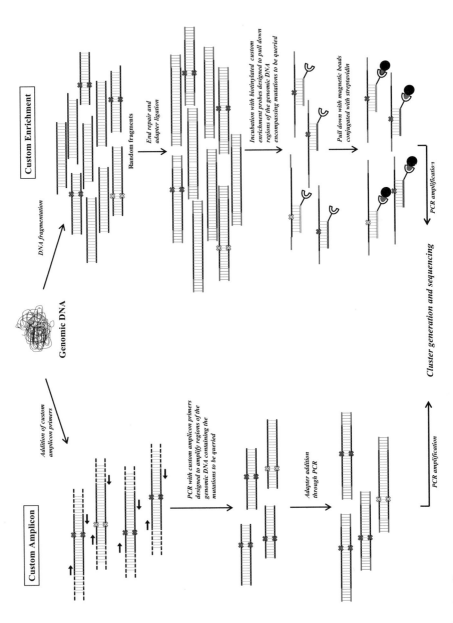

Fig. 7.1 (continued)

with adapter sequences to generate the targeted sequencing library. On the other hand, in *custom enrichment* method, the genomic DNA is fragmented and adapter ligated similar to WES library preparation. However, instead of genome-wide exon-specific enrichment probes, custom enrichment probes designed to pull down the regions of interest are used. These probes are biotinylated such that the library DNA hybridizing with the probes can be pulled down using magnetic beads conjugated with streptavidin. Both the libraries are PCR amplified and subjected to next generation sequencing (Fig. 7.1). Genomic DNA can be isolated from fresh frozen tumor tissue samples as well as formalin fixed paraffin embedded (FFPE) samples, although the DNA isolated from FFPE tissue sections are of poorer quality.

7.6.3   NGS Data Analysis

Data analysis is an integral requirement for uncovering genetic alterations from NGS data and particular computational skills are necessary which include knowledge of Linux operating system and any programming language such as PERL, PYTHON, JAVA, R etc. As an example, the data analysis pipeline for the sequencing output from Illumina's Solexa sequencing has been explained (Fig. 7.2). It is important to note that the following data analysis workflow is for calling single nucleotide variations (SNVs) or insertions/deletions (indels) following Genome Analysis Toolkit (GATK) guidelines (McKenna et al. 2010). The raw sequencing output comes as base intensities file or '.bcl' file which is not human readable and it consists of data from millions of DNA fragments. Additionally, since multiple samples are pooled in one reaction, de-multiplexing of different samples is essential. Hence in the first step, de-multiplexing as well as conversion of .bcl files to human readable text file format called FASTQ files is done by bcl2fastq (http://support.illumina.com/downloads/bcl2fastq_conversion_software_184.html). Each fragment of DNA sequenced is called as "read". The FASTQ file contains millions of reads as obtained from the sequencer. FastQC is a tool which determines the quality of sequencing on various parameters, such as average read quality, GC content, adapter contamination etc. (http://www.bioinformatics.babraham.ac.uk/projects/fastqc/). Read quality score is an average base quality score of each nucleotide in a

Fig. 7.1 Library preparation techniques for targeted sequencing of cancer-specific selected genes or genomic regions. In *Custom amplicon method* (*left*), the genomic DNA is subjected to PCR to amplify specific regions that may carry driver alterations to be sequenced. The single nucleotide variations (mutations) to be queried are denoted by colored crosses. Next, adapter sequences are added to the amplified fragments through PCR followed by cluster generation and next generation sequencing. In *Custom enrichment method* (*right*), the genomic DNA is subjected to fragmentation using acoustic waves. Adapter sequences are added to the fragments, followed by enrichment of regions of interest encompassing mutations using DNA probes complementary to those regions. As these probes are biotinylated, the fragments of interest are pulled down using streptavidin-coated magnetic beads (*red* and *black circles* respectively). Finally, the selected library fragments are PCR amplified, followed by cluster generation and next generation sequencing

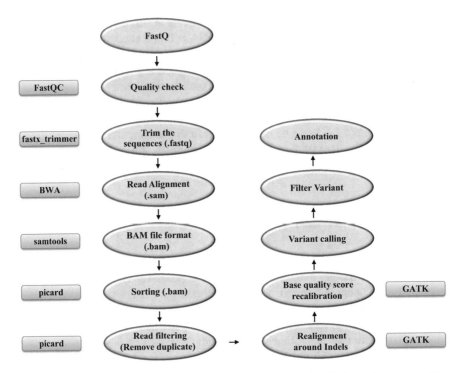

Fig. 7.2 Schematic of data analysis pipeline for targeted sequencing. Each step is represented by the *blue shapes* while the tools required by each step of data analysis are given in peach shapes. Base intensities file from the sequencing machine is first converted to human readable FastQ format. After various quality checking steps, the reads are aligned to the human reference genome. Finally, the positions of each base in the chromosome are determined and the files are converted to ready-to-use format for subsequent analyses

read. This quality score is called Phred quality score (Q score). Q scores are defined as a property that is logarithmically related to the base calling error probabilities (Ewing et al. 1998). For example, Q score 30 is equivalent to the probability of an incorrect base call being 1 in 1000 times. This means that base call accuracy is 99.9%. Reads where the peripheral bases have low quality scores are trimmed using FastX Trimmer (http://hannonlab.cshl.edu/fastx_toolkit/). Subsequently, the reads are mapped to the human reference genome using mapping tools like Burrows Wheeler Aligner (BWA) (http://bio-bwa.sourceforge.net/). The latest version of the human reference genome is GRCh38 (http://www.ncbi.nlm.nih.gov/projects/genome/assembly/grc/human/). Post-alignment, we obtain the '.sam' files which are very huge for further processing. These '.sam' files are converted to binary format or '.bam' files using Samtools (Li et al. 2009). Bam files are sorted by read name using Picard tool (http://broadinstitute.github.io/picard/). This step is important for optimizing further steps like searching or merging. An artifact of sequencing that is almost always encountered is read duplication or same read being sequenced more than once as different clusters. This usually arises during PCR amplification steps during library preparation. Duplicate reads are removed using Picard as these are non-informative and should not be counted as additional evidence for a variant. Due to presence of insertions and deletions in the genome, the algorithms that are used for read mapping give various types of artifacts. GATK is used for local realignment (McKenna et al. 2010). It is performed in two steps: first GATK's RealignerTargetCreator tool determines small suspicious intervals which are likely in need of realignment; in the second step IndelRealigner realigns reads over those intervals. Variant calling depends on the quality score of individual base in each read. Sequencing instruments produce per base quality score; this quality score is either over or under estimated due to systematic technical error. Base Quality Score Recalibration (BQSR) is done by using GATK's BaseRecalibrator tool (McKenna et al. 2010). This tool gives more accurate base qualities, which improves the accuracy of variant calls. The program initially builds a model of covariation based on known variants, and then it adjusts the base quality score.

SNVs are most abundant in a genome. Detection of SNVs is simple and reliable, whereas other genomic variants like indels are relatively difficult to identify. To identify SNVs in a sample as compared to reference genome, various tools can be used such as MuTect (Cibulskis et al. 2013), VarScan (Koboldt et al. 2012), SNVmix (Goya et al. 2010) and SomaticSniper (Larson et al. 2012). For indel identification various tools are available of which Pindel is noteworthy due to its accuracy (Ye et al. 2009).

7.6.4 Targeted Sequencing Panels

Targeted gene sequencing panels are useful tools for analyzing specific mutations in a given sample and such focused panels containing a select set of genes or gene regions having known or suspected associations with cancer have been developed through the past decade. There are various pan-cancer panels developed by different companies, e.g. FoundationOne™ from Foundation Medicine Inc., Illumina's Truseq-Amplicon Cancer Panel, Illumina's TruSight Cancer Panel, Personalized Cancer Mutation Panel (University of Pittsburgh Medical Centre), Cancer Gene Mutation Panel Version 2 (Baylor College of Medicine), AmpliSeq™Cancer Hotspot Panel v2 from Life Technologies, Qiagen's GeneRead DNAseq Targeted Panels V2 etc. Of note, FoundationOne™ is one of the most comprehensive targeted sequencing panels developed till date and it aims to find SNVs, indels, CNAs and gene arrangements in 315 selected cancer-related genes found to be altered in solid tumors (http://foundationone.com/). While Illumina's Truseq-Amplicon Cancer Panel is a custom amplicon based targeted sequencing panel that aims to query mutations in 48 cancer related genes (http://www.illumina.com/products/truseq_amplicon_cancer_panel.html), TruSight Cancer Panel is a custom enrichment based targeted sequencing panel that aims to investigate mutations in 94 genes associated mainly with breast and colorectal carcinoma (http://www.illumina.com/products/trusight_cancer.html). Although, the various available cancer panels are designed for multiple types of cancers, recent pan-cancer studies show that the genetic alteration landscape varies between different types of cancers (Kandoth et al. 2013; Tamborero et al. 2013). A targeted sequencing panel called GlioSeq has been formulated for all CNS tumors (Nikiforova et al. 2016). However, this does not cover many of the driver genes known to be altered in GBM (Brennan et al. 2013; Frattini et al. 2013). For example, genes that are highly altered in GBM such as PIK3R1, PDGFRA, KIT, VEGFR2, MDM2, CDK4, CDK6, LZTR1, MLL3 etc. are absent in the GlioSeq gene panel (Nikiforova et al. 2016). Hence, formulation of a targeted sequencing panel of clinical relevance for GBM patients is urgently required.

7.7 Current Status of Targeted Therapies for GBM

Enormous efforts have been undertaken through decades to understand molecular pathogenesis of GBM and there have been several attempts at developing targeted therapies for GBM. Over-expression of DNA repair gene, MGMT, in GBM leads to poor response to therapy. O6-Benzylguanine, an inhibitor of MGMT, was tested for combinatorial therapy along with temozolomide. However, the compound proved to be myelotoxic and hence studies were discontinued (Quinn et al. 2009). An inhibitor of $\alpha v\beta 3/5$ integrin, Cilengitide, was considered till phase III trial for use in GBM cases after which it was discontinued as it did not improve survival in patients (Reardon et al. 2011). Epigenetic modifiers such as histone de-acetylase enzymes (HDACs) have been found to be significantly mutated in GBM. HDAC inhibitor, Vorinostat, trial has recently entered phase II (Friday et al. 2012).

Two of the most profound examples of GBM targeted therapy are angiogenesis inhibitor, Bevacizumab and EGFR inhibitor therapies. GBM is characterized by extensive and sustained angiogenesis which is primarily regulated by vascular endothelial growth factor (VEGF) and its receptor (VEGFR) (Mao et al. 2015). Bevacizumab (Avastin), a humanized monoclonal antibody against VEGF, had been taken forward for clinical trial, but unfortunately it proved to be ineffective as it failed to improve survival in patients (Ferrara et al. 2004). This could be attributed to the fact that angiogenesis can be regulated by other molecules secreted by stromal cells (like microglial cells), and by transdifferentiated endothelial cells that arise from cancer stem cells (Mao et al. 2015; Nijaguna et al. 2015). EGFR is altered in >50% of GBM patients through mutations, CNAs and fusions that leads to cell proliferation and survival in cancer cells. Inhibitors of EGFR, erlotinib, lapatinib and nimotuzumab have been subjected to clinical trial which again was a failure (Mittal et al. 2015). A mutant form of EGFR called EGFRvIII is prevalent among GBM patients and it has been shown to reside primarily on small circular extrachromosomal fragments of DNA called double-minute chromosomes (Sanborn et al. 2013). In 2014, Nathanson et al. revealed that resistance to EGFR inhibitors occur by elimination of this mutant EGFR extrachromosomal DNA from the cancer cells (Nathanson et al. 2014). They additionally proved that, withdrawal of the inhibitors lead to re-emergence of clonal extrachromosomal EGFR mutants. Hence, it is evident that cancer cells can evade therapies by highly specific, dynamic, and adaptive mechanisms. From this, we understand that ample efforts have to be put to elucidate novel and effective therapeutic options for GBM patients. Additionally, knowledge about the entire clinically relevant driver genetic alteration spectrum can help in formulation of a cocktail of therapeutic drugs targeting multiple genes leading to the death of most of the cancer cells thus opening up possibilities of combating tumor recurrence.

7.8 Available Targeted Therapies and Other Novel Therapeutic Options

According to National Cancer Institute (NCI), USA, there are 473 cancer therapeutic drugs available which are being used for treatment of different types of cancers (http://www.cancer.gov/about-cancer/treatment/drugs). Although, the targeted therapeutic options available for GBM currently is disappointing, a significant number of targeted therapeutic molecules used for other types of cancers could be considered for the treatment of GBM. As explained earlier, multitude of molecules of the RTK/Ras/PI3K pathway gets altered in GBM by mutation, CNAs and gene fusions. These molecules play a vital role in cancer cell survival and proliferation and hence are important targets for personalized therapy. In fact, there are a number of humanized antibodies and small molecule inhibitors that have been approved by FDA and are being currently used for other types of cancers (Table 7.2) (Kotliarova and Fine 2012). Additionally, apart from Bevacizumab, other anti-angiogenic molecules have also been approved for other cancers which could be tested for GBM patients. Further, cell cycle regulatory kinases CDK4 and CDK6 get amplified in ~20% of GBM patients. Palbociclib is a CDK4/6 inhibitor which has been approved for breast cancers and can be considered for GBM therapy (Table 7.2).

Advancements in human genomics have created ways for gene therapy as novel therapeutic approaches to improve cancer regression and find a potential cure for the disease. This method comprises of transferring genetic material into a cancer cell through viral or non-viral vectors, production of oncolytic viruses to target cancer cells, immunomodulation of tumor cells or the host immune system, and manipulation of the tumor microenvironment to reduce tumor vasculature (Amer 2014). It is anticipated that gene therapy will play an important role in future cancer therapy as part of a multimodality treatment in combination with other forms of cancer therapy. This is due to the fact that these therapies have the potential to harm the cancer cells maximally with minimal effects on normal cells.

Oncolytic virotherapy is an emerging targeted therapy which involves generation of replication competent viruses that can target and destroy cancer cells with little or no harm to the normal cells. The basic principle behind oncolytic virotherapy is to genetically modify viruses such that they cannot replicate within normal cells but can undergo rapid replication within the cancer cells thus leading to lysis of the cell (Amer 2014). There are few oncolytic viruses generated to target GBM cells which

Table 7.2 List of targeted sequencing molecules

Sr. No.	Drug name	Active ingredient	Targets	Cancers
Antibody based				
1	Avastin	Bevacizumab	VEGF	Cervical cancer, colorectal cancer, glioblastoma, non-small cell lung cancer, primary peritoneal cancer, renal cell cancer
2	Cyramza	Ramucirumab	VEGFR2	Adenocarcinoma, clorectal cancer, non-small cell lung cancer
3	Erbitux	Cetuximab	EGFR, VEGFR2	Colorectal cancer, squamous cell carcinoma of the head and neck
4	Herceptin	Trastuzumab	ERRB2	Adenocarcinoma, breast cancer
5	Kadcyla	Ado-Trastuzumab Emtansine	ERRB2	Breast cancer
6	Perjeta	Pertuzumab	ERRB2	Breast cancer
7	Vectibix	Panitumumab	EGFR	Colorectal cancer
Small molecule inhibitor				
1	Bosulif	Bosutinib Monohydrate	BCR-ABL, SRC	Chronic myelogenous leukemia
2	Caprelsa	Vandetanib	EGFR, VEGFR2	Medullary thyroid cancer
3	Cometriq	Cabozantinib-S-Malate	MET, VEGFR2	Medullary thyroid cancer, Renal cell carcinoma
4	Eylea	Aflibercept	VEGFR2	Colorectal cancer
5	Farydak	Panobinostat Lactate	HDAC, HIF-1a, VEGF	Multiple myeloma
6	Gleevec	Imatinib Mesylate	PDGFR, KIT	Acute lymphoblastic leukemia, chronic eosinophilic leukemia, chronic myelogenous leukemia, dermatofibrosarcoma protuberans, gastrointestinal stromal tumor,myeloproliferative neoplasms, systemic mastocytosis
7	Ibrance	Palbociclib	CDK4, CDK6	Breast cancer
8	Inlyta	Axitinib	VEGFR, PDGFR, KIT	Renal cell carcinoma
9	Iressa	Gefitinib	EGFR, KIT	Non-small cell lung cancer
10	Jakafi	Ruxolitinib Phosphate	JAK1, JAK2	Myelofibrosis, polycythemia vera
11	Lapatinib	Lapatinib	EGFR, KIT	Breast cancer
12	Lenvima	Lenvatinib Mesylate	FGFR, KIT	Renal cell carcinoma, thyroid cancer
13	Mekinist	Trametinib Dimethyl Sulfoxide	MEK1 MEK2	Melanoma
14	Sorafenib	Sorafenib	RAF, MAPK, PDGFR	Hepatocellular carcinoma, renal cell carcinoma, thyroid cancer

(continued)

Table 7.2 (continued)

Sr. No.	Drug name	Active ingredient	Targets	Cancers
15	Sprycel	Dasatinib	SRC, KIT, Ephrin receptors	Acute lymphoblastic leukemia, chronic myelogenous leukemia
16	Sutent	Sunitinib Malate	PDGFR, VEGFR2	Gastrointestinal stromal tumor, pancreatic cancer, renal cell carcinoma
17	Tafinlar	Dabrafenib Mesylate	BRAF	Melanoma
18	Tarceva	Erlotinib Hydrochloride	EGFR, KIT	Non-small cell lung cancer, pancreatic cancer
19	Tasigna	Nilotinib Hydrochloride Monohydrate	KIT, ephrin receptors, DDR1, DDR2, PDGFRB, BCR_ABL, MAPK11	Chronic myelogenous leukemia
20	Torisel	Temsirolimus	mTOR, VEGFR2	Renal cell carcinoma
21	Velcade	Bortezomib	NF-κB	Multiple myeloma, mantle cell lymphoma
22	Votrient	Pazopanib Hydrochloride	KIT, FGFR, PDGFR, VEGFR	Renal cell carcinoma
23	Xalkori	Crizotinib	MET, ALK fusion	Non-small cell lung cancer
24	Zelboraf	Vemurafenib	BRAF	Melanoma
25	Zortress	Everolimus	mTOR	Breast cancer, pancreatic cancer, gastrointestinal cancer, lung cancer, renal cell carcinoma, subependymal giant cell astrocytoma
26	Zydelig	Idelalisib	PIK3CD	Chronic lymphocytic leukemia, non-Hodgkin lymphoma

http://www.cancer.gov/about-cancer/treatment/drugs
Kotliarova and Fine (2012)

are under clinical trials, for example, CRAdRGDflt-IL24 (Kaliberova et al. 2009) and ONYX-105 (Ries and Korn 2002). Another emerging targeted therapeutic approach which is gaining importance is the production of genetically modified chimeric antigen receptor (CAR) T lymphocytes. CAR T cells are reprogrammed to express monoclonal antibody-binding domains that trigger T-cell activation and effector function upon tumor antigen binding. Currently, clinical trials of CARs targeting EGFRvIII (NCT01454596) and HER2 (NCT01109095) are ongoing for GBM patients (Reardon et al. 2011). Vaccinations sensitize the immune system against target antigens and this technique can be utilized to kill cancer cells by regulating the host immune system. For example, Rindopepimut (Celldex Therapeutics) is a synthetic 14 amino acid peptide (mapping to the EGFRvIII-specific splice site) conjugated to the immune adjuvant keyhole limpet hemocyanin which has been developed as a potential vaccine to evoke the immune responses of a patient harboring EGFRvIII mutation to specifically target the GBM cells. In pre-clinical studies, EGFRvIII vaccination demonstrated survival benefit as well as EGFRvIII-specific humoral and cellular immune responses (Reardon et al. 2011). Hence, it is evident that GBM targeted therapy is under constant evolution through enormous research and this provides hope for the development of effective therapy to improve patient survival drastically and ultimately reach a point when the disease can be completely obliterated.

7.9 Conclusions and Future Directions

During the past decade, numerous groups have undertaken tremendous efforts to understand the genetics and epigenetics of GBM pathogenesis. Advancement in genomics technologies has paved the path for the development of NGS techniques which has led researchers to uncover the entire genetic alteration spectrum of GBM. Our understanding of GBM has progressed by leaps and bounds but the median survival achieved till date is only 15–17 months (Arvold and Reardon 2014; Stupp et al. 2009). Hence, it is evident that a change in the treatment strategy for these patients is required and personalized therapy is gaining importance in the field of cancer. Although patient stratification can help clinicians in determining the aggres-siveness of the therapy required for individual patients, the new promising approach for cancer treatment is targeted therapy which involves inhibition of specific altered molecules in the cancer cells through small molecule inhibitors or monoclonal anti-bodies. However, due to inter-tumoral heterogeneity, tumors from different indi-viduals show variable response to different targeted therapies. Moreover, intra-tumoral heterogeneity causes the tumor cells within a particular tumor to respond differently and treatment targeting a single molecule will not eradicate all tumor cells, thus leading to tumor recurrence (Almendro et al. 2013). For these reasons, identification of the entire milieu of driver genetic alterations within a tumor should be the priority. NGS based targeted sequencing paves the way for simultaneous sequencing of cancer-specific selected genes at very high coverage (Meldrum et al. 2011). Thus, a cocktail of targeted therapeutic molecules can be used as the novel therapeutic regime for eradication of GBM. Targeted sequencing is both cost and time effective and hence, can be used for target identification such that personalized therapy can be given to each patient. This proves that there is hope for better treatment options for GBM patients in the near future. However, much advancement in the formulation of effective tailored therapy for GBM is required and targeted therapy development has still a long way to go due to the following reasons. First, it is still unclear which driver genetic alterations have prominent roles to play in tumor development i.e., deregulated molecules on which cancer cells are more dependent for survival and proliferation. Moreover, the biology of GBM is still not completely understood and extensive research is required to understand various aspects such as, tumor-stroma interactions. For example, although GBM tumors show extensive angiogenesis, treatment with Bevacizumab, an inhibitor of angiogenic molecule VEGF, was found to be ineffective. This could be due to secretory molecules produced by stromal cells around the tumor and transdifferentiation of cancer stem cells to give rise to new blood vessels (Mao et al. 2015; Nijaguna et al. 2015). Additionally, understanding of cancer stem cells need much research as these cells are treatment refractory and thrive to give rise to recurrence (Nakano and Mangum 2011). Further, there is an urgent requirement for development of novel therapies for targeting GBM tumor cells. With the discovery of more driver genetic alterations, more number of inhibitors against the whole array of genetic alterations needs to be developed. Enormous efforts have to be put to promptly develop commercially available kits for identifying GBM specific driver genetic alterations. In conclusion, it is evident that personalized therapy is the future of GBM treatment and every effort needs to be made to make this available for application by clinicians and oncologists.

Acknowledgements JP and VP are thankful to DBT, Government of India, for scholarship. Infrastructural support by funding from DBT, DST and UGC to MCB is acknowledged. KS thanks DST and DBT, Government of India for financial support. KS is a J. C. Bose Fellow of the Department of Science and Technology.

References

American Brain Tumor Association. 2014. Glioblastoma and malignant astrocytoma USA.

Almendro, V., A. Marusyk, and K. Polyak. 2013. Cellular heterogeneity and molecular evolution in cancer. *Annual Review of Pathology* 8: 277–302.

Amer, M.H. 2014. Gene therapy for cancer: present status and future perspective. *Molecular and Cellular Therapies* 2: 27.

Arimappamagan, A., K. Somasundaram, K. Thennarasu, S. Peddagangannagari, H. Srinivasan, B.C. Shailaja, C. Samuel, I.R. Patric, S. Shukla, B. Thota, K.V. Prasanna, P. Pandey, A. Balasubramaniam, V. Santosh, B.A. Chandramouli, A.S. Hegde, P. Kondaiah, and M.R. Sathyanarayana Rao. 2013. A fourteen gene GBM prognostic signature identifies association of immune response pathway and mesenchymal subtype with high risk group. *PLoS One* 8: e62042.

Arita, H., Y. Narita, H. Takami, S. Fukushima, Y. Matsushita, A. Yoshida, Y. Miyakita, M. Ohno, S. Shibui, and K. Ichimura. 2013. TERT promoter mutations rather than methylation are the main mechanism for TERT upregulation in adult gliomas. *Acta Neuropathologica* 126: 939–941.

Arvold, N.D., and D.A. Reardon. 2014. Treatment options and outcomes for glioblastoma in the elderly patient. *Clinical Interventions in Aging* 9: 357–367.

Balduzzi, S., S. Mantarro, V. Guarneri, L. Tagliabue, V, Pistotti, L Moja, R. D'Amico. 2014. Trastuzumab-containing regimens for metastatic breast cancer. *The Cochrane Database of Systematic Reviews*: 12;(6): CD006242.

Bastien, J.I., K.A. McNeill, and H.A. Fine. 2015. Molecular characterizations of glioblastoma, targeted therapy, and clinical results to date. *Cancer* 121: 502–516.

Baudino, T.A. 2015. Targeted cancer therapy: The next generation of cancer treatment. *Current Drug Discovery Technologies* 12: 3–20.

Brennan, C.W., R.G. Verhaak, A. McKenna, B. Campos, H. Noushmehr, S.R. Salama, S. Zheng, D. Chakravarty, J.Z. Sanborn, S.H. Berman, R. Beroukhim, B. Bernard, C.J. Wu, G. Genovese, I. Shmulevich, J. Barnholtz-Sloan, L. Zou, R. Vegesna, S.A. Shukla, G. Ciriello, W.K. Yung, W. Zhang, C. Sougnez, T. Mikkelsen, K. Aldape, D.D. Bigner, E.G. Van Meir, M. Prados,

A. Sloan, K.L. Black, J. Eschbacher, G. Finocchiaro, W. Friedman, D.W. Andrews, A. Guha, M. Iacocca, B.P. O'Neill, G. Foltz, J. Myers, D.J. Weisenberger, R. Penny, R. Kucherlapati, C.M. Perou, D.N. Hayes, R. Gibbs, M. Marra, G.B. Mills, E. Lander, P. Spellman, R. Wilson, C. Sander, J. Weinstein, M. Meyerson, S. Gabriel, P.W. Laird, D. Haussler, G. Getz, L. Chin, and T.R. Network. 2013. The somatic genomic landscape of glioblastoma. *Cell* 155: 462–477.

Burger, P.C. 1995. Revising the World Health Organization (WHO) blue book–'Histological typing of tumours of the central nervous system'. *Journal of Neuro-Oncology* 24: 3–7.

Cai, J., P. Zhu, C. Zhang, Q. Li, Z. Wang, G. Li, G. Wang, P. Yang, J. Li, B. Han, C. Jiang, Y. Sun, and T. Jiang. 2016. Detection of ATRX and IDH1-R132H immunohistochemistry in the progression of 211 paired gliomas. *Oncotarget* 7: 16384–16395.

Cancer Genome Atlas Research N. 2008. Comprehensive genomic characterization defines human glioblastoma genes and core pathways. *Nature* 455: 1061–1068.

Chen, C.Y. 2014. DNA polymerases drive DNA sequencing-by-synthesis technologies: both past and present. *Frontiers in Microbiology* 5: 305.

Choe, G., S. Horvath, T.F. Cloughesy, K. Crosby, D. Seligson, A. Palotie, L. Inge, B.L. Smith, C.L. Sawyers, and P.S. Mischel. 2003. Analysis of the phosphatidylinositol 3′-kinase signaling pathway in glioblastoma patients in vivo. *Cancer Research* 63: 2742–2746.

Choi, M., U.I. Scholl, W. Ji, T. Liu, I.R. Tikhonova, P. Zumbo, A. Nayir, A. Bakkaloglu, S. Ozen, S. Sanjad, C. Nelson-Williams, A. Farhi, S. Mane, and R.P. Lifton. 2009. Genetic diagnosis by whole exome capture and massively parallel DNA sequencing. *Proceedings of the National Academy of Sciences of the United States of America* 106: 19096–19101.

Cibulskis, K., M.S. Lawrence, S.L. Carter, A. Sivachenko, D. Jaffe, C. Sougnez, S. Gabriel, M. Meyerson, E.S. Lander, and G. Getz. 2013. Sensitive detection of somatic point mutations in impure and heterogeneous cancer samples. *Nature Biotechnology* 31: 213–219.

Colman, H., L. Zhang, E.P. Sulman, J.M. McDonald, N.L. Shooshtari, A. Rivera, S. Popoff, C.L. Nutt, D.N. Louis, J.G. Cairncross, M.R. Gilbert, H.S. Phillips, M.P. Mehta, A. Chakravarti, C.E. Pelloski, K. Bhat, B.G. Feuerstein, R.B. Jenkins, and K. Aldape. 2010. A multigene predictor of outcome in glioblastoma. *Neuro-Oncology* 12: 49–57.

Doyle, D., G. Hanks and N. Cherny. 2005. *Oxford textbook of palliative medicine*. Oxford University Press PMID: 17618441; PMCID: PMC1929165.

Ewing, B., L. Hillier, M.C. Wendl, and P. Green. 1998. Base-calling of automated sequencer traces using phred I. Accuracy assessment. *Genome Research* 8: 175–185.

Ferrara, N., K.J. Hillan, H.P. Gerber, and W. Novotny. 2004. Discovery and development of bevacizumab, an anti-VEGF antibody for treating cancer. *Nature Reviews Drug Discovery* 3: 391–400.

Frattini, V., V. Trifonov, J.M. Chan, A. Castano, M. Lia, F. Abate, S.T. Keir, A.X. Ji, P. Zoppoli, F. Niola, C. Danussi, I. Dolgalev, P. Porrati, S. Pellegatta, A. Heguy, G. Gupta, D.J. Pisapia, P. Canoll, J.N. Bruce, R.E. McLendon, H. Yan, K. Aldape, G. Finocchiaro, T. Mikkelsen, G.G. Prive, D.D. Bigner, A. Lasorella, R. Rabadan, and A. Iavarone. 2013. The integrated landscape of driver genomic alterations in glioblastoma. *Nature Genetics* 45: 1141–1149.

Friday, B.B., S.K. Anderson, J. Buckner, C. Yu, C. Giannini, F. Geoffroy, J. Schwerkoske, M. Mazurczak, H. Gross, E. Pajon, K. Jaeckle, and E. Galanis. 2012. Phase II trial of vorinostat in combination with bortezomib in recurrent glioblastoma: A north central cancer treatment group study. *Neuro-Oncology* 14: 215–221.

Furnari, F.B., T. Fenton, R.M. Bachoo, A. Mukasa, J.M. Stommel, A. Stegh, W.C. Hahn, K.L. Ligon, D.N. Louis, C. Brennan, L. Chin, R.A. DePinho, and W.K. Cavenee. 2007. Malignant astrocytic glioma: Genetics, biology, and paths to treatment. *Genes & Development* 21: 2683–2710.

Giacinti, C., and A. Giordano. 2006. RB and cell cycle progression. *Oncogene* 25: 5220–5227.

Gilbert, M.R., J.J. Dignam, T.S. Armstrong, J.S. Wefel, D.T. Blumenthal, M.A. Vogelbaum, H. Colman, A. Chakravarti, S. Pugh, M. Won, R. Jeraj, P.D. Brown, K.A. Jaeckle, D. Schiff, V.W. Stieber, D.G. Brachman, M. Werner-Wasik, I.W. Tremont-Lukats, E.P. Sulman, K.D. Aldape, W.J. Curran Jr., and M.P. Mehta. 2014. A randomized trial of bevacizumab for newly diagnosed glioblastoma. *The New England Journal of Medicine* 370: 699–708.

Glantz, M., M. Chamberlain, Q. Liu, N.S. Litofsky, and L.D. Recht. 2003. Temozolomide as an alternative to irradiation for elderly patients with newly diagnosed malignant gliomas. *Cancer* 97: 2262–2266.

Goldman, J.M., and J.V. Melo. 2003. Chronic myeloid leukemia–advances in biology and new approaches to treatment. *The New England Journal of Medicine* 349: 1451–1464.

Goodwin, S., J.D. McPherson, and W.R. McCombie. 2016. Coming of age: Ten years of next-generation sequencing technologies. *Nature Reviews Genetics* 17: 333–351.

Goya, R., M.G. Sun, R.D. Morin, G. Leung, G. Ha, K.C. Wiegand, J. Senz, A. Crisan, M.A. Marra, M. Hirst, D. Huntsman, K.P. Murphy, S. Aparicio, and S.P. Shah. 2010. SNVMix: Predicting single nucleotide variants from next-generation sequencing of tumors. *Bioinformatics* 26: 730–736.

Guha, A., M.M. Feldkamp, N. Lau, G. Boss, and A. Pawson. 1997. Proliferation of human malignant astrocytomas is dependent on Ras activation. *Oncogene* 15: 2755–2765.

Herculano-Houzel, S. 2014. The glia/neuron ratio: How it varies uniformly across brain structures and species and what that means for brain physiology and evolution. *Glia* 62: 1377–1391.

Hermanson, M., K. Funa, M. Hartman, L. Claesson-Welsh, C.H. Heldin, B. Westermark, and M. Nister. 1992. Platelet-derived growth factor and its receptors in human glioma tissue: expression of messenger RNA and protein suggests the presence of autocrine and paracrine loops. *Cancer Research* 52: 3213–3219.

Holland, E.C., W.P. Hively, R.A. DePinho, and H.E. Varmus. 1998. A constitutively active epidermal growth factor receptor cooperates with disruption of G1 cell-cycle arrest pathways to induce glioma-like lesions in mice. *Genes and Development* 12: 3675–3685.

Kaliberova, L.N., V. Krendelchtchikova, D.K. Harmon, C.R. Stockard, A.S. Petersen, J.M. Markert, G.Y. Gillespie, W.E. Grizzle, D.J. Buchsbaum, and S.A. Kaliberov. 2009. CRAdRGDflt-IL24 virotherapy in combination with chemotherapy of experimental glioma. *Cancer Gene Therapy* 16: 794–805.

Kandoth, C., M.D. McLellan, F. Vandin, K. Ye, B. Niu, C. Lu, M. Xie, Q. Zhang, J.F. McMichael, M.A. Wyczalkowski, M.D. Leiserson, C.A. Miller, J.S. Welch, M.J. Walter, M.C. Wendl, T.J. Ley, R.K. Wilson, B.J. Raphael, and L. Ding. 2013. Mutational landscape and significance across 12 major cancer types. *Nature* 502: 333–339.

Keime-Guibert, F., O. Chinot, L. Taillandier, S. Cartalat-Carel, M. Frenay, G. Kantor, J.S. Guillamo, E. Jadaud, P. Colin, P.Y. Bondiau, P. Menei, H. Loiseau, V. Bernier, J. Honnorat, M. Barrie, K. Mokhtari, J.J. Mazeron, A. Bissery, J.Y. Delattre, and Association of French-Speaking N-O. 2007. Radiotherapy for glioblastoma in the elderly. *The New England Journal of Medicine* 356: 1527–1535.

Killela, P.J., Z.J. Reitman, Y. Jiao, C. Bettegowda, N. Agrawal, L.A. Diaz Jr., A.H. Friedman, H. Friedman, G.L. Gallia, B.C. Giovanella, A.P. Grollman, T.C. He, Y. He, R.H. Hruban, G.I. Jallo, N. Mandahl, A.K. Meeker, F. Mertens, G.J. Netto, B.A. Rasheed, G.J. Riggins, T.A. Rosenquist, M. Schiffman, M. Shih Ie, D. Theodorescu, M.S. Torbenson, V.E. Velculescu, T.L. Wang, N. Wentzensen, L.D. Wood, M. Zhang, R.E. McLendon, D.D. Bigner, K.W. Kinzler, B. Vogelstein, N. Papadopoulos, and H. Yan. 2013. TERT promoter mutations occur frequently in gliomas and a subset of tumors derived from cells with low rates of self-renewal. *Proceedings of the National Academy of Sciences of the United States of America* 110: 6021–6026.

Knobbe, C.B., and G. Reifenberger. 2003. Genetic alterations and aberrant expression of genes related to the phosphatidyl-inositol-3'-kinase/protein kinase B (Akt) signal transduction pathway in glioblastomas. *Brain Pathology* 13: 507–518.

Koboldt, D.C., Q. Zhang, D.E. Larson, D. Shen, M.D. McLellan, L. Lin, C.A. Miller, E.R. Mardis, L. Ding, and R.K. Wilson. 2012. VarScan 2: Somatic mutation and copy number alteration discovery in cancer by exome sequencing. *Genome Research* 22: 568–576.

Kotliarova, S., and H.A. Fine. 2012. SnapShot: Glioblastoma multiforme. *Cancer cell* 21: 710–710 e711.

Lander, E.S., L.M. Linton, B. Birren, C. Nusbaum, M.C. Zody, J. Baldwin, K. Devon, K. Dewar, M. Doyle, W. FitzHugh, R. Funke, D. Gage, K. Harris, A. Heaford, J. Howland, L. Kann, J. Lehoczky, R. LeVine, P. McEwan, K. McKernan, J. Meldrim, J.P. Mesirov, C. Miranda, W. Morris, J. Naylor, C. Raymond, M. Rosetti, R. Santos, A. Sheridan, C. Sougnez, Y. Stange-

Thomann, N. Stojanovic, A. Subramanian, D. Wyman, J. Rogers, J. Sulston, R. Ainscough, S. Beck, D. Bentley, J. Burton, C. Clee, N. Carter, A. Coulson, R. Deadman, P. Deloukas, A. Dunham, I. Dunham, R. Durbin, L. French, D. Grafham, S. Gregory, T. Hubbard, S. Humphray, A. Hunt, M. Jones, C. Lloyd, A. McMurray, L. Matthews, S. Mercer, S. Milne, J.C. Mullikin, A. Mungall, R. Plumb, M. Ross, R. Shownkeen, S. Sims, R.H. Waterston, R.K. Wilson, L.W. Hillier, J.D. McPherson, M.A. Marra, E.R. Mardis, L.A. Fulton, A.T. Chinwalla, K.H. Pepin, W.R. Gish, S.L. Chissoe, M.C. Wendl, K.D. Delehaunty, T.L. Miner, A. Delehaunty, J.B. Kramer, L.L. Cook, R.S. Fulton, D.L. Johnson, P.J. Minx, S.W. Clifton, T. Hawkins, E. Branscomb, P. Predki, P. Richardson, S. Wenning, T. Slezak, N. Doggett, J.F. Cheng, A. Olsen, S. Lucas, C. Elkin, E. Uberbacher, M. Frazier, R.A. Gibbs, D.M. Muzny, S.E. Scherer, J.B. Bouck, E.J. Sodergren, K.C. Worley, C.M. Rives, J.H. Gorrell, M.L. Metzker, S.L. Naylor, R.S. Kucherlapati, D.L. Nelson, G.M. Weinstock, Y. Sakaki, A. Fujiyama, M. Hattori, T. Yada, A. Toyoda, T. Itoh, C. Kawagoe, H. Watanabe, Y. Totoki, T. Taylor, J. Weissenbach, R. Heilig, W. Saurin, F. Artiguenave, P. Brottier, T. Bruls, E. Pelletier, C. Robert, P. Wincker, D.R. Smith, L. Doucette-Stamm, M. Rubenfield, K. Weinstock, H.M. Lee, J. Dubois, A. Rosenthal, M. Platzer, G. Nyakatura, S. Taudien, A. Rump, H. Yang, J. Yu, J. Wang, G. Huang, J. Gu, L. Hood, L. Rowen, A. Madan, S. Qin, R.W. Davis, N.A. Federspiel, A.P. Abola, M.J. Proctor, R.M. Myers, J. Schmutz, M. Dickson, J. Grimwood, D.R. Cox, M.V. Olson, R. Kaul, C. Raymond, N. Shimizu, K. Kawasaki, S. Minoshima, G.A. Evans, M. Athanasiou, R. Schultz, B.A. Roe, F. Chen, H. Pan, J. Ramser, H. Lehrach, R. Reinhardt, W.R. McCombie, M. de la Bastide, N. Dedhia, H. Blocker, K. Hornischer, G. Nordsiek, R. Agarwala, L. Aravind, J.A. Bailey, A. Bateman, S. Batzoglou, E. Birney, P. Bork, D.G. Brown, C.B. Burge, L. Cerutti, H.C. Chen, D. Church, M. Clamp, R.R. Copley, T. Doerks, S.R. Eddy, E.E. Eichler, T.S. Furey, J. Galagan, J.G. Gilbert, C. Harmon, Y. Hayashizaki, D. Haussler, H. Hermjakob, K. Hokamp, W. Jang, L.S. Johnson, T.A. Jones, S. Kasif, A. Kaspryzk, S. Kennedy, W.J. Kent, P. Kitts, E.V. Koonin, I. Korf, D. Kulp, D. Lancet, T.M. Lowe, A. McLysaght, T. Mikkelsen, J.V. Moran, N. Mulder, V.J. Pollara, C.P. Ponting, G. Schuler, J. Schultz, G. Slater, A.F. Smit, E. Stupka, J. Szustakowki, D. Thierry-Mieg, J. Thierry-Mieg, L. Wagner, J. Wallis, R. Wheeler, A. Williams, Y.I. Wolf, K.H. Wolfe, S.P. Yang, R.F. Yeh, F. Collins, M.S. Guyer, J. Peterson, A. Felsenfeld, K.A. Wetterstrand, A. Patrinos, M.J. Morgan, P. de Jong, J.J. Catanese, K. Osoegawa, H. Shizuya, S. Choi, Y.J. Chen, J. Szustakowki, and International Human Genome Sequencing C. 2001. Initial sequencing and analysis of the human genome. *Nature* 409: 860–921.

Larson, D.E., C.C. Harris, K. Chen, D.C. Koboldt, T.E. Abbott, D.J. Dooling, T.J. Ley, E.R. Mardis, R.K. Wilson, and L. Ding. 2012. SomaticSniper: Identification of somatic point mutations in whole genome sequencing data. *Bioinformatics* 28: 311–317.

Lathia, J.D., S.C. Mack, E.E. Mulkearns-Hubert, C.L.L. Valentim, and J.N. Rich. 2015. Cancer stem cells in glioblastoma. *Genes and Development* 29: 1203–1217.

Lavin, M.F., and N. Gueven. 2006. The complexity of p53 stabilization and activation. *Cell Death and Differentiation* 13: 941–950.

Levsky, J.M., and R.H. Singer. 2003. Fluorescence in situ hybridization: Past, present and future. *Journal of Cell Science* 116: 2833–2838.

Li, H., B. Handsaker, A. Wysoker, T. Fennell, J. Ruan, N. Homer, G. Marth, G. Abecasis, R. Durbin, and Genome Project Data Processing Subgroup. 2009. The sequence alignment/map format and SAMtools. *Bioinformatics* 25: 2078–2079.

Logan, J., K. Edwards, and N. Saunders. 2009. *Real-time PCR : Current technology and applications*. Norfolk: Caister Academic Press.

Louis, D.N., H. Ohgaki, O.D. Wiestler, W.K. Cavenee, P.C. Burger, A. Jouvet, B.W. Scheithauer, and P. Kleihues. 2007. The 2007 WHO classification of tumours of the central nervous system. *Acta Neuropathologica* 114: 97–109.

Louis, D.N., A. Perry, G. Reifenberger, A. von Deimling, D. Figarella-Branger, W.K. Cavenee, H. Ohgaki, O.D. Wiestler, P. Kleihues, and D.W. Ellison. 2016. The 2016 World Health Organization classification of tumors of the central nervous system: A summary. *Acta Neuropathologica* 131: 803–820.

Luckey, J.A., H. Drossman, A.J. Kostichka, D.A. Mead, J. D'Cunha, T.B. Norris, and L.M. Smith. 1990. High speed DNA sequencing by capillary electrophoresis. *Nucleic Acids Research* 18: 4417–4421.

Mangum, R. and Nakano, I. 2011. Glioma stem cells and their therapy resistance. *Journal of Carcinogene Mutagene* S1: 002.

Mao, J.M., J. Liu, G. Guo, X.G. Mao, and C.X. Li. 2015. Glioblastoma vasculogenic mimicry: Signaling pathways progression and potential anti-angiogenesis targets. *Biomarker Research* 3: 8.

Mardis, E.R. 2008. Next-generation DNA sequencing methods. *Annual Review of Genomics and Human Genetics* 9: 387–402.

Martinez, R., and M. Esteller. 2010. The DNA methylome of glioblastoma multiforme. *Neurobiology of Disease* 39: 40–46.

Maxam, A.M., and W. Gilbert. 1977. A new method for sequencing DNA. *Proceedings of the National Academy of Sciences of the United States of America* 74: 560–564.

McKenna, A., M. Hanna, E. Banks, A. Sivachenko, K. Cibulskis, A. Kernytsky, K. Garimella, D. Altshuler, S. Gabriel, M. Daly, and M.A. DePristo. 2010. The genome analysis toolkit: A MapReduce framework for analyzing next-generation DNA sequencing data. *Genome Research* 20: 1297–1303.

Mechtler, L. 2009. Neuroimaging in Neuro-Oncology. *Neurologic Clinics* 27: 171–201.

Meldrum, C., M.A. Doyle, and R.W. Tothill. 2011. Next-generation sequencing for cancer diagnostics: A practical perspective. *The Clinical Biochemist Reviews / Australian Association of Clinical Biochemists* 32: 177–195.

Mirebrahim, H., T.J. Close, and S. Lonardi. 2015. De novo meta-assembly of ultra-deep sequencing data. *Bioinformatics* 31: i9–16.

Mitchison, T.J. 2012. The proliferation rate paradox in antimitotic chemotherapy. *Molecular Biology of the Cell* 23: 1–6.

Mittal, S., S. Pradhan, and T. Srivastava. 2015. Recent advances in targeted therapy for glioblastoma. *Expert Review of Neurotherapeutics* 15: 935–946.

Morozova, O., and M.A. Marra. 2008. Applications of next-generation sequencing technologies in functional genomics. *Genomics* 92: 255–264.

Nathanson, D.A., B. Gini, J. Mottahedeh, K. Visnyei, T. Koga, G. Gomez, A. Eskin, K. Hwang, J. Wang, K. Masui, A. Paucar, H. Yang, M. Ohashi, S. Zhu, J. Wykosky, R. Reed, S.F. Nelson, T.F. Cloughesy, C.D. James, P.N. Rao, H.I. Kornblum, J.R. Heath, W.K. Cavenee, F.B. Furnari, and P.S. Mischel. 2014. Targeted therapy resistance mediated by dynamic regulation of extrachromosomal mutant EGFR DNA. *Science* 343: 72–76.

Ng, P.C., and E.F. Kirkness. 2010. Whole genome sequencing. *Methods in Molecular Biology* 628: 215–226.

Ng, S.B., E.H. Turner, P.D. Robertson, S.D. Flygare, A.W. Bigham, C. Lee, T. Shaffer, M. Wong, A. Bhattacharjee, E.E. Eichler, M. Bamshad, D.A. Nickerson, and J. Shendure. 2009. Targeted capture and massively parallel sequencing of 12 human exomes. *Nature* 461: 272–276.

Nieto-Sampedro, M., B. Valle-Argos, D. Gomez-Nicola, A. Fernandez-Mayoralas, and M. Nieto-Diaz. 2011. Inhibitors of glioma growth that reveal the tumour to the immune system. *Clinical Medicine Insights Oncology* 5: 265–314.

Nijaguna, M.B., V. Patil, S. Urbach, S.D. Shwetha, K. Sravani, A.S. Hegde, B.A. Chandramouli, A. Arivazhagan, P. Marin, V. Santosh, and K. Somasundaram. 2015. Glioblastoma-derived Macrophage Colony-stimulating Factor (MCSF) Induces Microglial Release of Insulin-like Growth Factor-binding Protein 1 (IGFBP1) to promote angiogenesis. *The Journal of Biological Chemistry* 290: 23401–23415.

Nikiforova, M.N., A.I. Wald, M.A. Melan, S. Roy, S. Zhong, R.L. Hamilton, F.S. Lieberman, J. Drappatz, N.M. Amankulor, I.F. Pollack, Y.E. Nikiforov, and C. Horbinski. 2016. Targeted next-generation sequencing panel (GlioSeq) provides comprehensive genetic profiling of central nervous system tumors. *Neuro-Oncology* 18: 379–387.

Nonoguchi, N., T. Ohta, J.E. Oh, Y.H. Kim, P. Kleihues, and H. Ohgaki. 2013. TERT promoter mutations in primary and secondary glioblastomas. *Acta Neuropathologica* 126: 931–937.

Noushmehr, H., D.J. Weisenberger, K. Diefes, H.S. Phillips, K. Pujara, B.P. Berman, F. Pan, C.E. Pelloski, E.P. Sulman, K.P. Bhat, R.G. Verhaak, K.A. Hoadley, D.N. Hayes, C.M. Perou, H.K. Schmidt, L. Ding, R.K. Wilson, D. Van Den Berg, H. Shen, H. Bengtsson, P. Neuvial, L.M. Cope, J. Buckley, J.G. Herman, S.B. Baylin, P.W. Laird, K. Aldape, and Cancer Genome Atlas Research Network. 2010. Identification of a CpG island methylator phenotype that defines a distinct subgroup of glioma. *Cancer cell* 17: 510–522.

Ohgaki, H., and P. Kleihues. 2013. The definition of primary and secondary glioblastoma. *Clinical Cancer Research: An Official Journal of the American Association for Cancer Research* 19: 764–772.

Osoegawa, K., A.G. Mammoser, C. Wu, E. Frengen, C. Zeng, J.J. Catanese, and P.J. de Jong. 2001. A bacterial artificial chromosome library for sequencing the complete human genome. *Genome Research* 11: 483–496.

Padfield, E., H.P. Ellis, and K.M. Kurian. 2015. Current therapeutic advances targeting EGFR and EGFRvIII in glioblastoma. *Frontiers in Oncology* 5: 5.

Quinn, J.A., S.X. Jiang, D.A. Reardon, A. Desjardins, J.J. Vredenburgh, J.N. Rich, S. Gururangan, A.H. Friedman, D.D. Bigner, J.H. Sampson, R.E. McLendon, J.E. Herndon 2nd, A. Walker, and H.S. Friedman. 2009. Phase II trial of temozolomide plus o6-benzylguanine in adults with recurrent, temozolomide-resistant malignant glioma. *Journal of Clinical Oncology: Official Journal of the American Society of Clinical Oncology* 27: 1262–1267.

Reardon, D.A., B. Neyns, M. Weller, J.C. Tonn, L.B. Nabors, and R. Stupp. 2011. Cilengitide: An RGD pentapeptide alphanubeta3 and alphanubeta5 integrin inhibitor in development for glioblastoma and other malignancies. *Future Oncology* 7: 339–354.

Ries, S., and W.M. Korn. 2002. ONYX-015: Mechanisms of action and clinical potential of a replication-selective adenovirus. *British Journal of Cancer* 86: 5–11.

Rizzo, T., and C. Rhonda. 2002. *Chemotherapy. Gale Encyclopedia of Cancer.* Farmington Hills, MI, USA

Rohlin, A., J. Wernersson, Y. Engwall, L. Wiklund, J. Bjork, and M. Nordling. 2009. Parallel sequencing used in detection of mosaic mutations: Comparison with four diagnostic DNA screening techniques. *Human Mutation* 30: 1012–1020.

Sanborn, J.Z., S.R. Salama, M. Grifford, C.W. Brennan, T. Mikkelsen, S. Jhanwar, S. Katzman, L. Chin, and D. Haussler. 2013. Double minute chromosomes in glioblastoma multiforme are revealed by precise reconstruction of oncogenic amplicons. *Cancer Research* 73: 6036–6045.

Sanger, F., S. Nicklen, and A.R. Coulson. 1977. DNA sequencing with chain-terminating inhibitors. *Proceedings of the National Academy of Sciences of the United States of America* 74: 5463–5467.

Sathornsumetee, S., J.N. Rich, and D.A. Reardon. 2007. Diagnosis and treatment of high-grade astrocytoma. *Neurologic Clinics* 25: 1111–1139. x.

Schadt, E.E., S. Turner, and A. Kasarskis. 2010. A window into third-generation sequencing. *Human Molecular Genetics* 19: R227–R240.

Schapira, A.H.V. 2007. *Neurology and clinical neuroscience*, 1336. Philadelphia: Mosby Elsevier.

See, W.L., I.L. Tan, J. Mukherjee, T. Nicolaides, and R.O. Pieper. 2012. Sensitivity of glioblastomas to clinically available MEK inhibitors is defined by neurofibromin 1 deficiency. *Cancer Research* 72: 3350–3359.

Shukla, S., S. Bhargava, and K. Somasundaram. 2014. Cancer gene signatures in risk stratification: Use in personalized medicine. *Current Science* 107: 815–823.

Shukla, S., I.R. Pia Patric, S. Thinagararjan, S. Srinivasan, B. Mondal, A.S. Hegde, B.A. Chandramouli, V. Santosh, A. Arivazhagan, and K. Somasundaram. 2013. A DNA methylation prognostic signature of glioblastoma: Identification of NPTX2-PTEN-NF-kappaB nexus. *Cancer Research* 73: 6563–6573.

Srinivasan, S., I.R. Patric, and K. Somasundaram. 2011. A ten-microRNA expression signature predicts survival in glioblastoma. *PLoS One* 6: e17438.

Stratton, M.R., P.J. Campbell, and P.A. Futreal. 2009. The cancer genome. *Nature* 458: 719–724.

Stupp, R., M.E. Hegi, W.P. Mason, M.J. van den Bent, M.J. Taphoorn, R.C. Janzer, S.K. Ludwin, A. Allgeier, B. Fisher, K. Belanger, P. Hau, A.A. Brandes, J. Gijtenbeek, C. Marosi, C.J. Vecht, K. Mokhtari, P. Wesseling, S. Villa, E. Eisenhauer, T. Gorlia, M. Weller, D. Lacombe, J.G. Cairncross, R.O. Mirimanoff, European Organisation for Research, Treatment of Cancer Brain Tumour, Radiation Oncology Groups, and National Cancer Institute of Canada Clinical Trials Groups. 2009. Effects of radiotherapy with concomitant and adjuvant temozolomide versus radiotherapy alone on survival in glioblastoma in a randomised phase III study: 5-year analysis of the EORTC-NCIC trial. *The Lancet Oncology* 10: 459–466.

Stupp, R., W.P. Mason, M.J. van den Bent, M. Weller, B. Fisher, M.J. Taphoorn, K. Belanger, A.A. Brandes, C. Marosi, U. Bogdahn, J. Curschmann, R.C. Janzer, S.K. Ludwin, T. Gorlia, A. Allgeier, D. Lacombe, J.G. Cairncross, E. Eisenhauer, R.O. Mirimanoff, European Organisation for Research, Treatment of Cancer Brain Tumour, Radiotherapy Groups, and National Cancer Institute of Canada Clinical Trials Group. 2005. Radiotherapy plus concomitant and adjuvant temozolomide for glioblastoma. *The New England Journal of Medicine* 352: 987–996.

Tamborero, D., A. Gonzalez-Perez, C. Perez-Llamas, J. Deu-Pons, C. Kandoth, J. Reimand, M.S. Lawrence, G. Getz, G.D. Bader, L. Ding, and N. Lopez-Bigas. 2013. Comprehensive identification of mutational cancer driver genes across 12 tumor types. *Scientific Reports* 3: 2650.

Thon, N., S. Kreth, and F.W. Kreth. 2013. Personalized treatment strategies in glioblastoma: MGMT promoter methylation status. *Oncotargets Therapy* 6: 1363–1372.

Tucker, T., M. Marra, and J.M. Friedman. 2009. Massively parallel sequencing: The next big thing in genetic medicine. *American Journal of Human Genetics* 85: 142–154.

Venter, J.C., M.D. Adams, E.W. Myers, P.W. Li, R.J. Mural, G.G. Sutton, H.O. Smith, M. Yandell, C.A. Evans, R.A. Holt, J.D. Gocayne, P. Amanatides, R.M. Ballew, D.H. Huson, J.R. Wortman, Q. Zhang, C.D. Kodira, X.H. Zheng, L. Chen, M. Skupski, G. Subramanian, P.D. Thomas, J. Zhang, G.L. Gabor Miklos, C. Nelson, S. Broder, A.G. Clark, J. Nadeau, V.A. McKusick, N. Zinder, A.J. Levine, R.J. Roberts, M. Simon, C. Slayman, M. Hunkapiller, R. Bolanos, A. Delcher, I. Dew, D. Fasulo, M. Flanigan, L. Florea, A. Halpern, S. Hannenhalli, S. Kravitz, S. Levy, C. Mobarry, K. Reinert, K. Remington, J. Abu-Threideh, E. Beasley, K. Biddick, V. Bonazzi, R. Brandon, M. Cargill, I. Chandramouliswaran, R. Charlab, K. Chaturvedi, Z. Deng, V. Di Francesco, P. Dunn, K. Eilbeck, C. Evangelista, A.E. Gabrielian, W. Gan, W. Ge, F. Gong, Z. Gu, P. Guan, T.J. Heiman, M.E. Higgins, R.R. Ji, Z. Ke, K.A. Ketchum, Z. Lai, Y. Lei, Z. Li, J. Li, Y. Liang, X. Lin, F. Lu, G.V. Merkulov, N. Milshina, H.M. Moore, A.K. Naik, V.A. Narayan, B. Neelam, D. Nusskern, D.B. Rusch, S. Salzberg, W. Shao, B. Shue, J. Sun, Z. Wang, A. Wang, X. Wang, J. Wang, M. Wei, R. Wides, C. Xiao, C. Yan, A. Yao, J. Ye, M. Zhan, W. Zhang, H. Zhang, Q. Zhao, L. Zheng, F. Zhong, W. Zhong, S. Zhu, S. Zhao, D. Gilbert, S. Baumhueter, G. Spier, C. Carter, A. Cravchik, T. Woodage, F. Ali, H. An, A. Awe, D. Baldwin, H. Baden, M. Barnstead, I. Barrow, K. Beeson, D. Busam, A. Carver, A. Center, M.L. Cheng, L. Curry, S. Danaher, L. Davenport, R. Desilets, S. Dietz, K. Dodson, L. Doup, S. Ferriera, N. Garg, A. Gluecksmann, B. Hart, J. Haynes, C. Haynes, C. Heiner, S. Hladun, D. Hostin, J. Houck, T. Howland, C. Ibegwam, J. Johnson, F. Kalush, L. Kline, S. Koduru, A. Love, F. Mann, D. May, S. McCawley, T. McIntosh, I. McMullen, M. Moy, L. Moy, B. Murphy, K. Nelson, C. Pfannkoch, E. Pratts, V. Puri, H. Qureshi, M. Reardon, R. Rodriguez, Y.H. Rogers, D. Romblad, B. Ruhfel, R. Scott, C. Sitter, M. Smallwood, E. Stewart, R. Strong, E. Suh, R. Thomas, N.N. Tint, S. Tse, C. Vech, G. Wang, J. Wetter, S. Williams, M. Williams, S. Windsor, E. Winn-Deen, K. Wolfe, J. Zaveri, K. Zaveri, J.F. Abril, R. Guigo, M.J. Campbell, K.V. Sjolander, B. Karlak, A. Kejariwal, H. Mi, B. Lazareva, T. Hatton, A. Narechania, K. Diemer, A. Muruganujan, N. Guo, S. Sato, V. Bafna, S. Istrail, R. Lippert, R. Schwartz, B. Walenz, S. Yooseph, D. Allen, A. Basu, J. Baxendale, L. Blick, M. Caminha, J. Carnes-Stine, P. Caulk, Y.H. Chiang, M. Coyne, C. Dahlke, A. Mays, M. Dombroski, M. Donnelly, D. Ely, S. Esparham, C. Fosler, H. Gire, S. Glanowski, K. Glasser, A. Glodek, M. Gorokhov, K. Graham, B. Gropman, M. Harris, J. Heil, S. Henderson, J. Hoover, D. Jennings, C. Jordan, J. Jordan, J. Kasha, L. Kagan, C. Kraft, A. Levitsky, M. Lewis, X. Liu, J. Lopez, D. Ma, W. Majoros, J. McDaniel, S. Murphy, M. Newman, T. Nguyen, N. Nguyen, M. Nodell, S. Pan,

J. Peck, M. Peterson, W. Rowe, R. Sanders, J. Scott, M. Simpson, T. Smith, A. Sprague, T. Stockwell, R. Turner, E. Venter, M. Wang, M. Wen, D. Wu, M. Wu, A. Xia, A. Zandieh, and X. Zhu. 2001. The sequence of the human genome. *Science* 291: 1304–1351.

Verhaak, R.G., K.A. Hoadley, E. Purdom, V. Wang, Y. Qi, M.D. Wilkerson, C.R. Miller, L. Ding, T. Golub, J.P. Mesirov, G. Alexe, M. Lawrence, M. O'Kelly, P. Tamayo, B.A. Weir, S. Gabriel, W. Winckler, S. Gupta, L. Jakkula, H.S. Feiler, J.G. Hodgson, C.D. James, J.N. Sarkaria, C. Brennan, A. Kahn, P.T. Spellman, R.K. Wilson, T.P. Speed, J.W. Gray, M. Meyerson, G. Getz, C.M. Perou, D.N. Hayes, and Network Cancer Genome Atlas Research. 2010. Integrated genomic analysis identifies clinically relevant subtypes of glioblastoma characterized by abnormalities in PDGFRA, IDH1, EGFR, and NF1. *Cancer Cell* 17: 98–110.

Vigneswaran, K., S. Neill, and C.G. Hadjipanayis. 2015. Beyond the World Health Organization grading of infiltrating gliomas: advances in the molecular genetics of glioma classification. *Annals of Translational Medicine* 3: 95.

Wang, H., T. Xu, Y. Jiang, H. Xu, Y. Yan, D. Fu, and J. Chen. 2015. The challenges and the promise of molecular targeted therapy in malignant gliomas. *Neoplasia* 17: 239–255.

Wang, J.L., Z.J. Zhang, M. Hartman, A. Smits, B. Westermark, C. Muhr, and M. Nister. 1995. Detection of TP53 gene mutation in human meningiomas: A study using immunohistochemistry, polymerase chain reaction/single-strand conformation polymorphism and DNA sequencing techniques on paraffin-embedded samples. *International Journal of Cancer Journal International du Cancer* 64: 223–228.

Warr, A., C. Robert, D. Hume, A. Archibald, N. Deeb, and M. Watson. 2015. Exome sequencing: Current and future perspectives. *G3* 5: 1543–1550.

Wen, P.Y., and S. Kesari. 2008. Malignant gliomas in adults. *The New England Journal of Medicine* 359: 492–507.

Ye, K., M.H. Schulz, Q. Long, R. Apweiler, and Z. Ning. 2009. Pindel: A pattern growth approach to detect break points of large deletions and medium sized insertions from paired-end short reads. *Bioinformatics* 25: 2865–2871.

Zhang, W., and H.T. Liu. 2002. MAPK signal pathways in the regulation of cell proliferation in mammalian cells. *Cell Research* 12: 9–18.

Chapter 8
Glioma Stem-Like Cells in Tumor Growth and Therapy Resistance of Glioblastoma

Abhirami Visvanathan and Kumaravel Somasundaram

Abstract Glioblastoma is detrimental brain tumor with less than 2 years of life expectancy. They are refractory to conventional therapy and show high relapse rate. GBM tumors exhibit diverse intra-tumoral heterogeneity with multidirectional evolution of clones created by plethora of genetic and epigenetic events. Plasticity being an obstacle in targeting the GBM cells, discovery of glioma stem like cells (GSCs) a decade ago shed light on the dark side of GBM. The intrinsic escape pathways and quiescence encoded within GSCs in combination with niche signals offer advantages like resistance to radio/chemotherapy, high invasion and migration capabilities, trans-differentiation and enhanced self-renewal to tumor. This chapter summarizes the recent advances in the field of GSCs including the distinct molecular characteristics and importance of GSCs in therapy resistance. Though enormous attempts to deduce the puzzle of GSCs were made, the perspective in conjunction with whole tumor studies is still at stake which emphasize the requirement of in-depth studies.

Keywords Glioblastoma • Glioma stem-like cells • Therapy resistance • Neurosphere • Temozolomide • Radiation

Abbreviations

CSC   Cancer stem cell
DGC   Differentiated glioma cell
GBM   Glioblastoma
GSC   Glioma stem-like cell
NSC   Neural stem cell
TMZ   Temozolomide

A. Visvanathan • K. Somasundaram (✉)
Department of Microbiology and Cell Biology, Indian Institute of Science,
Bangalore 560012, India
e-mail: skumar@mcbl.iisc.ernet.in; ksomasundaram1@gmail.com

© Springer International Publishing AG 2017   191
K. Somasundaram (ed.), *Advances in Biology and Treatment of Glioblastoma*,
Current Cancer Research, DOI 10.1007/978-3-319-56820-1_8

8.1 Introduction

Glioblastoma (GBM) is the most aggressive glioma in adults. It is classified as grade IV astrocytoma by World Health Organization with characteristics of intra-tumoral heterogeneity, high vasculature and infiltrative nature. GBM has a worse prognosis with less than 12–14 months of survival after diagnosis. Radiotherapy post-surgery has been shown to increase survival significantly from 3–4 months to 14.4 months in GBM patients and additional adjuvant temozolomide treatment pro-longs life expectancy up to 18.8 months (Stupp et al. 2009). Glioma stem like cells (GSC) which exist in small fraction, exhibit high self-renewal, and therapy resistant which leads to high propensity of recurrence.

8.2 Historical Perspective of Cancer Stem Cells (CSCs)

The cancer stem cell (CSC) hypothesis proposes that hierarchy of cells exists within a tumor with varying extent of proliferation, differentiation capability and *in vivo* tumorigenecity. A minor clonal population of cells on top of the hierarchy termed as "cancer stem cells" is necessary and sufficient for tumor expansion (Shapiro et al. 1981). The terms stem cell and progenitor are utilized interchangeably despite they belong to different states in the hierarchy and progenitors show restricted ability of self-renewal and unipotent (Bradshaw et al. 2016). CSCs have the ability to self-renew by symmetric divisions to expand pool of stem like cells while it can estab-lish another malignant stem cell and a progenitor cell by asymmetric cell division. The fate decision of CSCs depends on chromosomal aberrations or extra-cellular interactions with the niche/ microenvironment (Tang 2012). Tumor cells lacking stem cell properties fail to initiate self-propagating tumors regardless of their dif-ferentiation status or proliferative capacity which makes cancer stem cells as a lucrative drug target (Kreso and Dick 2014). Though glioma stem-like cells (GSCs) reflect characteristics of normal neural stem cells (NSC), unlike NSC they can give rise to glioma-like tumors when xenografted into subventricular striata of immune-compromised mice. The plasticity (differentiation and trans-differentiation) of nor-mal adult stem cells compared to CSC is limited.

Evidence for the cancer stem cell was first shown in human acute myeloid leuke-mia (AML). CD34$^+$/CD38$^-$ cancer initiating cells isolated from AML formed tumors *in vivo* when transplanted into nude mice (Dick et al. 1991). Breast cancer cells with profile of CD24$^+$CD44$^{-/low}$ distinguished tumorigenic from non tumorigenic cells (Yan et al. 2013). Initial identification of GSCs in whole tumor was proven by expansion of neurosphere cell clones under serum free culture conditions identical to normal neural stem cells (Ignatova et al. 2002) followed by Kondo et al. showed high incident of tumor formation by neurosphere cells sorted according to dye efflux capacity (Kondo et al. 2004). Discovery of CD133$^+$ GSC was a milestone in stem cell research since as few as 100 CD133$^+$ cells was able to form serially transplantable xenograft to recapitulate the pathology of patient tumor whereas 10^5 CD133$^-$ cells failed to initiate tumor (Singh et al. 2004). The tumor cells grown as neurosphere in limited numbers (1 cell/well) express stem related markers compared to the differentiated cells under serum condition for 2 weeks. Normal brain derived neurospheres failed to regain spheres post differentiation for 2 weeks which reiterates the enhanced self-renewal capability of GSC compared to NSC (Yuan et al. 2004). Followed by the breakthrough in GSC isolation, several groups have attempted to enrich GSCs as neurospheres from whole tumor using different surface markers and examined the tumor formation efficiency of this population by establishing intracranial xenografts with limited number of cells. Two reports have provided evidence that CD133$^-$ cells also exhibit stem like characteristics and tumor initiation (Beier et al. 2007; Wang et al. 2008). Later Gunther et al. has proven the existence of two distinct GSCs derived from GBM tumors with variable nature of invasive tumor formation and CD133 expression (Gunther et al. 2008).

8.3 Cancer Stem Cell Models

Glioma portraits high extent of heterogeneity and remain unrestrictive for standard therapy. Initiation and progression of GSCs are explained by continuous molecular evolution and whole tumor is composed of diverse types of GSCs with distinct expression signature. Investigating the underlying mechanism is beneficial for devising personalized clinical strategy and excludes unnecessary drugs. The proportions of GSC differ in various tumor types and grade. Hence evaluating the stoichiometry of GSCs in tumor serve the purpose of effective therapy as certain drugs are restricted to specific cell types. There are two models in current literature to explain the property and dynamics of GSCs. Hierarchical model emphasizes that each cell has predefined cell fate and GSCs belongs to the apex of hierarchy (Fig. 8.1a). They show distinct property of enhanced tumorigenesis and therapy resistance (Dick 2009; Nguyen et al. 2012). Stochastic model show randomized population of tumor cells where any cell can acquire or lose the tumorigenic property and the dynamic events rely on intrinsic and extrinsic factors. It portrays tumor as homogenous population with clonal expansion and it allows bi-directional transitions among different epigenetic/transcriptomic phenotypes due to genomic instability created by irreversible genetic aberrations (Fig. 8.1b).

Several experimental and theoretical approaches were employed to solve the dilemma on stem cell theory. Studies in hematopoietic system show that despite cells belongs to distinct functional profile, any isolated subpopulation will regain the proportions of heterogeneity over time under physiological condition and stem cells undergo transition stochastically between progenitor and transit amplifying cell states (Gupta et al. 2011). Due to plasticity, GSCs give rise to non GSC by differentiation or asymmetric cell division while non –GSCs can also revert to stem-like cells under physiological condition (Fig. 8.1c). To experimentally test the models, GSCs and non-GSCs sorted on the basis of cell surface marker (CD133) and were cultured

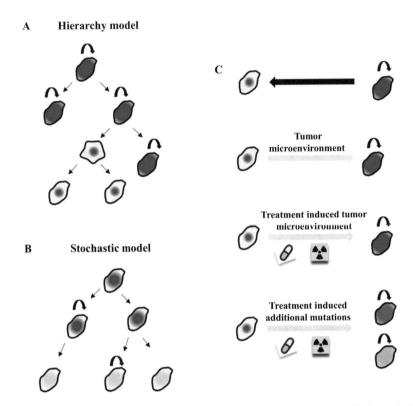

Fig. 8.1 Cancer stem cell models (**a**) Hierarchy/elite model describes tumor as biologically distinct clones of cells with varying efficiency of tumorigenicity. A small subset of cells possesses high self-renewal capacity and act as a reservoir (⬤) for tumor. Different stages of differentiation lead to emergence of progenitors (◉) and differentiated cells (◉) with limited self-propagation and restricted tumorigenicity. (**b**) Stochastic model explains a flexible system of cells where every cell has the potential to become a GSC and at any point a population of cells can impart GSC-like property (◉ ◉). (**c**) The transition of GSC to non-GSC is a pre-dominant event happening all the time (*black arrow*), while the formation of GSC from non-GSC may happen occasionally (*grey arrow*), when the cells are exposed to appropriate tumor niche related cues like hypoxia (Skjellegrind et al. 2016) and endothelial cells (Fessler et al. 2015). Treatment (TMZ/radiation) also enhances the stochastic switching (Auffinger et al. 2014; Dahan et al. 2014) via the metabolomic reprogramming by alterations in glycolysis (Mao et al. 2012), Reactive oxygen species (Hsieh et al. 2011), Nitric oxide (Altieri et al. 2015) or by intrinsic acquisition of additional mutation. These events result in the transition of non-GSCs to GSCs with a same or varying genetic make-up (⬤ ◉ ◉)

separately in order to track transition dynamics of parent and sub-clones. Though GSCs and non-GSC are organized within restricted compartment, the inter-conversion of non-GSC to GSC is a stochastic event (Wang et al. 2014). Mathematical modeling and lineage tracking by limited dilution tumorigenesis in vivo in other cancers provide additional support to the unified stem theory (Chaffer et al. 2011; Gupta et al. 2011; Morel et al. 2008; Quintana et al. 2010; Sottoriva et al. 2013). Chen and colleagues have established that regardless of predetermined fate decision or genetic background, low probability of spontaneous GSC transition from bulk cells occur and it relies on epigenetic reprogramming by regulation of histone modifiers (Kozono et al. 2015). Normal somatic cells can be reversed to pluripotent state by introducing Yamanaka factors SOX2, OCT4, MYC and KLF4. Similarly fate of non GSCs to GSC is reconstructed by altered epigenetic barriers encoded in DNA and histones. The activation of four factors SOX2, SALL2, OLIG2 and POU3F2 rewire histone marks and transcriptome profile of differentiated cells back to GSCs. Induced stem-like cells from differentiated cells recapitulate the H3K27 acetylation profile of GSCs and tumorigenecity (Suva et al. 2014). Differentiated cells were successfully reprogrammed to form neurospheres *in vitro* with comparable spherogenecity as of GSC culture and gene expression profile by over expression of four transcription factors. An independent study by Olmez et al. has obtained induced GSCs by introducing OCT4, SOX2 and Nanog to differentiated cells and they were able to sustain stem property independent of exogenous mitogens (Olmez et al. 2015). Different GSCs possess varying capability of differentiation and permanent cell cycle exit when exposed to BMP. Re-exposure to EGF/FGF leads to cell cycle re-entry and proliferation regardless of long term non-cycling state. The incomplete differentiation and quiescence of specific clones are due to the partial DNA methylation coupled with abrupt SOX2 occupancy in stem specific promoters is the limitation which locks the cells in hyper quiescent stem like cells (Caren et al. 2015).

Therapy resistance of tumor is partially due to GSCs and high order hierarchy tumors are refractory to drugs. In contrary to hierarchy model, during standard therapy, dedifferentiation of non-stem cells to stem compartment occur which reiterates the existence of stochastic transition model (Wang et al. 2014). Enhanced reprogramming of non-GSC to GSC when exposed to radiation (Bao et al. 2006a) and temozolomide (enrichment for CD133/Nestin OCT4, SOX2) (Auffinger et al. 2014) were additional proof for the operation of stochastic model (Fig. 8.1c).

8.4 Tumor Heterogeneity and Cancer Stem Cells

Recent studies have interrogated the existence of diversity among GSCs within a single tumor. Single cell sequencing coupled with CNV analysis enabled molecular profiling of individual cells derived from five different tumors demonstrated the presence of an intra-tumoral expression gradient (Patel et al. 2014). In addition to the variable expression of genes related to oncogenic signaling, proliferation, complement/immune response, and hypoxia, stem cell specific gene signature also showed variation within different regions of tumor. Further, it has been shown that a single GBM tumor contains heterogeneous clones of GSCs with different morphologies, self-renewal and proliferative capacities (Soeda et al. 2015).

The origin of GSCs remains paradoxical as they can arise either from NSCs or differentiated glial cells. Since previous reports suggest intra-tumoral heterogeneity exists within stem cell population, it gives hint that multiple stem cell clones would have evolved during the tumorigenesis which further expand to establish a complex system. Failed DNA aberration surveillance within NSCs may lead to initial seed of tumor initiating cell. Multiple mutant clones might evolve within a span of time

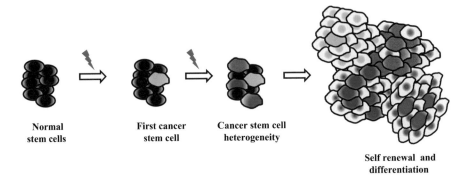

Fig. 8.2 Heterogeneity of cancer initiation and progression Exposure to carcinogens (↯) creates a rare cancer stem cell (◐) from a normal stem cell (●) due to genetic aberration. Additional clones of new cancer stem cells (◐ ◐ ◐) are formed either from the first formed cancer stem cell due to its genetic instability or directly from another normal stem cell due to another new genetic aberration. Further epigenetic changes results in creation of a large number of differentiated bulk cells (◌ ◌ ◌ ◌) thus forming a tumor

directly from different NSCs. Due to genomic instability, the previously formed tumor initiating cells may also acquire additional genetic alterations thus resulting in wide heterogeneity (Fig. 8.2).

Initial studies revealed inactivation of tumor suppressors Nf1, p53, Pten in normal neural progenitors is sufficient and indispensible to initiate astrocytoma (Alcantara Llaguno et al. 2009). In addition, adenoviral injection of Cre recombinase into sub ventricular zone (SVZ), an NSC reservoir of Nf1/p53 floxed mice induced grade III/IV glioma at post natal and adult ages. Independent report showed deletion of p53 and Pten in murine neural stem cells forms aggressive GBM and the cells are resistant for differentiation (Zheng et al. 2008). The above work was extended in astrocytes/neurons/SVZ NSCs by introducing shNF1-shp53 or H-RasV12-shp53 genetic aberrations and proved dedifferentiation of cells in order to initiate and maintain the tumor (Friedmann-Morvinski et al. 2012). Additional support for NSC driven tumorigenesis was provided by PTEN deletion in normal neural stem cells which creates GSCs by derepressing PAX7 transcription (Duan et al. 2015).

As the whole tumor study widen the spectrum of heterogeneity by dividing GBM into neural, proneural, mesenchymal and classical tumors on the basis of transcriptome, recent research extended the classification to GSCs. Mesenchymal GSCs with (NF1 alteration and WT IDH1) high CD44/low Olig2 expression cause aggressive intracranial tumors with resistant phenotype to radiation compared to proneural GSC (mutant IDH with GCIMP) (Bhat et al. 2013; Mao et al. 2013). Chandran et al. provided support for distinct expression and metabolic profiles exist between proneural and mesenchymal GSCs and they report mesenchymal GSC portray profound radioresistance than other classes with high ALDH1A3 (Aldehyde Dehydrogenase 1 Family Member A3) expression (Chandran et al. 2015). Radiation induces shift in gene expression towards mesenchymal like profile and inhibition of ALDH1A3 attenuates the shift (Mao et al. 2013).

8.5   Cancer Stem Cell Isolation

8.5.1   Neurospheres

Whole tumor and cell line based studies do not portray the molecular mechanisms specific to CSCs as they are of small population and the alterations are masked by the bulk differentiated cells. Hence it is necessary to explore the effects in such a system where stem cells are enriched by selective stem specific growth factors. GSCs are able to form clonal structures named as "neurospheres," *in vitro* that recapitulate the intra-clonal diversity which exists within tumor. The initial evidence of neurosphere culture was provided by maintaining stem like cells with self-renewal and multipotent property on methyl-cellulose matrix in presence of EGF (Epidermal growth factor) and FGF (fibroblast growth factor) (Ignatova et al. 2002). Serum free medium supplemented with growth factors EGF, N2, B27 and FGF with anchorage withdrawal condition, cells are allowed to propagate as heterogeneous population of cancer stem and progenitor cells. Neurospheres is a mixture of committed progenitors, stem and differentiated cells. Enzymatic/chemical or mechanical disruption methods are used to passage neurospheres cells. Approximately after 7–10 days of dissociation, the spheroid reaches the size of 100–200 μM with an average of 3000–5000 cells per sphere. Passaging efficiency and size of the sphere are measures for self-renewability and proliferation respectively. Different combination of growth factors and dissociation protocols are followed to propagate neurospheres and hence it is essential to validate the stem properties during the passages. As with increasing passages self-renewal and differentiation capacity were altered and induced chromosomal instability occur in neurospheres culture (Vukicevic et al. 2010).

Limitations of neurosphere culture: neurospheres cells expand more slowly in suspension culture *in vitro* than their *in vivo* counterparts. It is difficult to identify the precise cellular targets and real-time monitoring of cellular responses due to the presence of restricted progenitors and differentiated cell types along with neural stem cells (Pastrana et al. 2011). The diffusion of growth factors is limited in sphere condition and it might disrupt the uniformity of GSC phenotype. Disrupted neurosphere derived single cells were captured by time lapse microscope and they form adventitious clumps or fused multi-clones as they were motile. Since the composition of neurosphere was assumed as clonal cells arise from a founder cell it is crucial to complement the assay by limited number of cells (1–10 cell per well) (Ladiwala et al. 2012). Cell density, medium volume and surface area of the culture dish are limiting factors in determining clonal proliferation and intercellular fusion. In addition presence of EGF and FGF in neurosphere culture condition renders selective pressure for progenitor pool with high EGFR/FGFR and it fails to recreate the heterogeneity and histological features in xenograft as of GSCs isolated fresh from tumor (Lathia et al. 2015). To overcome the uneven distribution of growth factors adherent stem culture on laminin coated culture ware was developed and studies on stem like characteristics show the cells portray positivity for stem specific markers and they selectively enrich for proliferative neural progenitors with high Nestin (Sun et al. 2009).

8.5.2   De Novo Isolation of GSCs Using Markers

GSCs can be identified on the basis of their expression of cell surface markers. The markers which define the cancer stem cell population remain controversial. CD133 membrane glycoprotein is a marker for glial neuronal progenitors and stem cells. CD133[+]cells represent a subpopulation of cells in brain tumors with a frequency of as low as 1% or less in low-grade tumors and high as 30% in highly aggressive glioblastomas (Dirks 2006; Hemmati et al. 2003). Selection for CD133[+] cells enriched the populations of cells with stem-like properties, though evidences suggest the existence of CD133[-] glioma stem cells and both CD133[+] and CD133[-] cells isolated from the same tumor specimen can be cultured as neurospheres (Sun et al. 2009). Both populations of cells are able to self-renew and initiate tumors upon xenotransplantation (Beier and Beier 2011). The discrepancy is explained by Brescia et al. that due to CD133 localization changes from cell surface to cytoplasm the physiological importance of cellular compartment specific CD133 is underestimated. Further glycosylated membrane localized AC133 antigen instead of mRNA of CD133 is reliable in identifying the stem phenotype (Lathia et al. 2015). In addition by exploiting the enhanced expression of detoxifying molecules like ALDH1A (aldefluor) and ABCG2 (side population and dye retention) in stem cells they can be purified from a heterogeneous population. Exploiting the high efflux capability of stem cells, a side population (SP) which shows low DNA binding fluorescent dye content can be purified. 0.2–0.8% of neurosphere cells of mouse forebrain falls in to SP and they disappear with ABC transporter inhibition by verapamil (Kim and Morshead 2003). SSEA1 (CD15) (Son et al. 2009), ABCG2 (Jin et al. 2009), CD44 (Liu et al. 2006) and L1CAM (Bao et al. 2008), Nanog (Ben-Porath et al. 2008; Suva et al. 2014) and A2B5 (Tchoghandjian et al. 2010) are few other markers which define the identity of GSCs. Regardless of the methods used the resultant will be a mixture of progenitors and primitive stem cells with varying level of tumorigenic potential. To get a stringent separation a set of markers combined with functional assays *in vivo* (tumor formation with limited number of GSCs and the serial transplantation) is reliable. Independent of mutation background of GSCs, the markers CD133, CD15, L1CAM are widely expressed and it reveals that GSC signature profile is recreated via different mutations. The selection of markers for whole tumor studies should be selected with care as cytosolic SOX2, Nestin, and CD133 are expressed in NSCs and aberrant expression should be scored for CSCs.

8.6   Characterization of GSCs

(1) **Multipotency-** In the presence of serum and adherent support GSCs can differentiate in to glial, neural, oligodendrocytic lineages accompanied by increased expression of lineage restrictive genes (MAP2, Tubulin beta III, O4, Tuj1, GFAP) confirms the multipotent nature of GSCs. (2) **Limited dilution assay (LDA)**-Small number (1–50) of cells is plated in multiple wells in order to test the clonogenecity

and to ensure the sphere formation is not due to aggregation. In addition to neurosphere assay, LDA examines the incidents of wells with no sphere formation at higher dilutions of cells. Particular size limit is usually defined to consider a clump as neurosphere to eliminate the cell clones with limiting self-renewal (Rahman et al. 2015). (**3**) *In vivo* **serial transplantation**- Formation of aggressive GBM like tumor with the characteristics such as high necrotic regions vasculature nuclear atypia pseudopalisading cells with limited number of GSCs. It supports the fact that GSCs are capable to initiate and repopulate a whole tumor which reflects the histology of GBM patient tumors (deCarvalho et al. 2010).

8.7 Role of GSCs in Therapy Resistance

8.7.1 Perspective on GSC Treatment Response

GSCs were reported to exhibit high drug resistance with migratory potential and the enriched proportion of GSCs aggravates the tumor. Parada group, using ΔTK-IRES-GFP (Nes-ΔTK-GFP) mouse model showed that Nestin positive cells were remnant post temozolomide (TMZ) treatment and could reinitiate tumor (Chen et al. 2012). Post TMZ treatment, the residual tumor mass showed endogenous high Nestin and characteristics of GSCs. CD133$^+$ GSCs promptly activate DNA double strand break repair pathways via ATM/ATR and ChK1 phosphorylation post TMZ treatment which results in the efficient killing of CD133$^-$ cells compared to CD133$^+$ cells. Further, cytotoxicity of TMZ was high in differentiated cells maintained in serum containing media compared to the matched GSCs (Ghods et al. 2007). Long term TMZ treatment as 2 weeks increased the percentage of side population which is characteristic of GSCs and in vivo tumorigenecity (Chua et al. 2008). An independent report suggests that hypoxic core derived CD133$^+$ cells are intrinsically resistance to TMZ compared to peripheral cells (Pistollato et al. 2010). Studies on clinical efficacy of TMZ in targeting GSCs show selective dose-dependent decrease in proliferation of CD133$^+$ cells with minor cell death (Clement et al. 2007). As shown in differentiated glioma cells, the promoter methylation and transcript/protein levels of MGMT partially determine the TMZ sensitivity in GSCs (Blough et al. 2010).

In contrast to previous reports, Beier and colleagues have concluded that CD133$^+$clonal cells are selectively depleted by TMZ compared to CD133$^-$ cells and the lethality relies on MGMT levels. The dosage given to patients is sufficient to eliminate MGMT negative GSCs and not MGMT positive GSCs which are similar as CD133$^-$ cells. Authors explained the discordance to previous studies by limitation of using short term metabolic viability assays over prolong observation of cytotoxicity. CD133 being an ambiguous stem marker, the physiological effects needs further scrutiny. Pharmacokinetics of TMZ shows a maximum concentration of 5 μM in the cerebrospinal fluid of GBM patients post treatment which is far below the concentration required to kill GSCs, hence maintaining 50 μM within tumor cells is required to eliminate GSCs (Beier et al. 2008). Several attempts on synergizing the cytotoxicity by using specific pathway inhibitors with TMZ were taken to overcome the dosage limitation. Drugs targeting IGF1/Shh pathway (Hsieh et al. 2011), STAT3 (Villalva et al. 2011) and NOTCH (Gilbert et al. 2010) were proved to make GSCs susceptible to sub optimal TMZ concentrations.

Post high dose gamma irradiation, the percentage of CD133$^+$ cells were found to be high compared to surgically resected tumors before treatment (Tamura et al. 2010). Clonogenic assay showed high CD133$^+$ cells were resistant to radiation compared to the CD133$^-$ cells. In addition, the minimal number of cells required to establish a xenograft is less when the cells were exposed to irradiation as irradiation selectively enriches CD133$^+$ cells (Bao et al. 2006a). Similar physiopathology was showed in vivo when a mixed population of independently labeled CD133$^+$/CD133$^-$ cells implanted and the ratio of CD133$^+$:CD133$^-$ increased post irradiation. Efforts were taken to radiosensitize GSCs by inhibition of specific set of genes (De Bacco et al. 2011; Kim et al. 2015; Lomonaco et al. 2009; Wang et al. 2010).

8.7.2 Mechanisms Behind GSC Therapy Resistance

Several other mechanisms in GSCs apart from MGMT expression operate to safeguard from standard therapy. **(1) Successful efflux of drugs**: High expression of ABC transporters (ABCB1, ABCG) (Schaich et al. 2009) which pump out the drugs across membrane in ATP dependent manner help GSCs to escape from chemotherapy. The failure in clinical trial of Erlotinib (EGFR inhibitor) and Vincristine (mitotic toxin) are due to high expression of multidrug resistant ABC transporter p-GP and BCRP (de Vries et al. 2012). **(2) DNA repair**: TMZ cytotoxicity relies on active mismatch repair pathway and mutation in MSH6 leads to TMZ resistance in recurrent GBM (Yip et al. 2009). Active G2-M checkpoint during DNA damage lends sufficient time for tumor cells to overcome genotoxicity and intrinsic levels of active DNA repair protein forms of p-Chk1, p-Chk2 and RAD17 are maintained high in CD133$^+$ GSC compared to CD133$^-$ cells. Multiple DNA repair pathways show cumulative effect on GSC radio sensitivity with enhanced cell cycle checkpoint activation (Ahmed et al. 2015). Chk1 inhibitor debromohymenialdisine was proven to sensitize GSCs to radiation (Huang et al. 2010). In addition, inhibition of ATM showed pronounced radio sensitization in GSCs than independent blockade of Chk1, ATR or PARP (Ahmed et al. 2015). Lim et al., showed that homologous recombination was augmented in GSCs compared to differentiated cells (Lim et al. 2012). Further, the inhibition of PARP1, which is required for single strand base repair and GSC growth, leads to radiosensitization (Venere et al. 2014). Contradictory reports suggest that CD133$^+$ cells are sensitive than differentiated cells due to a defective S-check point despite intact G2-M check point in CD133$^+$ cells (McCord et al. 2009). Slow cell cycle progression with less efficient base excision and single strand base repair was observed in CD133$^+$ cells (Ropolo et al. 2009). The controversy is attributed to the heterogeneous genetic and epigenetic background of GSCs and the specificity of stem cell specific marker CD133. **(3) Anti apoptotic pathway**: Anti apoptotic genes BCL2L1a, BCL-2 and MCL1 are abundant in chemo resistant GSCs compared to the differentiated counterpart which help in evading cell death (Yamada et al. 2011). Hedgehog pathway, a master regulator in GSCs, switch on the transcription of these genes (Hsieh et al. 2011). Intrinsic family of inhibitor of apoptosis (IAP), cIAP2 and XIAP are maintained high in GSCs and antagonizer for XIAP sensitizes GSCs to radiation (Vellanki et al. 2009). In addition over expression of miRNAs which target proapoptotic genes was observed in GSCs. miRNA 582-5p and 363 directly degrade Caspase 3, Caspase 9 and Bim proteins and escape self-destruction during therapy (Floyd et al. 2014) **(4) Hypoxia and high redox potential**: The cells embedded far from vasculature show hypoxic nature and are resistant to TMZ. Hypoxic niche is enriched for GSCs and it induces the expression of p-GP transporters due to high anaerobic glycolysis combined with low reactive oxygen species (ROS) (Wartenberg et al. 2003). A free radical generator tirapazamine which causes DNA single strand breaks showed promising results in TMZ treatment in hypoxic niche *in vitro* (Del Rowe et al. 2000). **(5) Vascular nich**: Tumor microenvironment includes stroma, matrix and blood vessels which influences GSC adaptation in response to hypoxia, radiation, drugs and metabolic scarcity. Autocrine and paracrine immune circuits induce and recruit/guide GSCs towards perivascular and hypoxic niche. The chemo-attractant SDF1α expressed in vascular and hypoxic regions of brain recruit CD133$^+$ GSCs with high CXCR4 (Cheng et al. 2013). (SCF)/c-Kit (Sun et al. 2004), VEGF/VEGFR (Schmidt et al. 2005) are other few receptor ligand interactions which enhance niche formation. Rich and colleagues showed that GSCs preferentially localize near vasculature by using tagged CD133$^+$ GSCs and CD133$^-$ in three dimensional architecture of tumor within mouse brain (Lathia et al. 2011). GSCs produce high levels of VEGF and SDF1 (stromal-derived factor-1) which involve in angiogenesis and therapy resistance (Bao et al. 2009; Folkins et al. 2009). Tumors established using C6 GSCs show intense micro-vessels and enhanced migration of bone marrow derived endothelial progenitor cells (EPCs) compared to tumors formed by adherent C6 cell (Folkins et al. 2009). CD133$^+$ cells xenografts show distinct profile of angiogenic factors including high VEGF with enhanced angiogenesis and hemorrhage compared to CD133$^-$cells. CD133$^+$ GSC conditioned medium supports endothelial cell migration and tube formation *in vitro* and inhibition of VEGF by Bevacizumab inhibits GSC derived tumor significantly than non-GSC tumors (Bao et al. 2006b). Diminishing angiogenesis using VEGF inhibitors create a vicious loop of events including new hypoxic regions with high HIF1α expression which further aggravates the tumor (Mancuso et al. 2006). Re-establishment of vasculature by pericyte recruitment followed by VEGF inhibition creates an opportunity window for better drug delivery (Jain 2003). Anti VEGF therapy combined with radiation in vivo showed significant tumor load reduction within a restricted time window by redistributing oxygen to radio resistant core and increasing DNA damage (Winkler et al. 2004). In addition to aggressive related phenotype, a subpopulation of GSCs is known to carry EMT related markers with high migratory ability and can cause secondary tumors. By using fluorescent dye tracking Myung Lee group showed infiltrating front of tumor cells into normal tissue and few cells migrated far from tumor mass (Jeon et al. 2008b). In addition, they provided evidence that human normal neural stem cells were shown to migrate towards C6 tumor and within 7 days they entered in to tumor core. **(6) Metabolic circuit**- GSCs portray heterogeneity in metabolic program depend on genetic background and the microenvironment they reside in. Contrary to existing literature on Warburg effect, GSCs consume less glucose and depend on oxidative phosphorylation (OXPHOS) than glycolysis compared to differentiated glioma cells. Production of lactate was minimal while ATP levels were maintained high in GSCs. Further inhibition of glycolysis or OXPHOS independently showed less extent of alterations on energy production of GSCs (Vlashi et al. 2011). High mitochondrial oxidative potential correlates with resistant phenotype of GSCs compared to differentiated cells. Radio resistant GSCs display low glucose uptake, inactive Akt pathway and high lipid catabolism. Fatty acid oxidation and ROS production was enhanced in resistant clones combined with high SIRT1-PGCα expression (Ye et al. 2013). **(7) Quiescence and GSCs**- Majority of standard therapy includes anti proliferative/mitotic drugs and they are incapable in successful removal of quiescent population GSCs. Releasing the brake on cell cycle is considered as a strategy to sensitize GSCs. As long term self-renewal correlates to quiescence or slow cycling kinetics, GSCs were characterized for Nanog and HIF1-alpha positivity which are markers for quiescence in hematopoietic SC in different grades of glioma. GBM, but not lower grades have enriched segments enriched for quiescent cells between necrotic regions and blood vessels with moderate hypoxic condition. Above observation was reflected in different regions of neurospheres established from GBM tissue (Ishii et al. 2016). GSCs might portray altered quiescence phenotype than NSCs and differentiated glioma cells. In adult mouse NSCs, p21 deletion leads to aberrant activation of quiescent cells to proliferative phase in vivo and reduce longevity of NSCs (Kippin et al. 2005). Pten deletion which is prevalent in GBM tumorigenesis, recapitulate the active proliferation phenotype by increased number of neurospheres formation with larger size and shows high extent of BrdU incorporation (Groszer et al. 2001). The collective signals of extracellular matrix and secreted factors within the niche determine the quiescence state of GSCs (Glaser et al. 2007). Study on mitotic spindle formation of GSCs show compared to differentiated cells they exhibit monopolar or multipolar abnormalities and high incidence of matured centrosomes with polyploidy (Mannino et al. 2014). Deleyrolle et al. showed the dye retaining cells (slow cycling) isolated from primary GBM exhibit high tumorigenesis in limited dilution transplantation and enhanced expression of CD133, CD15 and ABCG2 compared to bulk cells (Deleyrolle et al. 2011). Additional insight into quiescence against proliferative subset of GSCs and their differential properties is required which may have important clinical inferences on therapy response.

GBMs recur at a high rate and GSCs are one of the causes of relapse as they have high potential of resisting treatment and migration into non-tumor sites. GSCs isolated from recurrent tumor show enhanced stem like property (High CD133) and aggressive in vivo xenograft formation compared to matched primary tumor (Huang et al. 2008). Tumors enriched in high self-renewal GSC clones might lead to high risk of recurrence with shorter period to reinitiate the tumor (Fig. 8.3). The quiescence nature in subset of GSCs implicates the resistance of cells for routine therapy and they remain untreatable to reinitiate the tumor.

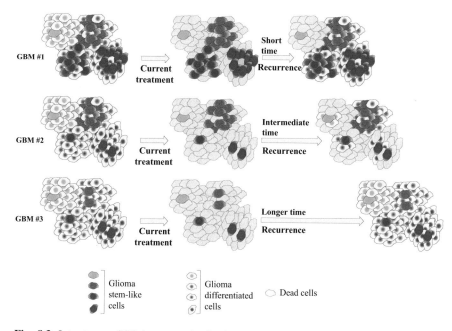

Fig. 8.3 Intra tumor GSC heterogeneity in therapy resistance and recurrence Self-renewing capacity of GSCs determines the recurrence rate. Tumor consists of several GSCs with different genetic alterations which determine their self-renewal capacity. GSCs with high self-renewal capacity grows back fast with the resultant faster recurrence. *While GBM #1* tumor has three kinds of GSCs with high self-renewal capacity and hence recur in a short time, *GBM#3* tumor has four kinds of GSCs with low self-renewal capacity and hence takes long time for recurrence. *GBM# 2* tumor has one GSC with high self-renewal capacity and hence takes intermediate time to recur

8.8   Targeting GSCs as a Therapy Modality

The intra- and inter-tumoral heterogeneity has paved the way for identifying cancer-specific driver alteration(s) so that an individual specific targeted therapy in combination with standard therapy could be considered. With the help of transcriptome and exome sequencing of large clinical cohort of glioma tumors, the probable candidates of drug designing have been selected further for trials. In combination with routine therapy, personalized drugs can enhance the efficacy of tumor removal and reduce side effects. Since GSCs display therapy resistance and they are responsible for expansion of tumor, it is a necessity to eradicate them for improved survival of patients. Several trials were undertaken aiming to eliminate GSCs using the prevalent mutations or gene expression signature of GSCs.

Iron oxide nanoparticles conjugated with EGFRvIII antibody treatment successfully induced apoptosis in neurospheres with EGFRvIII amplification. Further, it showed promising results in mouse implanted xenograft carrying EGFRvIII with high penetration into tumor and infiltrating zones (Hadjipanayis et al. 2010). miRNA145, a tumor suppressor which targets GSC specific genes OCT4 and SOX2 was delivered using cationic polyethylenimine (PU-PEI) to tumor sites in vivo and it leads to sensitization of GSCs to radio and chemotherapy in vitro (Yang et al. 2012). The CXCL12-CXCR4 interaction active in CD133⁺ GSCs enhances migration and infiltrative potential and hence blocking CXCR4 surface receptor significantly inhibited in vivo xenograft by attenuating angiogenesis (Ping et al. 2011).

NSCs are currently speculated as better drug vehicle as they selectively migrate to tumor sites with high dispersal rate. Carboxyl esterase expressing NSCs in combination with a pro-drug Irinitecan (CPT-11) migrate specifically to tumor sites and induce high concentration of antineoplastic effects with minimal side effects (Metz et al. 2013). Genetically modified oncolytic viral therapy selectively allows successful replication of virus in tumor site and not in normal brain cells. In order to achieve this, gene which is common for tumor maintenance and adenoviral life cycle is deleted in the recombinant adenovirus which makes it specific weapon for tumor cells. It leads to oncolysis which occur due to virus replication-mediated cell lysis (Sonabend et al. 2006). In GSCs, a modified recombinant adenovirus, Ad-Delo3-RGD which contains E1A and E1B deletion and a RGD-modified fiber showed efficient cytotoxicity against tumor cell with high YB-1(Y-Box protein) expression (Mantwill et al. 2013). As remnant GSCs impart radio-chemoresistance and cause recurrence, phase II trial termed as Stem cell radiotherapy (ScRT) is underway where radiation is given to GSC niche post-surgery in addition to surgical areas (https://clinicaltrials.gov/ct2/show/NCT02039778).

The application of immunotherapy for glioma is extended to selectively kill GSCs. Adoptive T cell therapy to eliminate GSCs is an emerging sector and researchers have engineered stem-like memory T cells to recognize specific chimeric antigen receptor (CAR) present on GSCs in order to get long term cytotoxicity effects. Treatment with IL13-zetakine, a CAR which detects GSCs and differentiated cells with high IL13Rα2, leads to cytolysis and in vivo xenograft reduction (Brown et al. 2012). GSC specific antigen induced T-cell response eliminates GSCs in tumor. Activation of HER2-targeting T-cells by HER2-positive GBM cells induce secretion of INF-γ and interleukin-2 which leads to depletion of CD133⁺ cells besides CD133⁻ cells (Ahmed et al. 2010). Phase I trial is initiated for vaccination with dendritic cells derived post exposure to lysate derived from an allogenic GSC line (Xu et al. 2012). In addition, BMP4 treatment was shown to reduce tumorigenecity of CD133⁺ by enhancing differentiation of GSCs (Piccirillo and Vescovi 2007). Intradermal -infusion of dendritic cells activated by peptides of CD133 antigen is currently tested on GBM patients (https://clinicaltrials.gov/ct2/show/NCT02049489).

8.9 Pathways Crucial for GSC Maintenance

Targeting GSCs enhances the efficacy of standard therapy as they impart high drug resistance and invasive potential. Regardless of chemo-radio therapy, the incidents of GBM recurrence are of 90% and it is due to incomplete removal of GSCs post treatment. Antagonizing agents for essential GSC related pathway genes can be combined with routine therapy. Plethora of molecular pathways have been identified for GSCs including NOTCH, HEDGEHOG, NFkB, WNT and several attempts are being tried to disrupt GSC maintenance by using specific chemical inhibitors. Table 8.1 provides an overview of reports about various altered signaling pathways in GSCs.

Table 8.1 Overview of pathways essential for GSCs

Pathway	Member	Reference
Wnt	SFRP1, SFRP4 and FZD7	Kierulf-Vieira et al. (2016)
	LEF1	Gao et al. (2014)
	sFRP4	Bhuvanalakshmi et al. (2015)
	GSK-3β	Rathod et al. (2014), Sandberg et al. (2013)
	sFRP4	Warrier et al. (2013)
	Wnt3a	Riganti et al. (2013)
	Axin	Xia et al. (2013)
	ASCL1	Rheinbay et al. (2013)
	β-catenin	Chen et al. (2014), Gong and Huang (2012), Kim et al. (2013), Nakata et al. (2013), Shi et al. (2015)
Hedgehog	Gli 1, Gli2	Fareh et al. (2012), Xu et al. (2008), Zbinden et al. (2010)
	Shh	Clement et al. (2007), Gopinath et al. (2013)
NFκB	P-IKB/P-IKKA/B	Kim et al. (2016)
	NFκB	Dixit et al. (2013), Gupta et al. (2013), Hu et al. (2013), Kaufhold et al. (2016), Nogueira et al. (2011)
	RelB	Ohtsu et al. (2016)
	p50	Zhang et al. (2014)
	p52	Tchoghandjian et al. (2014)
	p65/p50	Annabi et al. (2009), Garner et al. (2013), Kaus et al. (2010)
Notch	NOTCH1	Cenciarelli et al. (2014), Mukherjee et al. (2016), Shen et al. (2015), Wang et al. (2012, 2016)
	NOTCH1, HES1	Saito et al. (2015)
	γ-secretase	Dai et al. (2011), Hovinga et al. (2010), Hu et al. (2011), Kristoffersen et al. (2014), Natsumeda et al. (2015); Tanaka et al. 2015; Yahyanejad et al. (2016)
	HES1	Charles et al. (2010), Ding et al. (2014), Yin et al. (2014)
NOTCH	NOTCH	Wang et al. (2014), Wu et al. (2013)
	Notch1, JAG1, HEY2 Survivin	Liu et al. (2014)
	NOTCH1, HEY1/2	Guichet et al. (2015)
	NICD	Hu et al. (2014), Qiang et al. (2012)
	NOTCH1, NOTCH3, HES1, MAML1, DLL-3, JAG2	Saito et al. (2014)
	γ-secretase, NOTCH1	Kristoffersen et al. (2013), Ulasov et al. (2011)
	DLL3	Turchi et al. (2013)
	CBF1	Floyd et al. (2012)
	Numb4d7	Jiang et al. (2012)
	Jagged-Notch	Jeon et al. (2008a), Jin et al. (2012)
	Notch-2	Yoon et al. (2012)
	DLL1/4, JAG1	Zhu et al. (2011)
	HES/HEY	Ying et al. (2011)
	Mastermind-like protein 3	Seidel et al. (2010)
	Notch1 and Hes1	Zhen et al. (2010)
	Notch1, Notch2	Wang et al. (2010)
	γ-secretase, NOTCH2	Fan et al. (2010)
	NOTCH1/2/3/4, JAG1/2, DLL1, HES1/5	Zhang et al. (2008)
	NOTCH1/2/3, HES1/2/4	Shiras et al. (2007)
	γ-secretase, HES1	Fan et al. (2006)

8.10 Applying GSC Findings to Whole Tumor Studies

The debate on stem cell markers and prognosis remain unresolved. Several clinical investigations were attempted to dissect the prognostic value of many stem markers. Since they act as reservoir of tumor and refractory to therapy modalities, they are expected to behave as poor prognostic markers. CD133 positivity showed significant poor overall survival in multivariate survival analysis involving grade, age and resection (Pallini et al. 2008; Zeppernick et al. 2008). In support to the above notion, neurosphere formation from patient tumor samples *in vitro* acts as yardstick regardless of p53 or MGMT status for predicting survival in patients. Independent reports prove that high Nestin with CD133 correlates with poor survival (Strojnik et al. 2007; Zhang et al. 2008). In contrast, the study conducted on 153 glioma patients show no significant dependency of overall survival or progression free survival on Nestin expression (Chinnaiyan et al. 2008). Musashi-1, an RNA binding protein enriched in GSCs was shown to positively correlate with tumor grade though it fails to stand as prognostic marker (Strojnik et al. 2007). Several independent IHC based studies of major stem specific genes (BMI,SOX2, OCT4, Id1) in different cohorts of grade IV tumor demonstrate neither prognostic value nor correlation to grades of tumor (Dahlrot et al. 2013). In order to decipher the prognostic value of GSC specific markers, we carried out a comprehensive analysis wherein we attempted an univariate cox regression analysis of stem cell markers, SOX2, SALL2, POU3F2, OLIG2, MYC, BMP4, BMI1, NESTIN, SSEA1, CD133, CD44, OCT4, Musashi 1, Nanog, IL6 and L1CAM using TCGA transcriptome data. As GSCs cause therapy resistance, we have examined the prognostic value in patient cohorts divided on the basis of various therapy methods, radiation only, radiation +TMZ, radiation + any chemotherapy). While patient age predicted poor prognosis in all three cohorts, majority of the stem cell markers failed to show prognostic value in whole tumor data (data not shown). CD44, SSEA1 and IL6 predicted poor prognosis in one or more cohorts. In contrast, SOX2, Nanog and MYC expression was found associated with better prognosis in one or more cohorts. While we do not have any explanation why most stem cell markers failed to predict prognosis, we believe that as GSCs belong to a small subset, the whole tumor RNA data might not reflect the true proportion of GSCs and their contribution to therapy resistance. Further studies are required to get a deeper insight into these aspects.

8.11 Conclusions and Future Directions

Promiscuous nature and heterogeneity of GSCs are major challenges in understanding the characteristics of these cells. In addition, obtaining specific targeting strategies of GSCs, improved isolation and expansion methodologies should be developed as they restrict the characterization of GSCs. The markers which define GSCs remain controversial for past decade and the existing literature supports the fact that heterogeneity exists within GSCs derived from a tumor. Current discoveries on

GSC specific pathways have paved a way to clinical drug trials to eliminate GSCs in combination with standard therapy. Recent reports have provided support that the neurosphere formation *in vitro* from resected tumor sample is a predictive marker of poor prognosis. As the GSCs and their microenvironment being key players in deciding the drug efficacy 3D scaffold glioma cultures are near future system of study for screening the drugs or target genes. Introducing suicidal genes which destabilize GSC maintenance by viral/nano particle delivery into tumor site is an emerging field of clinical application. Another avenue open for therapeutic scope of GSC is to induce differentiation and make it susceptible for standard therapy. Identification of four reprogramming factors in proneural GSCs instigated the novel identification of gene therapy targets. Generalization of GSC behavior or molecular profile from restricted cohort of GSCs is misleading since the emerging data suggests high plasticity and adaptability of GSCs. Personalized therapy tailored for patient specific GSC signature can be a better option in future. Further molecular profiling studies assisted by mathematical modeling are required to predict functions and target GSCs.

Acknowledgement KS thanks DST and DBT, Government of India for financial support. Infrastructural support by funding by funding from DBT, DST and UGC to MCB is acknowledged. KS is a JC Bose Fellow of the Department of Science and Technology. We thank Vikas Patil for performing the bioinformatics analysis. AV acknowledges IISc for the fellowship.

References

Ahmed, N., V.S. Salsman, Y. Kew, D. Shaffer, S. Powell, Y.J. Zhang, R.G. Grossman, H.E. Heslop, and S. Gottschalk. 2010. HER2-specific T cells target primary glioblastoma stem cells and induce regression of autologous experimental tumors. *Clinical Cancer Research : An Official Journal of the American Association for Cancer Research* 16: 474–485.

Ahmed, S.U., R. Carruthers, L. Gilmour, S. Yildirim, C. Watts, and A.J. Chalmers. 2015. Selective inhibition of parallel DNA damage response pathways optimizes radiosensitization of glioblastoma stem-like cells. *Cancer Research* 75: 4416–4428.

Alcantara Llaguno, S., J. Chen, C.H. Kwon, E.L. Jackson, Y. Li, D.K. Burns, A. Alvarez-Buylla, and L.F. Parada. 2009. Malignant astrocytomas originate from neural stem/progenitor cells in a somatic tumor suppressor mouse model. *Cancer cell* 15: 45–56.

Altieri, R., M. Fontanella, A. Agnoletti, P.P. Panciani, G. Spena, E. Crobeddu, G. Pilloni, V. Tardivo, M. Lanotte, F. Zenga, A. Ducati, and D. Garbossa. 2015. Role of nitric oxide in glioblastoma therapy: Another step to resolve the terrible puzzle ? *Translational Medicine @ UniSa* 12: 54–59.

Annabi, B., C. Laflamme, A. Sina, M.P. Lachambre, and R. Beliveau. 2009. A MT1-MMP/ NF-kappaB signaling axis as a checkpoint controller of COX-2 expression in CD133+ U87 glioblastoma cells. *Journal of Neuroinflammation* 6: 8.

Auffinger, B., A.L. Tobias, Y. Han, G. Lee, D. Guo, M. Dey, M.S. Lesniak, and A.U. Ahmed. 2014. Conversion of differentiated cancer cells into cancer stem-like cells in a glioblastoma model after primary chemotherapy. *Cell Death and Differentiation* 21: 1119–1131.

Bao, P., A. Kodra, M. Tomic-Canic, M.S. Golinko, H.P. Ehrlich, and H. Brem. 2009. The role of vascular endothelial growth factor in wound healing. *The Journal of Surgical Research* 153: 347–358.

Bao, S., Q. Wu, Z. Li, S. Sathornsumetee, H. Wang, R.E. McLendon, A.B. Hjelmeland, and J.N. Rich. 2008. Targeting cancer stem cells through L1CAM suppresses glioma growth. *Cancer Research* 68: 6043–6048.

Bao, S., Q. Wu, R.E. McLendon, Y. Hao, Q. Shi, A.B. Hjelmeland, M.W. Dewhirst, D.D. Bigner, and J.N. Rich. 2006a. Glioma stem cells promote radioresistance by preferential activation of the DNA damage response. *Nature* 444: 756–760.

Bao, S., Q. Wu, S. Sathornsumetee, Y. Hao, Z. Li, A.B. Hjelmeland, Q. Shi, R.E. McLendon, D.D. Bigner, and J.N. Rich. 2006b. Stem cell-like glioma cells promote tumor angiogenesis through vascular endothelial growth factor. *Cancer Research* 66: 7843–7848.

Beier, C.P., and D. Beier. 2011. CD133 negative cancer stem cells in glioblastoma. *Frontiers in Bioscience* 3: 701–710.

Beier, D., P. Hau, M. Proescholdt, A. Lohmeier, J. Wischhusen, P.J. Oefner, L. Aigner, A. Brawanski, U. Bogdahn, and C.P. Beier. 2007. CD133(+) and CD133(−) glioblastoma-derived cancer stem cells show differential growth characteristics and molecular profiles. *Cancer Research* 67: 4010–4015.

Beier, D., S. Rohrl, D.R. Pillai, S. Schwarz, L.A. Kunz-Schughart, P. Leukel, M. Proescholdt, A. Brawanski, U. Bogdahn, A. Trampe-Kieslich, B. Giebel, J. Wischhusen, G. Reifenberger, P. Hau, and C.P. Beier. 2008. Temozolomide preferentially depletes cancer stem cells in glioblastoma. *Cancer Research* 68: 5706–5715.

Ben-Porath, I., M.W. Thomson, V.J. Carey, R. Ge, G.W. Bell, A. Regev, and R.A. Weinberg. 2008. An embryonic stem cell-like gene expression signature in poorly differentiated aggressive human tumors. *Nature Genetics* 40: 499–507.

Bhat, K.P., V. Balasubramaniyan, B. Vaillant, R. Ezhilarasan, K. Hummelink, F. Hollingsworth, K. Wani, L. Heathcock, J.D. James, L.D. Goodman, S. Conroy, L. Long, N. Lelic, S. Wang, J. Gumin, D. Raj, Y. Kodama, A. Raghunathan, A. Olar, K. Joshi, C.E. Pelloski, A. Heimberger, S.H. Kim, D.P. Cahill, G. Rao, W.F. Den Dunnen, H.W. Boddeke, H.S. Phillips, I. Nakano, F.F. Lang, H. Colman, E.P. Sulman, and K. Aldape. 2013. Mesenchymal differentiation mediated by NF-kappaB promotes radiation resistance in glioblastoma. *Cancer Cell* 24: 331–346.

Bhuvanalakshmi, G., F. Arfuso, M. Millward, A. Dharmarajan, and S. Warrier. 2015. Secreted frizzled-related protein 4 inhibits glioma stem-like cells by reversing epithelial to mesenchymal transition, inducing apoptosis and decreasing cancer stem cell properties. *PLoS One* 10: e0127517.

Blough, M.D., M.R. Westgate, D. Beauchamp, J.J. Kelly, O. Stechishin, A.L. Ramirez, S. Weiss, and J.G. Cairncross. 2010. Sensitivity to temozolomide in brain tumor initiating cells. *Neuro-Oncology* 12: 756–760.

Bradshaw, A., A. Wickremsekera, S.T. Tan, L. Peng, P.F. Davis, and T. Itinteang. 2016. Cancer stem cell hierarchy in glioblastoma multiforme. *Frontiers in Surgery* 3: 21.

Brown, C.E., R. Starr, B. Aguilar, A.F. Shami, C. Martinez, M. D'Apuzzo, M.E. Barish, S.J. Forman, and M.C. Jensen. 2012. Stem-like tumor-initiating cells isolated from IL13Ralpha2 expressing gliomas are targeted and killed by IL13-zetakine-redirected T Cells. *Clinical Cancer Research: An Official Journal of the American Association for Cancer Research* 18: 2199–2209.

Caren, H., S.H. Stricker, H. Bulstrode, S. Gagrica, E. Johnstone, T.E. Bartlett, A. Feber, G. Wilson, A.E. Teschendorff, P. Bertone, S. Beck, and S.M. Pollard. 2015. Glioblastoma stem cells respond to differentiation cues but fail to undergo commitment and terminal cell-cycle arrest. *Stem Cell Reports* 5: 829–842.

Cenciarelli, C., H.E. Marei, M. Zonfrillo, P. Pierimarchi, E. Paldino, P. Casalbore, A. Felsani, A.L. Vescovi, G. Maira, and A. Mangiola. 2014. PDGF receptor alpha inhibition induces apoptosis in glioblastoma cancer stem cells refractory to anti-Notch and anti-EGFR treatment. *Molecular Cancer* 13: 247.

Chaffer, C.L., I. Brueckmann, C. Scheel, A.J. Kaestli, P.A. Wiggins, L.O. Rodrigues, M. Brooks, F. Reinhardt, Y. Su, K. Polyak, L.M. Arendt, C. Kuperwasser, B. Bierie, and R.A. Weinberg. 2011. Normal and neoplastic nonstem cells can spontaneously convert to a stem-like state. *Proceedings of the National Academy of Sciences of the United States of America* 108: 7950–7955.

Chandran, U.R., S. Luthra, L. Santana-Santos, P. Mao, S.H. Kim, M. Minata, J. Li, P.V. Benos, M. DeWang, B. Hu, S.Y. Cheng, I. Nakano, and R.W. Sobol. 2015. Gene expression profiling distinguishes proneural glioma stem cells from mesenchymal glioma stem cells. *Genomics Data* 5: 333–336.

Charles, N., T. Ozawa, M. Squatrito, A.M. Bleau, C.W. Brennan, D. Hambardzumyan, and E.C. Holland. 2010. Perivascular nitric oxide activates notch signaling and promotes stem-like character in PDGF-induced glioma cells. *Cell Stem Cell* 6: 141–152.

Chen, J., Y. Li, T.S. Yu, R.M. McKay, D.K. Burns, S.G. Kernie, and L.F. Parada. 2012. A restricted cell population propagates glioblastoma growth after chemotherapy. *Nature* 488: 522–526.

Chen, X., W. Hu, B. Xie, H. Gao, C. Xu, and J. Chen. 2014. Downregulation of SCAI enhances glioma cell invasion and stem cell like phenotype by activating Wnt/beta-catenin signaling. *Biochemical and Biophysical Research Communications* 448: 206–211.

Cheng, L., Z. Huang, W. Zhou, Q. Wu, S. Donnola, J.K. Liu, X. Fang, A.E. Sloan, Y. Mao, J.D. Lathia, W. Min, R.E. McLendon, J.N. Rich, and S. Bao. 2013. Glioblastoma stem cells generate vascular pericytes to support vessel function and tumor growth. *Cell* 153: 139–152.

Chinnaiyan, P., M. Wang, A.M. Rojiani, P.J. Tofilon, A. Chakravarti, K.K. Ang, H.Z. Zhang, E. Hammond, W. Curran Jr., and M.P. Mehta. 2008. The prognostic value of nestin expression in newly diagnosed glioblastoma: report from the radiation therapy oncology group. *Radiation Oncology* 3: 32.

Chua, C., N. Zaiden, K.H. Chong, S.J. See, M.C. Wong, B.T. Ang, and C. Tang. 2008. Characterization of a side population of astrocytoma cells in response to temozolomide. *Journal of Neurosurgery* 109: 856–866.

Clement, V., P. Sanchez, N. de Tribolet, I. Radovanovic, and A. Ruiz i Altaba. 2007. HEDGEHOG-GLI1 signaling regulates human glioma growth, cancer stem cell self-renewal, and tumorigenicity. *Current Biology* 17: 165–172.

Dahan, P., J. Martinez Gala, C. Delmas, S. Monferran, L. Malric, D. Zentkowski, V. Lubrano, C. Toulas, E. Cohen-Jonathan Moyal, and A. Lemarie. 2014. Ionizing radiations sustain glioblastoma cell dedifferentiation to a stem-like phenotype through survivin: possible involvement in radioresistance. *Cell Death & Disease* 5: e1543.

Dahlrot, R.H., S.K. Hermansen, S. Hansen, and B.W. Kristensen. 2013. What is the clinical value of cancer stem cell markers in gliomas? *International Journal of Clinical and Experimental Pathology* 6: 334–348.

Dai, L., J. He, Y. Liu, J. Byun, A. Vivekanandan, S. Pennathur, X. Fan, and D.M. Lubman. 2011. Dose-dependent proteomic analysis of glioblastoma cancer stem cells upon treatment with gamma-secretase inhibitor. *Proteomics* 11: 4529–4540.

De Bacco, F., P. Luraghi, E. Medico, G. Reato, F. Girolami, T. Perera, P. Gabriele, P.M. Comoglio, and C. Boccaccio. 2011. Induction of MET by ionizing radiation and its role in radioresistance and invasive growth of cancer. *Journal of the National Cancer Institute* 103: 645–661.

de Vries, N.A., T. Buckle, J. Zhao, J.H. Beijnen, J.H. Schellens, and O. van Tellingen. 2012. Restricted brain penetration of the tyrosine kinase inhibitor erlotinib due to the drug transporters P-gp and BCRP. *Investigational New Drugs* 30: 443–449.

deCarvalho, A.C., K. Nelson, N. Lemke, N.L. Lehman, A.S. Arbab, S. Kalkanis, and T. Mikkelsen. 2010. Gliosarcoma stem cells undergo glial and mesenchymal differentiation in vivo. *Stem Cells* 28: 181–190.

Del Rowe, J., C. Scott, M. Werner-Wasik, J.P. Bahary, W.J. Curran, R.C. Urtasun, and B. Fisher. 2000. Single-arm, open-label phase II study of intravenously administered tirapazamine and radiation therapy for glioblastoma multiforme. *Journal of Clinical Oncology : Official Journal of the American Society of Clinical Oncology* 18: 1254–1259.

Deleyrolle, L.P., A. Harding, K. Cato, F.A. Siebzehnrubl, M. Rahman, H. Azari, S. Olson, B. Gabrielli, G. Osborne, A. Vescovi, and B.A. Reynolds. 2011. Evidence for label-retaining tumour-initiating cells in human glioblastoma. *Brain : A Journal of Neurology* 134: 1331–1343.

Dick, J.E. 2009. Looking ahead in cancer stem cell research. *Nature Biotechnology* 27: 44–46.

Dick, J.E., T. Lapidot, and F. Pflumio. 1991. Transplantation of normal and leukemic human bone marrow into immune-deficient mice: Development of animal models for human hematopoiesis. *Immunological Reviews* 124: 25–43.

Ding, D., K.S. Lim, and C.G. Eberhart. 2014. Arsenic trioxide inhibits Hedgehog, Notch and stem cell properties in glioblastoma neurospheres. *Acta Neuropathologica Communications* 2: 31.

Dirks, P.B. 2006. Cancer: Stem cells and brain tumours. *Nature* 444: 687–688.

Dixit, D., R. Ghildiyal, N.P. Anto, S. Ghosh, V. Sharma, and E. Sen. 2013. Guggulsterone sensitizes glioblastoma cells to Sonic hedgehog inhibitor SANT-1 induced apoptosis in a Ras/NFkappaB dependent manner. *Cancer Letters* 336: 347–358.

Duan, S., G. Yuan, X. Liu, R. Ren, J. Li, W. Zhang, J. Wu, X. Xu, L. Fu, Y. Li, J. Yang, W. Zhang, R. Bai, F. Yi, K. Suzuki, H. Gao, C.R. Esteban, C. Zhang, J.C. Izpisua Belmonte, Z. Chen, X. Wang, T. Jiang, J. Qu, F. Tang, and G.H. Liu. 2015. PTEN deficiency reprogrammes human neural stem cells towards a glioblastoma stem cell-like phenotype. *Nature Communications* 6: 10068.

Fan, X., L. Khaki, T.S. Zhu, M.E. Soules, C.E. Talsma, N. Gul, C. Koh, J. Zhang, Y.M. Li, J. Maciaczyk, G. Nikkhah, F. Dimeco, S. Piccirillo, A.L. Vescovi, and C.G. Eberhart. 2010. NOTCH pathway blockade depletes CD133-positive glioblastoma cells and inhibits growth of tumor neurospheres and xenografts. *Stem Cells* 28: 5–16.

Fan, X., W. Matsui, L. Khaki, D. Stearns, J. Chun, Y.M. Li, and C.G. Eberhart. 2006. Notch pathway inhibition depletes stem-like cells and blocks engraftment in embryonal brain tumors. *Cancer Research* 66: 7445–7452.

Fareh, M., L. Turchi, V. Virolle, D. Debruyne, F. Almairac, S. de-la-Forest Divonne, P. Paquis, O. Preynat-Seauve, K.H. Krause, H. Chneiweiss, and T. Virolle. 2012. The miR 302-367 cluster drastically affects self-renewal and infiltration properties of glioma-initiating cells through CXCR4 repression and consequent disruption of the SHH-GLI-NANOG network. *Cell Death and Differentiation* 19: 232–244.

Fessler, E., T. Borovski, and J.P. Medema. 2015. Endothelial cells induce cancer stem cell features in differentiated glioblastoma cells via bFGF. *Molecular Cancer* 14: 157.

Floyd, D.H., B. Kefas, O. Seleverstov, O. Mykhaylyk, C. Dominguez, L. Comeau, C. Plank, and B. Purow. 2012. Alpha-secretase inhibition reduces human glioblastoma stem cell growth in vitro and in vivo by inhibiting Notch. *Neuro-Oncology* 14: 1215–1226.

Floyd, D.H., Y. Zhang, B.K. Dey, B. Kefas, H. Breit, K. Marks, A. Dutta, C. Herold-Mende, M. Synowitz, R. Glass, R. Abounader, and B.W. Purow. 2014. Novel anti-apoptotic microRNAs 582-5p and 363 promote human glioblastoma stem cell survival via direct inhibition of caspase 3, caspase 9, and Bim. *PLoS One* 9: e96239.

Folkins, C., Y. Shaked, S. Man, T. Tang, C.R. Lee, Z. Zhu, R.M. Hoffman, and R.S. Kerbel. 2009. Glioma tumor stem-like cells promote tumor angiogenesis and vasculogenesis via vascular endothelial growth factor and stromal-derived factor 1. *Cancer Research* 69: 7243–7251.

Friedmann-Morvinski, D., E.A. Bushong, E. Ke, Y. Soda, T. Marumoto, O. Singer, M.H. Ellisman, and I.M. Verma. 2012. Dedifferentiation of neurons and astrocytes by oncogenes can induce gliomas in mice. *Science* 338: 1080–1084.

Gao, X., Y. Mi, Y. Ma, and W. Jin. 2014. LEF1 regulates glioblastoma cell proliferation, migration, invasion, and cancer stem-like cell self-renewal. *Tumour Biology : The Journal of the International Society for Oncodevelopmental Biology and Medicine* 35: 11505–11511.

Garner, J.M., M. Fan, C.H. Yang, Z. Du, M. Sims, A.M. Davidoff, and L.M. Pfeffer. 2013. Constitutive activation of signal transducer and activator of transcription 3 (STAT3) and nuclear factor kappaB signaling in glioblastoma cancer stem cells regulates the Notch pathway. *The Journal of Biological Chemistry* 288: 26167–26176.

Ghods, A.J., D. Irvin, G. Liu, X. Yuan, I.R. Abdulkadir, P. Tunici, B. Konda, S. Wachsmann-Hogiu, K.L. Black, and J.S. Yu. 2007. Spheres isolated from 9L gliosarcoma rat cell line possess chemoresistant and aggressive cancer stem-like cells. *Stem Cells* 25: 1645–1653.

Gilbert, C.A., M.C. Daou, R.P. Moser, and A.H. Ross. 2010. Gamma-secretase inhibitors enhance temozolomide treatment of human gliomas by inhibiting neurosphere repopulation and xenograft recurrence. *Cancer Research* 70: 6870–6879.

Glaser, T., S.M. Pollard, A. Smith, and O. Brustle. 2007. Tripotential differentiation of adherently expandable neural stem (NS) cells. *PLoS one* 2: e298.

Gong, A., and S. Huang. 2012. FoxM1 and Wnt/beta-catenin signaling in glioma stem cells. *Cancer Research* 72: 5658–5662.

Gopinath, S., R. Malla, K. Alapati, B. Gorantla, M. Gujrati, D.H. Dinh, and J.S. Rao. 2013. Cathepsin B and uPAR regulate self-renewal of glioma-initiating cells through GLI-regulated Sox2 and Bmi1 expression. *Carcinogenesis* 34: 550–559.

Groszer, M., R. Erickson, D.D. Scripture-Adams, R. Lesche, A. Trumpp, J.A. Zack, H.I. Kornblum, X. Liu, and H. Wu. 2001. Negative regulation of neural stem/progenitor cell proliferation by the Pten tumor suppressor gene in vivo. *Science* 294: 2186–2189.

Guichet, P.O., S. Guelfi, M. Teigell, L. Hoppe, N. Bakalara, L. Bauchet, H. Duffau, K. Lamszus, B. Rothhut, and J.P. Hugnot. 2015. Notch1 stimulation induces a vascularization switch with pericyte-like cell differentiation of glioblastoma stem cells. *Stem Cells* 33: 21–34.

Gunther, H.S., N.O. Schmidt, H.S. Phillips, D. Kemming, S. Kharbanda, R. Soriano, Z. Modrusan, H. Meissner, M. Westphal, and K. Lamszus. 2008. Glioblastoma-derived stem cell-enriched cultures form distinct subgroups according to molecular and phenotypic criteria. *Oncogene* 27: 2897–2909.

Gupta, P., D. Dixit, and E. Sen. 2013. Oncrasin targets the JNK-NF-kappaB axis to sensitize glioma cells to TNFalpha-induced apoptosis. *Carcinogenesis* 34: 388–396.

Gupta, P.B., C.M. Fillmore, G. Jiang, S.D. Shapira, K. Tao, C. Kuperwasser, and E.S. Lander. 2011. Stochastic state transitions give rise to phenotypic equilibrium in populations of cancer cells. *Cell* 146: 633–644.

Hadjipanayis, C.G., R. Machaidze, M. Kaluzova, L. Wang, A.J. Schuette, H. Chen, X. Wu, and H. Mao. 2010. EGFRvIII antibody-conjugated iron oxide nanoparticles for magnetic resonance imaging-guided convection-enhanced delivery and targeted therapy of glioblastoma. *Cancer Research* 70: 6303–6312.

Hemmati, H.D., I. Nakano, J.A. Lazareff, M. Masterman-Smith, D.H. Geschwind, M. Bronner-Fraser, and H.I. Kornblum. 2003. Cancerous stem cells can arise from pediatric brain tumors. *Proceedings of the National Academy of Sciences of the United States of America* 100: 15178–15183.

Hovinga, K.E., F. Shimizu, R. Wang, G. Panagiotakos, M. Van Der Heijden, H. Moayedpardazi, A.S. Correia, D. Soulet, T. Major, J. Menon, and V. Tabar. 2010. Inhibition of notch signaling in glioblastoma targets cancer stem cells via an endothelial cell intermediate. *Stem Cells* 28: 1019–1029.

Hsieh, C.H., W.C. Shyu, C.Y. Chiang, J.W. Kuo, W.C. Shen, and R.S. Liu. 2011. NADPH oxidase subunit 4-mediated reactive oxygen species contribute to cycling hypoxia-promoted tumor progression in glioblastoma multiforme. *PloS One* 6: e23945.

Hu, Y., P. Cheng, J.C. Ma, Y.X. Xue, and Y.H. Liu. 2013. Platelet-derived growth factor BB mediates the glioma-induced migration of bone marrow-derived mesenchymal stem cells by promoting the expression of vascular cell adhesion molecule-1 through the PI3K, P38 MAPK and NF-kappaB pathways. *Oncology Reports* 30: 2755–2764.

Hu, Y.Y., L.A. Fu, S.Z. Li, Y. Chen, J.C. Li, J. Han, L. Liang, L. Li, C.C. Ji, M.H. Zheng, and H. Han. 2014. Hif-1alpha and Hif-2alpha differentially regulate Notch signaling through competitive interaction with the intracellular domain of Notch receptors in glioma stem cells. *Cancer Letters* 349: 67–76.

Hu, Y.Y., M.H. Zheng, G. Cheng, L. Li, L. Liang, F. Gao, Y.N. Wei, L.A. Fu, and H. Han. 2011. Notch signaling contributes to the maintenance of both normal neural stem cells and patient-derived glioma stem cells. *BMC Cancer* 11: 82.

Huang, Q., Q.B. Zhang, J. Dong, Y.Y. Wu, Y.T. Shen, Y.D. Zhao, Y.D. Zhu, Y. Diao, A.D. Wang, and Q. Lan. 2008. Glioma stem cells are more aggressive in recurrent tumors with malignant progression than in the primary tumor, and both can be maintained long-term in vitro. *BMC Cancer* 8: 304.

Huang, Z., L. Cheng, O.A. Guryanova, Q. Wu, and S. Bao. 2010. Cancer stem cells in glioblastoma--molecular signaling and therapeutic targeting. *Protein & Cell* 1: 638–655.

Ignatova, T.N., V.G. Kukekov, E.D. Laywell, O.N. Suslov, F.D. Vrionis, and D.A. Steindler. 2002. Human cortical glial tumors contain neural stem-like cells expressing astroglial and neuronal markers in vitro. *Glia* 39: 193–206.

Ishii, A., T. Kimura, H. Sadahiro, H. Kawano, K. Takubo, M. Suzuki, and E. Ikeda. 2016. Histological Characterization of the Tumorigenic "Peri-Necrotic Niche" Harboring Quiescent Stem-Like Tumor Cells in Glioblastoma. *PloS One* 11: e0147366.

Jain, R.K. 2003. Molecular regulation of vessel maturation. *Nature Medicine* 9: 685–693.

Jeon, H.M., X. Jin, J.S. Lee, S.Y. Oh, Y.W. Sohn, H.J. Park, K.M. Joo, W.Y. Park, D.H. Nam, R.A. DePinho, L. Chin, and H. Kim. 2008a. Inhibitor of differentiation 4 drives brain tumor-initiating cell genesis through cyclin E and notch signaling. *Genes & Development* 22: 2028–2033.

Jeon, J.Y., J.H. An, S.U. Kim, H.G. Park, and M.A. Lee. 2008b. Migration of human neural stem cells toward an intracranial glioma. *Experimental & Molecular Medicine* 40: 84–91.

Jiang, X., H. Xing, T.M. Kim, Y. Jung, W. Huang, H.W. Yang, S. Song, P.J. Park, R.S. Carroll, and M.D. Johnson. 2012. Numb regulates glioma stem cell fate and growth by altering epidermal growth factor receptor and Skp1-Cullin-F-box ubiquitin ligase activity. *Stem Cells* 30: 1313–1326.

Jin, X., S.H. Kim, H.M. Jeon, S. Beck, Y.W. Sohn, J. Yin, J.K. Kim, Y.C. Lim, J.H. Lee, S.H. Kim, S.H. Kang, X. Pian, M.S. Song, J.B. Park, Y.S. Chae, Y.G. Chung, S.H. Lee, Y.J. Choi, D.H. Nam, Y.K. Choi, and H. Kim. 2012. Interferon regulatory factor 7 regulates glioma stem cells via interleukin 6 and Notch signalling. *Brain : A Journal of Neurology* 135: 1055–1069.

Jin, Y., Z.Q. Bin, H. Qiang, C. Liang, C. Hua, D. Jun, W.A. Dong, and L. Qing. 2009. ABCG2 is related with the grade of glioma and resistance to mitoxantone, a chemotherapeutic drug for glioma. *Journal of Cancer Research and Clinical Oncology* 135: 1369–1376.

Kaufhold, S., H. Garban, and B. Bonavida. 2016. Yin Yang 1 is associated with cancer stem cell transcription factors (SOX2, OCT4, BMI1) and clinical implication. *Journal of Experimental & Clinical Cancer Research* 35: 84.

Kaus, A., D. Widera, S. Kassmer, J. Peter, K. Zaenker, C. Kaltschmidt, and B. Kaltschmidt. 2010. Neural stem cells adopt tumorigenic properties by constitutively activated NF-kappaB and subsequent VEGF up-regulation. *Stem Cells and Development* 19: 999–1015.

Kierulf-Vieira, K.S., C.J. Sandberg, Z. Grieg, C.C. Gunther, I.A. Langmoen, and E.O. Vik-Mo. 2016. Wnt inhibition is dysregulated in gliomas and its re-establishment inhibits proliferation and tumor sphere formation. *Experimental Cell Research* 340: 53–61.

Kim, K.H., H.J. Seol, E.H. Kim, J. Rheey, H.J. Jin, Y. Lee, K.M. Joo, J. Lee, and D.H. Nam. 2013. Wnt/beta-catenin signaling is a key downstream mediator of MET signaling in glioblastoma stem cells. *Neuro-Oncology* 15: 161–171.

Kim, M., and C.M. Morshead. 2003. Distinct populations of forebrain neural stem and progenitor cells can be isolated using side-population analysis. *The Journal of Neuroscience : The Official journal of the Society for Neuroscience* 23: 10703–10709.

Kim, S.H., R. Ezhilarasan, E. Phillips, D. Gallego-Perez, A. Sparks, D. Taylor, K. Ladner, T. Furuta, H. Sabit, R. Chhipa, J.H. Cho, A. Mohyeldin, S. Beck, K. Kurozumi, T. Kuroiwa, R. Iwata, A. Asai, J. Kim, E.P. Sulman, S.Y. Cheng, L.J. Lee, M. Nakada, D. Guttridge, B. DasGupta, V. Goidts, K.P. Bhat, and I. Nakano. 2016. Serine/threonine kinase MLK4 determines mesenchymal identity in glioma stem cells in an NF-kappaB-dependent manner. *Cancer Cell* 29: 201–213.

Kim, S.H., K. Joshi, R. Ezhilarasan, T.R. Myers, J. Siu, C. Gu, M. Nakano-Okuno, D. Taylor, M. Minata, E.P. Sulman, J. Lee, K.P. Bhat, A.E. Salcini, and I. Nakano. 2015. EZH2 protects glioma stem cells from radiation-induced cell death in a MELK/FOXM1-dependent manner. *Stem Cell Reports* 4: 226–238.

Kippin, T.E., D.J. Martens, and D. van der Kooy. 2005. p21 loss compromises the relative quiescence of forebrain stem cell proliferation leading to exhaustion of their proliferation capacity. *Genes & Development* 19: 756–767.

Kondo, T., T. Setoguchi, and T. Taga. 2004. Persistence of a small subpopulation of cancer stem-like cells in the C6 glioma cell line. *Proceedings of the National Academy of Sciences of the United States of America* 101: 781–786.

Kozono, D., J. Li, M. Nitta, O. Sampetrean, D. Gonda, D.S. Kushwaha, D. Merzon, V. Ramakrishnan, S. Zhu, K. Zhu, H. Matsui, O. Harismendy, W. Hua, Y. Mao, C.H. Kwon, H. Saya, I. Nakano, D.P. Pizzo, S.R. VandenBerg, and C.C. Chen. 2015. Dynamic epigenetic regulation of glioblastoma tumorigenicity through LSD1 modulation of MYC expression. *Proceedings of the National Academy of Sciences of the United States of America* 112: E4055–E4064.

Kreso, A., and J.E. Dick. 2014. Evolution of the cancer stem cell model. *Cell Stem Cell* 14: 275–291.

Kristoffersen, K., M.K. Nedergaard, M. Villingshoj, R. Borup, H. Broholm, A. Kjaer, H.S. Poulsen, and M.T. Stockhausen. 2014. Inhibition of Notch signaling alters the phenotype of orthotopic tumors formed from glioblastoma multiforme neurosphere cells but does not hamper intracranial tumor growth regardless of endogene Notch pathway signature. *Cancer Biology & Therapy* 15: 862–877.

Kristoffersen, K., M. Villingshoj, H.S. Poulsen, and M.T. Stockhausen. 2013. Level of Notch activation determines the effect on growth and stem cell-like features in glioblastoma multiforme neurosphere cultures. *Cancer Biology & Therapy* 14: 625–637.

Ladiwala, U., H. Basu, and D. Mathur. 2012. Assembling neurospheres: dynamics of neural progenitor/stem cell aggregation probed using an optical trap. *PloS One* 7: e38613.

Lathia, J.D., J.M. Heddleston, M. Venere, and J.N. Rich. 2011. Deadly teamwork: Neural cancer stem cells and the tumor microenvironment. *Cell Stem Cell* 8: 482–485.

Lathia, J.D., S.C. Mack, E.E. Mulkearns-Hubert, C.L. Valentim, and J.N. Rich. 2015. Cancer stem cells in glioblastoma. *Genes & Development* 29: 1203–1217.

Lim, Y.C., T.L. Roberts, B.W. Day, A. Harding, S. Kozlov, A.W. Kijas, K.S. Ensbey, D.G. Walker, and M.F. Lavin. 2012. A role for homologous recombination and abnormal cell-cycle progression in radioresistance of glioma-initiating cells. *Molecular Cancer Therapeutics* 11: 1863–1872.

Liu, G., X. Yuan, Z. Zeng, P. Tunici, H. Ng, I.R. Abdulkadir, L. Lu, D. Irvin, K.L. Black, and J.S. Yu. 2006. Analysis of gene expression and chemoresistance of CD133+ cancer stem cells in glioblastoma. *Molecular Cancer* 5: 67.

Liu, M., K. Inoue, T. Leng, S. Guo, and Z.G. Xiong. 2014. TRPM7 channels regulate glioma stem cell through STAT3 and Notch signaling pathways. *Cellular Signalling* 26: 2773–2781.

Lomonaco, S.L., S. Finniss, C. Xiang, A. Decarvalho, F. Umansky, S.N. Kalkanis, T. Mikkelsen, and C. Brodie. 2009. The induction of autophagy by gamma-radiation contributes to the radioresistance of glioma stem cells. *International Journal of Cancer* 125: 717–722.

Mancuso, M.R., R. Davis, S.M. Norberg, S. O'Brien, B. Sennino, T. Nakahara, V.J. Yao, T. Inai, P. Brooks, B. Freimark, D.R. Shalinsky, D.D. Hu-Lowe, and D.M. McDonald. 2006. Rapid vascular regrowth in tumors after reversal of VEGF inhibition. *The Journal of Clinical Investigation* 116: 2610–2621.

Mannino, M., N. Gomez-Roman, H. Hochegger, and A.J. Chalmers. 2014. Differential sensitivity of Glioma stem cells to Aurora kinase A inhibitors: Implications for stem cell mitosis and centrosome dynamics. *Stem Cell Research* 13: 135–143.

Mantwill, K., U. Naumann, J. Seznec, V. Girbinger, H. Lage, P. Surowiak, D. Beier, M. Mittelbronn, J. Schlegel, and P.S. Holm. 2013. YB-1 dependent oncolytic adenovirus efficiently inhibits tumor growth of glioma cancer stem like cells. *Journal of Translational Medicine* 11: 216.

Mao, P., K. Joshi, J. Li, S.H. Kim, P. Li, L. Santana-Santos, S. Luthra, U.R. Chandran, P.V. Benos, L. Smith, M. Wang, B. Hu, S.Y. Cheng, R.W. Sobol, and I. Nakano. 2013. Mesenchymal glioma stem cells are maintained by activated glycolytic metabolism involving aldehyde dehydrogenase 1A3. *Proceedings of the National Academy of Sciences of the United States of America* 110: 8644–8649.

Mao, Z., X. Tian, M. Van Meter, Z. Ke, V. Gorbunova, and A. Seluanov. 2012. Sirtuin 6 (SIRT6) rescues the decline of homologous recombination repair during replicative senescence. *Proceedings of the National Academy of Sciences of the United States of America* 109: 11800–11805.

McCord, A.M., M. Jamal, E.S. Williams, K. Camphausen, and P.J. Tofilon. 2009. CD133+ glioblastoma stem-like cells are radiosensitive with a defective DNA damage response compared with established cell lines. *Clinical Cancer Research : An Official Journal of the American Association for Cancer Research* 15: 5145–5153.

Metz, M.Z., M. Gutova, S.F. Lacey, Y. Abramyants, T. Vo, M. Gilchrist, R. Tirughana, L.Y. Ghoda, M.E. Barish, C.E. Brown, J. Najbauer, P.M. Potter, J. Portnow, T.W. Synold, and K.S. Aboody. 2013. Neural stem cell-mediated delivery of irinotecan-activating carboxylesterases to glioma: implications for clinical use. *Stem Cells Translational Medicine* 2: 983–992.

Morel, A.P., M. Lievre, C. Thomas, G. Hinkal, S. Ansieau, and A. Puisieux. 2008. Generation of breast cancer stem cells through epithelial-mesenchymal transition. *PloS One* 3: e2888.

Mukherjee, S., C. Tucker-Burden, C. Zhang, K. Moberg, R. Read, C. Hadjipanayis, and D.J. Brat. 2016. Drosophila Brat and Human Ortholog TRIM3 Maintain Stem Cell Equilibrium and Suppress Brain Tumorigenesis by Attenuating Notch Nuclear Transport. *Cancer Research* 76: 2443–2452.

Nakata, S., B. Campos, J. Bageritz, J.L. Bermejo, N. Becker, F. Engel, T. Acker, S. Momma, C. Herold-Mende, P. Lichter, B. Radlwimmer, and V. Goidts. 2013. LGR5 is a marker of poor prognosis in glioblastoma and is required for survival of brain cancer stem-like cells. *Brain Pathology* 23: 60–72.

Natsumeda, M., K. Maitani, Y. Liu, H. Miyahara, H. Kaur, Q. Chu, H. Zhang, U. Kahlert, and C.G. Eberhart. 2015. Targeting notch signaling and autophagy increases cytotoxicity in glioblastoma neurospheres. *Brain Pathology* 26 (6): 713–723.

Nguyen, L.V., R. Vanner, P. Dirks, and C.J. Eaves. 2012. Cancer stem cells: An evolving concept. *Nature Reviews Cancer* 12: 133–143.

Nogueira, L., P. Ruiz-Ontanon, A. Vazquez-Barquero, M. Lafarga, M.T. Berciano, B. Aldaz, L. Grande, I. Casafont, V. Segura, E.F. Robles, D. Suarez, L.F. Garcia, J.A. Martinez-Climent, and J.L. Fernandez-Luna. 2011. Blockade of the NFkappaB pathway drives differentiating glioblastoma-initiating cells into senescence both in vitro and in vivo. *Oncogene* 30: 3537–3548.

Ohtsu, N., Y. Nakatani, D. Yamashita, S. Ohue, T. Ohnishi, and T. Kondo. 2016. Eva1 maintains the stem-like character of glioblastoma-initiating cells by activating the noncanonical NF-kappaB signaling pathway. *Cancer Research* 76: 171–181.

Olmez, I., W. Shen, H. McDonald, and B. Ozpolat. 2015. Dedifferentiation of patient-derived glioblastoma multiforme cell lines results in a cancer stem cell-like state with mitogen-independent growth. *Journal of Cellular and Molecular Medicine* 19: 1262–1272.

Pallini, R., L. Ricci-Vitiani, G.L. Banna, M. Signore, D. Lombardi, M. Todaro, G. Stassi, M. Martini, G. Maira, L.M. Larocca, and R. De Maria. 2008. Cancer stem cell analysis and clinical outcome in patients with glioblastoma multiforme. *Clinical Cancer Research : An Official Journal of the American Association for Cancer Research* 14: 8205–8212.

Pastrana, E., V. Silva-Vargas, and F. Doetsch. 2011. Eyes wide open: A critical review of sphere-formation as an assay for stem cells. *Cell Stem Cell* 8: 486–498.

Patel, A.P., I. Tirosh, J.J. Trombetta, A.K. Shalek, S.M. Gillespie, H. Wakimoto, D.P. Cahill, B.V. Nahed, W.T. Curry, R.L. Martuza, D.N. Louis, O. Rozenblatt-Rosen, M.L. Suva, A. Regev, and B.E. Bernstein. 2014. Single-cell RNA-seq highlights intratumoral heterogeneity in primary glioblastoma. *Science* 344: 1396–1401.

Piccirillo, S.G., and A.L. Vescovi. 2007. Brain tumour stem cells: Possibilities of new therapeutic strategies. *Expert Opinion on Biological Therapy* 7: 1129–1135.

Ping, Y.F., X.H. Yao, J.Y. Jiang, L.T. Zhao, S.C. Yu, T. Jiang, M.C. Lin, J.H. Chen, B. Wang, R. Zhang, Y.H. Cui, C. Qian, J. Wang, and X.W. Bian. 2011. The chemokine CXCL12 and its receptor CXCR4 promote glioma stem cell-mediated VEGF production and tumour angiogenesis via PI3K/AKT signalling. *The Journal of Pathology* 224: 344–354.

Pistollato, F., S. Abbadi, E. Rampazzo, L. Persano, A. Della Puppa, C. Frasson, E. Sarto, R. Scienza, D. D'Avella, and G. Basso. 2010. Intratumoral hypoxic gradient drives stem cells distribution and MGMT expression in glioblastoma. *Stem Cells* 28: 851–862.

Qiang, L., T. Wu, H.W. Zhang, N. Lu, R. Hu, Y.J. Wang, L. Zhao, F.H. Chen, X.T. Wang, Q.D. You, and Q.L. Guo. 2012. HIF-1alpha is critical for hypoxia-mediated maintenance of glioblastoma stem cells by activating Notch signaling pathway. *Cell Death and Differentiation* 19: 284–294.

Quintana, E., M. Shackleton, H.R. Foster, D.R. Fullen, M.S. Sabel, T.M. Johnson, and S.J. Morrison. 2010. Phenotypic heterogeneity among tumorigenic melanoma cells from patients that is reversible and not hierarchically organized. *Cancer Cell* 18: 510–523.

Rahman, M., K. Reyner, L. Deleyrolle, S. Millette, H. Azari, B.W. Day, B.W. Stringer, A.W. Boyd, T.G. Johns, V. Blot, R. Duggal, and B.A. Reynolds. 2015. Neurosphere and adherent culture conditions are equivalent for malignant glioma stem cell lines. *Anatomy and Cell Biology* 48: 25–35.

Rathod, S.S., S.B. Rani, M. Khan, D. Muzumdar, and A. Shiras. 2014. Tumor suppressive miRNA-34a suppresses cell proliferation and tumor growth of glioma stem cells by targeting Akt and Wnt signaling pathways. *FEBS Open Bio* 4: 485–495.

Rheinbay, E., M.L. Suva, S.M. Gillespie, H. Wakimoto, A.P. Patel, M. Shahid, O. Oksuz, S.D. Rabkin, R.L. Martuza, M.N. Rivera, D.N. Louis, S. Kasif, A.S. Chi, and B.E. Bernstein. 2013. An aberrant transcription factor network essential for Wnt signaling and stem cell maintenance in glioblastoma. *Cell Reports* 3: 1567–1579.

Riganti, C., I.C. Salaroglio, V. Caldera, I. Campia, J. Kopecka, M. Mellai, L. Annovazzi, A. Bosia, D. Ghigo, and D. Schiffer. 2013. Temozolomide downregulates P-glycoprotein expression in glioblastoma stem cells by interfering with the Wnt3a/glycogen synthase-3 kinase/beta-catenin pathway. *Neuro-Oncology* 15: 1502–1517.

Ropolo, M., A. Daga, F. Griffero, M. Foresta, G. Casartelli, A. Zunino, A. Poggi, E. Cappelli, G. Zona, R. Spaziante, G. Corte, and G. Frosina. 2009. Comparative analysis of DNA repair in stem and nonstem glioma cell cultures. *Molecular Cancer Research* 7: 383–392.

Saito, N., K. Aoki, N. Hirai, S. Fujita, J. Iwama, Y. Hiramoto, M. Ishii, K. Sato, H. Nakayama, J. Harashina, M. Hayashi, H. Izukura, H. Kimura, K. Ito, T. Sakurai, Y. Yokouchi, T. Oharazeki, K. Takahashi, and S. Iwabuchi. 2015. Effect of Notch expression in glioma stem cells on therapeutic response to chemo-radiotherapy in recurrent glioblastoma. *Brain Tumor Pathology* 32: 176–183.

Saito, N., J. Fu, S. Zheng, J. Yao, S. Wang, D.D. Liu, Y. Yuan, E.P. Sulman, F.F. Lang, H. Colman, R.G. Verhaak, W.K. Yung, and D. Koul. 2014. A high Notch pathway activation predicts response to gamma secretase inhibitors in proneural subtype of glioma tumor-initiating cells. *Stem Cells* 32: 301–312.

Sandberg, C.J., G. Altschuler, J. Jeong, K.K. Stromme, B. Stangeland, W. Murrell, U.H. Grasmo-Wendler, O. Myklebost, E. Helseth, E.O. Vik-Mo, W. Hide, and I.A. Langmoen. 2013. Comparison of glioma stem cells to neural stem cells from the adult human brain identifies dysregulated Wnt- signaling and a fingerprint associated with clinical outcome. *Experimental Cell Research* 319: 2230–2243.

Schaich, M., L. Kestel, M. Pfirrmann, K. Robel, T. Illmer, M. Kramer, C. Dill, G. Ehninger, G. Schackert, and D. Krex. 2009. A MDR1 (ABCB1) gene single nucleotide polymorphism predicts outcome of temozolomide treatment in glioblastoma patients. *Annals of Oncology : Official Journal of the European Society for Medical Oncology / ESMO* 20: 175–181.

Schmidt, N.O., W. Przylecki, W. Yang, M. Ziu, Y. Teng, S.U. Kim, P.M. Black, K.S. Aboody, and R.S. Carroll. 2005. Brain tumor tropism of transplanted human neural stem cells is induced by vascular endothelial growth factor. *Neoplasia* 7: 623–629.

Seidel, S., B.K. Garvalov, V. Wirta, L. von Stechow, A. Schanzer, K. Meletis, M. Wolter, D. Sommerlad, A.T. Henze, M. Nister, G. Reifenberger, J. Lundeberg, J. Frisen, and T. Acker. 2010. A hypoxic niche regulates glioblastoma stem cells through hypoxia inducible factor 2 alpha. *Brain : A Journal of Neurology* 133: 983–995.

Shapiro, J.R., W.K. Yung, and W.R. Shapiro. 1981. Isolation, karyotype, and clonal growth of heterogeneous subpopulations of human malignant gliomas. *Cancer Research* 41: 2349–2359.

Shen, Y., H. Chen, J. Zhang, Y. Chen, M. Wang, J. Ma, L. Hong, N. Liu, Q. Fan, X. Lu, Y. Tian, A. Wang, J. Dong, Q. Lan, and Q. Huang. 2015. Increased Notch Signaling Enhances Radioresistance of Malignant Stromal Cells Induced by Glioma Stem/ Progenitor Cells. *PloS One* 10: e0142594.

Shi, L., X. Fei, Z. Wang, and Y. You. 2015. PI3K inhibitor combined with miR-125b inhibitor sensitize TMZ-induced anti-glioma stem cancer effects through inactivation of Wnt/beta-catenin signaling pathway. *In vitro cellular & developmental biology Animal* 51: 1047–1055.

Shiras, A., S.T. Chettiar, V. Shepal, G. Rajendran, G.R. Prasad, and P. Shastry. 2007. Spontaneous transformation of human adult nontumorigenic stem cells to cancer stem cells is driven by genomic instability in a human model of glioblastoma. *Stem Cells* 25: 1478–1489.

Singh, S.K., C. Hawkins, I.D. Clarke, J.A. Squire, J. Bayani, T. Hide, R.M. Henkelman, M.D. Cusimano, and P.B. Dirks. 2004. Identification of human brain tumour initiating cells. *Nature* 432: 396–401.

Skjellegrind, H.K., A. Fayzullin, E.O. Johnsen, L. Eide, I.A. Langmoen, M.C. Moe, and E.O. Vik-Mo. 2016. Short-term differentiation of glioblastoma stem cells induces hypoxia tolerance. *Neurochemical Research* 41: 1545–1558.

Soeda, A., A. Hara, T. Kunisada, S. Yoshimura, T. Iwama, and D.M. Park. 2015. The evidence of glioblastoma heterogeneity. *Scientific Reports* 5: 7979.

Son, M.J., K. Woolard, D.H. Nam, J. Lee, and H.A. Fine. 2009. SSEA-1 is an enrichment marker for tumor-initiating cells in human glioblastoma. *Cell Stem Cell* 4: 440–452.

Sonabend, A.M., I.V. Ulasov, and M.S. Lesniak. 2006. Conditionally replicative adenoviral vectors for malignant glioma. *Reviews in Medical Virology* 16: 99–115.

Sottoriva, A., I. Spiteri, D. Shibata, C. Curtis, and S. Tavare. 2013. Single-molecule genomic data delineate patient-specific tumor profiles and cancer stem cell organization. *Cancer Research* 73: 41–49.

Strojnik, T., G.V. Rosland, P.O. Sakariassen, R. Kavalar, and T. Lah. 2007. Neural stem cell markers, nestin and musashi proteins, in the progression of human glioma: correlation of nestin with prognosis of patient survival. *Surgical Neurology* 68: 133–143. discussion 143–134.

Stupp, R., M.E. Hegi, W.P. Mason, M.J. van den Bent, M.J. Taphoorn, R.C. Janzer, S.K. Ludwin, A. Allgeier, B. Fisher, K. Belanger, P. Hau, A.A. Brandes, J. Gijtenbeek, C. Marosi, C.J. Vecht, K. Mokhtari, P. Wesseling, S. Villa, E. Eisenhauer, T. Gorlia, M. Weller, D. Lacombe, J.G. Cairncross, R.O. Mirimanoff, European Organisation for R, Treatment of Cancer Brain T, Radiation Oncology G, and National Cancer Institute of Canada Clinical Trials G. 2009. Effects of radiotherapy with concomitant and adjuvant temozolomide versus radiotherapy alone on survival in glioblastoma in a randomised phase III study: 5-year analysis of the EORTC-NCIC trial. *The Lancet Oncology* 10: 459–466.

Sun, L., J. Lee, and H.A. Fine. 2004. Neuronally expressed stem cell factor induces neural stem cell migration to areas of brain injury. *The Journal of Clinical Investigation* 113: 1364–1374.

Sun, Y., W. Kong, A. Falk, J. Hu, L. Zhou, S. Pollard, and A. Smith. 2009. CD133 (Prominin) negative human neural stem cells are clonogenic and tripotent. *PloS One* 4: e5498.

Suva, M.L., E. Rheinbay, S.M. Gillespie, A.P. Patel, H. Wakimoto, S.D. Rabkin, N. Riggi, A.S. Chi, D.P. Cahill, B.V. Nahed, W.T. Curry, R.L. Martuza, M.N. Rivera, N. Rossetti, S. Kasif, S. Beik, S. Kadri, I. Tirosh, I. Wortman, A.K. Shalek, O. Rozenblatt-Rosen, A. Regev, D.N. Louis, and B.E. Bernstein. 2014. Reconstructing and reprogramming the tumor-propagating potential of glioblastoma stem-like cells. *Cell* 157: 580–594.

Tamura, K., M. Aoyagi, H. Wakimoto, N. Ando, T. Nariai, M. Yamamoto, and K. Ohno. 2010. Accumulation of CD133-positive glioma cells after high-dose irradiation by Gamma Knife surgery plus external beam radiation. *Journal of Neurosurgery* 113: 310–318.

Tanaka, S., M. Nakada, D. Yamada, I. Nakano, T. Todo, Y. Ino, T. Hoshii, Y. Tadokoro, K. Ohta, M.A. Ali, Y. Hayashi, J. Hamada, and A. Hirao. 2015. Strong therapeutic potential of gamma-secretase inhibitor MRK003 for CD44-high and CD133-low glioblastoma initiating cells. *Journal of Neuro-Oncology* 121: 239–250.

Tang, D.G. 2012. Understanding cancer stem cell heterogeneity and plasticity. *Cell Research* 22: 457–472.

Tchoghandjian, A., N. Baeza, C. Colin, M. Cayre, P. Metellus, C. Beclin, L. Ouafik, and D. Figarella-Branger. 2010. A2B5 cells from human glioblastoma have cancer stem cell properties. *Brain Pathology* 20: 211–221.

Tchoghandjian, A., C. Jennewein, I. Eckhardt, S. Momma, D. Figarella-Branger, and S. Fulda. 2014. Smac mimetic promotes glioblastoma cancer stem-like cell differentiation by activating NF-kappaB. *Cell Death and Differentiation* 21: 735–747.

Turchi, L., D.N. Debruyne, F. Almairac, V. Virolle, M. Fareh, Y. Neirijnck, F. Burel-Vandenbos, P. Paquis, M.P. Junier, E. Van Obberghen-Schilling, H. Chneiweiss, and T. Virolle. 2013. Tumorigenic potential of miR-18A* in glioma initiating cells requires NOTCH-1 signaling. *Stem Cells* 31: 1252–1265.

Ulasov, I.V., S. Nandi, M. Dey, A.M. Sonabend, and M.S. Lesniak. 2011. Inhibition of Sonic hedgehog and Notch pathways enhances sensitivity of CD133(+) glioma stem cells to temozolomide therapy. *Molecular Medicine* 17: 103–112.

Vellanki, S.H., A. Grabrucker, S. Liebau, C. Proepper, A. Eramo, V. Braun, T. Boeckers, K.M. Debatin, and S. Fulda. 2009. Small-molecule XIAP inhibitors enhance gamma-irradiation-induced apoptosis in glioblastoma. *Neoplasia* 11: 743–752.

Venere, M., P. Hamerlik, Q. Wu, R.D. Rasmussen, L.A. Song, A. Vasanji, N. Tenley, W.A. Flavahan, A.B. Hjelmeland, J. Bartek, and J.N. Rich. 2014. Therapeutic targeting of constitutive PARP activation compromises stem cell phenotype and survival of glioblastoma-initiating cells. *Cell Death and Differentiation* 21: 258–269.

Villalva, C., S. Martin-Lanneree, U. Cortes, F. Dkhissi, M. Wager, A. Le Corf, J.M. Tourani, I. Dusanter-Fourt, A.G. Turhan, and L. Karayan-Tapon. 2011. STAT3 is essential for the maintenance of neurosphere-initiating tumor cells in patients with glioblastomas: A potential for targeted therapy? *International Journal of Cancer* 128: 826–838.

Vlashi, E., C. Lagadec, L. Vergnes, T. Matsutani, K. Masui, M. Poulou, R. Popescu, L. Della Donna, P. Evers, C. Dekmezian, K. Reue, H. Christofk, P.S. Mischel, and F. Pajonk. 2011. Metabolic state of glioma stem cells and nontumorigenic cells. *Proceedings of the National Academy of Sciences of the United States of America* 108: 16062–16067.

Vukicevic, V., A. Jauch, T.C. Dinger, L. Gebauer, V. Hornich, S.R. Bornstein, M. Ehrhart-Bornstein, and A.M. Muller. 2010. Genetic instability and diminished differentiation capacity in long-term cultured mouse neurosphere cells. *Mechanisms of Ageing and Development* 131: 124–132.

Wang, J., P.O. Sakariassen, O. Tsinkalovsky, H. Immervoll, S.O. Boe, A. Svendsen, L. Prestegarden, G. Rosland, F. Thorsen, L. Stuhr, A. Molven, R. Bjerkvig, and P.O. Enger. 2008. CD133 negative glioma cells form tumors in nude rats and give rise to CD133 positive cells. *International Journal of Cancer* 122: 761–768.

Wang, J., T.P. Wakeman, J.D. Lathia, A.B. Hjelmeland, X.F. Wang, R.R. White, J.N. Rich, and B.A. Sullenger. 2010. Notch promotes radioresistance of glioma stem cells. *Stem Cells* 28: 17–28.

Wang, J., C. Wang, Q. Meng, S. Li, X. Sun, Y. Bo, and W. Yao. 2012. siRNA targeting Notch-1 decreases glioma stem cell proliferation and tumor growth. *Molecular Biology Reports* 39: 2497–2503.

Wang, J., Z. Yan, X. Liu, S. Che, C. Wang, and W. Yao. 2016. Alpinetin targets glioma stem cells by suppressing Notch pathway. *Tumour Biology : The Journal of the International Society for Oncodevelopmental Biology and Medicine* 37: 9243–9248.

Wang, W., Y. Quan, Q. Fu, Y. Liu, Y. Liang, J. Wu, G. Yang, C. Luo, Q. Ouyang, and Y. Wang. 2014. Dynamics between cancer cell subpopulations reveals a model coordinating with both hierarchical and stochastic concepts. *PloS One* 9: e84654.

Warrier, S., S.K. Balu, A.P. Kumar, M. Millward, and A. Dharmarajan. 2013. Wnt antagonist, secreted frizzled-related protein 4 (sFRP4), increases chemotherapeutic response of glioma stem-like cells. *Oncology Research* 21: 93–102.

Wartenberg, M., P. Budde, M. De Marees, F. Grunheck, S.Y. Tsang, Y. Huang, Z.Y. Chen, J. Hescheler, and H. Sauer. 2003. Inhibition of tumor-induced angiogenesis and matrix-metalloproteinase expression in confrontation cultures of embryoid bodies and tumor spheroids by plant ingredients used in traditional chinese medicine. *Laboratory Investigation; A Journal of Technical Methods and Pathology* 83: 87–98.

Winkler, F., S.V. Kozin, R.T. Tong, S.S. Chae, M.F. Booth, I. Garkavtsev, L. Xu, D.J. Hicklin, D. Fukumura, E. di Tomaso, L.L. Munn, and R.K. Jain. 2004. Kinetics of vascular normalization by VEGFR2 blockade governs brain tumor response to radiation: role of oxygenation, angiopoietin-1, and matrix metalloproteinases. *Cancer Cell* 6: 553–563.

Wu, J., Z. Ji, H. Liu, Y. Liu, D. Han, C. Shi, C. Shi, C. Wang, G. Yang, X. Chen, C. Shen, H. Li, Y. Bi, D. Zhang, and S. Zhao. 2013. Arsenic trioxide depletes cancer stem-like cells and inhibits repopulation of neurosphere derived from glioblastoma by downregulation of Notch pathway. *Toxicology Letters* 220: 61–69.

Xia, Z., P. Wei, H. Zhang, Z. Ding, L. Yang, Z. Huang, and N. Zhang. 2013. AURKA governs self-renewal capacity in glioma-initiating cells via stabilization/activation of beta-catenin/Wnt signaling. *Molecular Cancer Research : MCR* 11: 1101–1111.

Xu, Q., X. Yuan, G. Liu, K.L. Black, and J.S. Yu. 2008. Hedgehog signaling regulates brain tumor-initiating cell proliferation and portends shorter survival for patients with PTEN-coexpressing glioblastomas. *Stem Cells* 26: 3018–3026.

Xu, X., F. Stockhammer, and M. Schmitt. 2012. Cellular-based immunotherapies for patients with glioblastoma multiforme. *Clinical & Developmental Immunology* 2012: 764213.

Yahyanejad, S., H. King, V.S. Iglesias, P.V. Granton, L.M. Barbeau, S.J. van Hoof, A.J. Groot, R. Habets, J. Prickaerts, A.J. Chalmers, D.B. Eekers, J. Theys, S.C. Short, F. Verhaegen, and M. Vooijs. 2016. NOTCH blockade combined with radiation therapy and temozolomide prolongs survival of orthotopic glioblastoma. *Oncotarget* 7 (27): 41251–41264.

Yamada, K., J. Tso, F. Ye, J. Choe, Y. Liu, L.M. Liau, and C.L. Tso. 2011. Essential gene pathways for glioblastoma stem cells: clinical implications for prevention of tumor recurrence. *Cancers* 3: 1975–1995.

Yan, W., Y. Chen, Y. Yao, H. Zhang, and T. Wang. 2013. Increased invasion and tumorigenicity capacity of CD44+/CD24- breast cancer MCF7 cells in vitro and in nude mice. *Cancer Cell International* 13: 62.

Yang, Y.P., Y. Chien, G.Y. Chiou, J.Y. Cherng, M.L. Wang, W.L. Lo, Y.L. Chang, P.I. Huang, Y.W. Chen, Y.H. Shih, M.T. Chen, and S.H. Chiou. 2012. Inhibition of cancer stem cell-like properties and reduced chemoradioresistance of glioblastoma using microRNA145 with cationic polyurethane-short branch PEI. *Biomaterials* 33: 1462–1476.

Ye, F., Y. Zhang, Y. Liu, K. Yamada, J.L. Tso, J.C. Menjivar, J.Y. Tian, W.H. Yong, D. Schaue, P.S. Mischel, T.F. Cloughesy, S.F. Nelson, L.M. Liau, W. McBride, and C.L. Tso. 2013. Protective properties of radio-chemoresistant glioblastoma stem cell clones are associated with metabolic adaptation to reduced glucose dependence. *PloS One* 8: e80397.

Yin, J., G. Park, J.E. Lee, J.Y. Park, T.H. Kim, Y.J. Kim, S.H. Lee, H. Yoo, J.H. Kim, and J.B. Park. 2014. CPEB1 modulates differentiation of glioma stem cells via downregulation of HES1 and SIRT1 expression. *Oncotarget* 5: 6756–6769.

Ying, M., S. Wang, Y. Sang, P. Sun, B. Lal, C.R. Goodwin, H. Guerrero-Cazares, A. Quinones-Hinojosa, J. Laterra, and S. Xia. 2011. Regulation of glioblastoma stem cells by retinoic acid: Role for Notch pathway inhibition. *Oncogene* 30: 3454–3467.

Yip, S., J. Miao, D.P. Cahill, A.J. Iafrate, K. Aldape, C.L. Nutt, and D.N. Louis. 2009. MSH6 mutations arise in glioblastomas during temozolomide therapy and mediate temozolomide resistance. *Clinical Cancer Research : An Official Journal of the American Association for Cancer Research* 15: 4622–4629.

Yoon, C.H., M.J. Kim, R.K. Kim, E.J. Lim, K.S. Choi, S. An, S.G. Hwang, S.G. Kang, Y. Suh, M.J. Park, and S.J. Lee. 2012. c-Jun N-terminal kinase has a pivotal role in the maintenance of self-renewal and tumorigenicity in glioma stem-like cells. *Oncogene* 31: 4655–4666.

Yuan, X., J. Curtin, Y. Xiong, G. Liu, S. Waschsmann-Hogiu, D.L. Farkas, K.L. Black, and J.S. Yu. 2004. Isolation of cancer stem cells from adult glioblastoma multiforme. *Oncogene* 23: 9392–9400.

Zbinden, M., A. Duquet, A. Lorente-Trigos, S.N. Ngwabyt, I. Borges, and A. Ruiz i Altaba. 2010. NANOG regulates glioma stem cells and is essential in vivo acting in a cross-functional network with GLI1 and p53. *The EMBO Journal* 29: 2659–2674.

Zeppernick, F., R. Ahmadi, B. Campos, C. Dictus, B.M. Helmke, N. Becker, P. Lichter, A. Unterberg, B. Radlwimmer, and C.C. Herold-Mende. 2008. Stem cell marker CD133 affects clinical outcome in glioma patients. *Clinical Cancer Research : An Official Journal of the American Association for Cancer Research* 14: 123–129.

Zhang, L., X. Ren, Y. Cheng, X. Liu, J.E. Allen, Y. Zhang, Y. Yuan, S.Y. Huang, W. Yang, A. Berg, B.S. Webb, J. Connor, C.G. Liu, Z. Lu, W.S. El-Deiry, and J.M. Yang. 2014. The NFkappaB inhibitor, SN50, induces differentiation of glioma stem cells and suppresses their oncogenic phenotype. *Cancer Biology & Therapy* 15: 602–611.

Zhang, M., T. Song, L. Yang, R. Chen, L. Wu, Z. Yang, and J. Fang. 2008. Nestin and CD133: Valuable stem cell-specific markers for determining clinical outcome of glioma patients. *Journal of Experimental & Clinical Cancer Research : CR* 27: 85.

Zhen, Y., S. Zhao, Q. Li, Y. Li, and K. Kawamoto. 2010. Arsenic trioxide-mediated Notch pathway inhibition depletes the cancer stem-like cell population in gliomas. *Cancer Letters* 292: 64–72.

Zheng, H., H. Ying, H. Yan, A.C. Kimmelman, D.J. Hiller, A.J. Chen, S.R. Perry, G. Tonon, G.C. Chu, Z. Ding, J.M. Stommel, K.L. Dunn, R. Wiedemeyer, M.J. You, C. Brennan, Y.A. Wang, K.L. Ligon, W.H. Wong, L. Chin, and R.A. DePinho. 2008. p53 and Pten control neural and glioma stem/progenitor cell renewal and differentiation. *Nature* 455: 1129–1133.

Zhu, T.S., M.A. Costello, C.E. Talsma, C.G. Flack, J.G. Crowley, L.L. Hamm, X. He, S.L. Hervey-Jumper, J.A. Heth, K.M. Muraszko, F. DiMeco, A.L. Vescovi, and X. Fan. 2011. Endothelial cells create a stem cell niche in glioblastoma by providing NOTCH ligands that nurture self-renewal of cancer stem-like cells. *Cancer Research* 71: 6061–6072.

Chapter 9
Animal Models in Glioblastoma: Use in Biology and Developing Therapeutic Strategies

A.J. Schuhmacher and M. Squatrito

Abstract The gliomas are a large group of brain tumors and Glioblastoma Multiforme (GBM) is the most common and lethal primary central nervous system tumor in adults. Despite the recent advances in treatment modalities, GBM patients generally respond poorly to all therapeutic approaches and prognosis remain dismal. Gaining insights into the pathways that determine this poor treatment response and the generation of more relevant animal models that recapitulate a patient's tumor will be instrumental for the elaboration of new therapeutic modalities.

Here we will focus on the available animal models for adult GBM and their use in preclinical drug development. We will be examining the recent advances in genetically engineered mouse models and discuss how such models may offer specific advantages over cell culture and xenograft systems for validating drug targets and prioritizing candidates for clinical trials. Lastly we will briefly examine the clinical relevance in glioma research of other animal models such as fruit fly, zebrafish and canine.

Keywords Glioma • Glioblastoma • GBM • Animal models • GEMM

9.1 Introduction

The gliomas are a large group of brain tumors and within gliomas the Glioblastoma Multiforme (GBM) is the most frequent form of the disease and overall the most common and lethal primary central nervous system (CNS) tumor in adults.

A.J. Schuhmacher • M. Squatrito (✉)
Cancer Cell Biology Programme, Seve Ballesteros Foundation Brain Tumor Group,
Centro Nacional de Investigaciones Oncológicas, CNIO, 28029 Madrid, Spain
e-mail: msquatrito@cnio.es

© Springer International Publishing AG 2017
K. Somasundaram (ed.), *Advances in Biology and Treatment of Glioblastoma*,
Current Cancer Research, DOI 10.1007/978-3-319-56820-1_9

219

GBMs are divided in two subtypes on the basis of clinical history: "primary GBMs" that arise *de novo*, with no evidences of precursor lesions, and "secondary GBMs", evolving from a lower grade tumor over time (Ohgaki and Kleihues 2013). Irrespectively of their primary or secondary origin, histologically GBMs are characterized by tumor cells invading adjacent normal brain parenchyma, by vascular proliferation and by the presence of area of necrosis and haemorrhage. Necrotic regions are typically surrounded by dense cellular zones known to be highly hypoxic, commonly referred as pseudopalisades.

On a molecular basis, a decade of studies, including the most recent large-scale genomic analysis (Verhaak et al. 2010; Noushmehr et al. 2010; Parsons et al. 2008; Ceccarelli et al. 2016; TCGA Network 2008; Brennan et al. 2013) has underlined the complexity of the genetic events that characterize the glioblastoma genome. However, the functional significance of the vast majority of these alterations remains elusive.

The initial publication by The Cancer Genome Atlas (TCGA) described biologically significant alterations in three core signaling cascades: (1) the TP53 pathway, (2) the G1/S cell cycle checkpoint coordinated by the Rb family, and (3) the receptor tyrosine kinases (RTKs) and their RAS-mitogen activated protein kinase (MAPK) and phosphoinositide 3-kinase (PI3K) downstream effector pathways (TCGA Network 2008). Moreover, genome-wide mutational analysis of GBMs uncovered somatic mutations of the isocitrate dehydrogenase 1 gene (*IDH1*) in a fraction of tumors, most commonly secondary glioblastomas (Parsons et al. 2008; Yan et al. 2009). Various molecular characterization studies have subsequently linked such genetic alterations, gene expression, and DNA methylation signatures with prognosis (Noushmehr et al. 2010; Verhaak et al. 2010; Ceccarelli et al. 2016). In particular, mutations in the *IDH1* and *IDH2* genes have been shown to depict a separate subset of GBM with a hypermethylation phenotype (G-CIMP) and a more favorable prognosis (Noushmehr et al. 2010; Yan et al. 2009). On the contrary, the lack of *IDH* mutations in low-grade gliomas characterizes a clinically distinct IDH-wild-type subclass with poor, GBM-like outcome (Ceccarelli et al. 2016; Eckel-Passow et al. 2015; TCGA Network 2015).

Over the past century, the classification of brain tumors has been centered mostly on the notion that tumors can be classified according to their microscopic resemblances with distinctive putative cells of origin and their supposed levels of differentiation (Louis et al. 2016a; Ramaswamy and Taylor 2016). It has become apparent that such morphologically centered classification lacks accuracy and is accompanied by remarkable inter-observer variability (van den Bent 2010). Moreover, histologically indistinguishable tumors assigned to equal "pathological entity" can show extremely diverse responses to therapy and have very different outcomes (Ramaswamy and Taylor 2016). Consequently, a recent update of the World Health Organization (WHO) classification of brain tumors (2016 CNS WHO) drops the century-old standard of diagnosis based exclusively on microscopy and integrates molecular factors into the classification of CNS tumor entities (Louis et al. 2016b).

According to the 2016 CNS WHO, GBMs are now grouped into (1) GBM IDH-wild-type (approximately 90% of cases), which mainly affects patients over 55 years of age and coincides commonly with the clinically defined primary or de novo glioblastoma; (2)

GBM IDH-mutant (approximately 10% of cases), which conversely occurs in younger patients and coincides with secondary glioblastoma with clinical or histologic evidence of a less malignant precursor lesion; and (3) GBM NOS (not otherwise specified), a diagnosis that is used for those tumors for which full IDH evaluation cannot be assessed (Louis et al. 2016b).

Standard therapy for GBMs includes resection of the tumor mass, followed by concurrent radiotherapy and chemotherapy. Although the last decade highlighted enormous advances in treating other solid cancers, such as lung and breast, the median survival for GBM stayed nearly the same over the last 50 years, averaging 15 months (Stupp et al. 2005; Stupp et al. 2009; Theeler and Gilbert 2015). Regardless of the improvements in surgical and imaging techniques, we still face multiple problems when treating brain tumors, some because of extensive infiltration of tumors cells, their invasion into normal brain parenchyma or other sites, and resistance to standard radiation and chemotherapy. Nevertheless, the therapeutic strategy for gliomas has remained essentially unchanged for decades due to a limited understanding of the biology of the disease. Radiation and chemo-resistance are characteristic of various cancers, however it is not clear if this therapy resistance is a consequence of tumor progression or it is intrinsically associated with the genetic events that lead to the tumor formation in the first place (Squatrito and Holland 2011). Gaining insights into the pathways that determine this poor treatment response and developing more relevant animal models that recapitulate a patient's GBM tumor will be instrumental for the development of new therapeutic modalities (Jue and McDonald 2016).

Here will focus on the currently available animal models for adult GBM and their use in preclinical drug development. We will be discussing the recent advances in genetically engineered mouse models (GEMMs) and how such models may offer specific advantages over cell culture and xenograft systems for validating drug targets and prioritizing candidates for clinical trials. We will also briefly examine the clinical relevance in glioma research of other animal models such as fruit fly, zebrafish and canine.

9.2 Mouse Models

9.2.1 Implantation Models

In vivo models fall into two main categories: those that implant tumor cells or biopsies into host animals and those that develop *de novo* by genetic manipulation. Among the implantation models we can discriminate between *allografts* where tumor cells are derived and implanted into the same species, and *xenografts* when they are different and the recipient is immunosuppressed. These models can be either *orthotopic* when they are implanted in the native site or *heterotypic* if they are implanted in a non-original site.

Implantation models have been informative but display several limitations. In these models "initiation" occurs by injection of a large number of cells, therefore differing from endogenous spontaneous tumor development where presumably a cell is transformed and evolves *in situ*. Moreover, the tumor implantation location can impact the response to therapies such as radiation (Camphausen et al. 2005b).

The traditional allograft models consist of glioma cell lines generated by chemical carcinogenesis that have been maintained in culture for long time periods. When implanted into a syngeneic host these tumors do not resemble the histology of human gliomas. These models lack the microvascular abnormalities and, despite they display some invasion, are deficient of single cell infiltration characteristic of GBM (Huszthy et al. 2012). While these models might have a value to study and target the tumor-stroma interactions, allograft models have a limited value in predicting Phase II clinical trial performance (Voskoglou-Nomikos et al. 2003).

Xenograft models require that the host animals lack an intact immune system to allow implantation. This is a major concern as these tumors are missing the pressure to evade immune destruction, a hallmark of cancer. In these models the tumor microenvironment (TME) belongs to a different species and frequently implanted cells fail to excite a normal stromal response due in part to the heterotypic human-mouse exchange of growth factors and receptors. Another drawback to consider when using immunocompromised mouse strains is that many of them carry DNA repair defects limiting their use to test novel treatments including radiation (Biedermann et al. 1991).

Subcutaneous xenografts of glioblastoma cell lines remain a popular method of assessing tumorigenesis and drug efficacy because they are highly penetrant, easy to implant and to monitor growth kinetics. However, these models have several caveats including the lack a blood brain barrier (BBB) and a native TME that influence the tumor and drug response. Moreover, molecular profiles of subcutaneous and orthotopic tumors are different (Camphausen et al. 2005a, b). When culturing established lines for a long time in presence of serum a clonal selection and culture adaptation is primed. Cell lines adapt to this non-physiological condition with abundant nutrients in a Petri dish by increasing proliferation and metabolism and decreasing cell adhesion. When intracranially injected these tumors are well defined and rarely infiltrate.

In the past years xenografts models have evolved with the development of the cancer stem cell (CSC) field. CSCs have been proposed to be capable of tumor maintenance, neurosphere (NS) formation, hierarchical differentiation, therapeutic resistance and tumor recurrence. Tumor cells derived from freshly isolated GBM can be cultured with new cell culture tools optimized for propagating CSCs under serum-free neurobasal growth media, supplemented with growth factors. Renewable NS formation in culture is a defining characteristic of certain brain tumor initiating cells and a predictor of increased hazard of patient death and more rapid tumor progression in malignant glioma (Laks et al. 2009).

Molecular profiles of glioma derived NS are stable over time and more closely mirror the phenotype and genotype of the original patient (Lee et al. 2006; Günther et al. 2008). When orthotopically implanted they show extensive infiltrative lesions. This is a major improvement in xenograft modeling, however, these models do not exhibit the microvascular proliferation and pseudopalisading necrosis observed in GBM (Hambardzumyan et al. 2011; Huszthy et al. 2012).

Generation and preservation of glioma derived NS lines can be a challenge for many laboratories. Recently a Human Glioblastoma Cell Culture (HGCC) open resource for *in vitro* and *in vivo* modeling of a large part GBM diversity has been generated (Xie et al. 2015). HGCC consists of a bio bank of 48 GBM cell lines and an associated database containing high-resolution molecular data. These lines have been derived from surgical samples of GBM patients, harbor genomic lesions characteristic of GBMs, represent all four transcriptional subtypes and have been maintained under conditions to preserve their glioma stem cell characteristics. HGCC represents a valuable resource for *in vitro* and *in vivo* modeling of GBM variety to both basic and translational GBM research.

Patient derived xenograft (PDX) models also known as "*avatar*" models are very popular for many cancer types. To generate them, fresh tumor fragments are injected orthotopically or serially passaged subcutaneaously in immunodeficient mice. These models show biological consistency with the tumor of origin. They are phenotypically stable at the histological, transcriptomic, proteomic and genomic level for several rounds of transplantation (Aparicio et al. 2015). Of important consideration to study drug response is that polyclonality is mirrowed even if the original clonality differs. These tumors are derived from human gliomas and could serve to predict therapeutic responses for individual patients as they recapitulate drug sensitivity patterns seen in patients for other cancer types (Zhang et al. 2013).

As all xenografts, PDX models lack complete native antitumor immune response. While PDX excite a stromal reaction, there is a replacement of stromal elements by murine. Incompatibilities of cytokines and integrins between species impede to fully mimic the natural TME of human tumors. These models show polyclonality, however, PDX models show changes in the clonal composition of the tumor. Engraftment of tumor cells into a foreign host exerts a selection pressure for the less differentiated cells to grow (Aparicio et al. 2015).

Intracranial implantation of a fresh GBM fragment is technically challenging. Tiny fragments of surgical tumors can be implanted into the mice brain by surgical implantation via craniotomy (Antunes et al. 2000; Taillandier et al. 2003) or with a trocar system (Fei et al. 2010). These models maintain several clones as well as other TME components. These derived tumors resemble the growth and invasion of GBM and develop other characteristics of human GBM, such as pseudopalisading necrosis, dilated vessels and angiogenesis. These features are maintained upon passaging in immunocompromised animals.

An alternative method is the dissociation of GBM as spheroids or cell suspension. In the biopsy spheroid model a GBM biopsy is minced and transferred to agar-coated plates containing standard serum supplemented cell culture media. Cellular aggregates (spheroids) are formed under these conditions (Bjerkvig et al. 1990). The spheroids contained preserved vessels, connective tissue, and macrophages, revealing a close resemblance to the conditions in the original tumor. When intracranially implanted biopsy spheroids display diffuse invasion. Trough repeated transplantation cycles to favor adaptation to the rodent brain an increased proliferation, angiogenesis necrotic areas and microvascular proliferation appear

(Wang et al. 2009; Sakariassen et al. 2006). A cell suspension from a given patient biopsy can be generated and stereotactically injected them into the mouse brains (Joo et al. 2013). Invasiveness, microvessel density, and proliferation index of the patient GBM and corresponding orthotopic xenograft correlate. *In vivo* tumor formation and invasion capacities of dissociated GBM cells correlate with worse clinical outcome.

Tumor implantation provides several advantages over cell suspension: when a similar volume is transplanted solid tumor cells contain more cells than cell suspension; more importantly tumor cells and stroma are implanted, maintaining the original microenvironment structure thus favoring cell growth and maintenance of tumor biology (Fei et al. 2010). However, success rates of tumor engraftment are low (16%–24%) but can be increased with indirect transplantation growing the tumors subcutaneously prior orthotopic implatation (Antunes et al. 2000). Extracranial expansion and scalp soft tissue infiltration is often observed upon tumor implantation by craniotomy. These inconveniences can be partially overcame with tumor implantation with a trocar system (Fei et al. 2010).

In the precision medicine era implantation biopsy models can be informative as human cancer surrogates for therapeutic purposes, some of them have been able to predict differential results of clinical treatment of the parental tumors (Joo et al. 2013). Intratumoral heterogeneity to therapeutic modalities can be modeled with some limitations that include the lack a proper immune response. Future analysis of genetic differences between responding and non-responding xenograft tumors can help to identify predictive-response biomarkers to stratify patients.

Different strains, with a range of alterations of adaptive and innate immunity for implantation models have been generated as hosts for implantation models (Shultz et al. 2007). An important advance for cancer immunotherapy would be the establishment of a functional human immune system in these mice that generates robust primary and secondary immune responses. Attempts to achieve this goal rely on: (1) the transgenic expression of human molecules such as human MHC, (2) adoptive transfer of such molecules or different immune cell types and (3) patient bone marrow/ human haematopoietic stem cells transplantation (Morgan 2012).

9.2.2 Genetically Engineered Models

Recent developments in the GEM modelling have contributed to the understanding of the molecular pathways responsible for tumor initiation and progression, to elucidate the role of various components of the TME and to provide a platform for testing new therapeutic strategies. The ideal conditions for a mouse model to mimic the natural history of a tumor are: (1) to carry the same mutations found in human tumors; (2) these mutations have to be introduced in their endogenous loci; (3) mutant genes must be silent during embryonic and early postnatal development (except for models of inherited or pediatric tumors); (4) mutant genes must be expressed in specific target tissues or in selected cell types and (5) mutations must take place in a limited number of cells.

Sophisticated models can be biologically informative but challenging to effectively implement in therapeutic trials. From a drug development point of view, in addition to faithfully recapitulate the tumor genetics, further characteristics are desirable such as: short tumor latency, high penetrance, to be easy to use and simple to generate and to incorporate a built-in mechanism such as a non invasive *in vivo* imaging reporter to monitor tumor burden and to measure therapeutic efficacy. Unfortunately fulfilling some of these characteristics might go against others. For example, a rapid tumor formation can impact the acquisition of additional stochastic events and a proper evolution of the TME (Huse and Holland 2009).

A number of excellent reviews related to GEM modelling have been recently published (Candolfi et al. 2007; Chen et al. 2012; de Vries et al. 2009; Fomchenko and Holland 2006; Huse and Holland 2009; Schmid et al. 2012; Huszthy et al. 2012; McNeill et al. 2015; Hambardzumyan et al. 2011). In this book chapter we will highlight the major improvements of these models.

Several models with considerable promise for preclinical testing have been generated in the past two decades by altering key signalling pathways known to be disrupted in human GBM including *PDGFR, EGFR, RB, TP53, RAS* and *AKT* (Holland et al. 2000; Guha 1998; Ueki et al. 1996; Henson et al. 1994). An overview of GEMMs for gliomas is depicted in Table 9.1. The type of model can determine the experimental outcome in certain situations. From a genetically point of view we can distinguish within germ line/prenatal, somatic/postnatal and gene transfer mouse models (Frese and Tuveson 2007; Cook et al. 2012). Independently of the technical approach, GEM can be classified as either transgenic or endogenous.

Classical transgenic mice for cancer are generated by pronuclear injection of cDNA constructs expressing oncogenes or dominant-negative tumor-suppressor genes in a non-physiological manner. The construct contains promoter elements designed to restrict tissue tropism such an ectopic promoter and enhancer elements. These models present several caveats: transgenes often integrate randomly in the genome as large concatamers, leading to overexpression (non-physiological levels of mutated genes), and their chromosomal positional effects can result in mosaicism and incomplete penetrance producing potentially confounding phenotypes (Robertson et al. 1995). The first GEMMs for brain tumors were models that overexpressed oncogenes (Brinster et al. 1984). Transgenic models have been upgraded taking advantage of genetic tools that allow to reversibly control target transgene expression with exogenous ligands, such as doxycycline (Schönig et al. 2002), interferon (Kühn et al. 1995) or 4-hydroxitamoxifen (Frese and Tuveson 2007).

With the appearance of gene targeting by means of homologous recombination into embryonic stem cells, strategies to develop mouse models of gain and loss of function for specific genes revolutionized the field. Endogenous GEMMs represent mutant mice that lose the expression of tumor suppressor genes or express oncogenes or dominant-negative tumor suppressor genes from their native promoters. First models generated by gene targeting consisted in the replacement of endogenous locus by a targeting vector that disrupts this allele. Such models are termed as 'knockout'. The first astrocytic glioma model initiated by loss of tumor suppressors, rather than overexpression of transgenic oncogenes, was established combining *Nf1* and *Trp53* deficient mutants (Reilly et al. 2000).

Table 9.1 Genetic engineering mouse models of glioma

Genes involved	Promoter	Mouse system	Histology	Incidence	Reference
$Nf1^{+/-}$; $p53^{+/-}$		Classical KO	A/AA/HG	92% by 6 months	Reilly et al. (2000)
$Nf1^{+/lox}$; $p53^{+/-}$	GFAP	Classical and conditional KO (GFAP-Cre)	A/AA/HG,L, S	100% by 5–10 months	Zhu et al. (2005)
$Nf1^{+/lox}$; $p53^{+/lox}$, $Pten^{+/lox}$	GFAP	Conditional KO (GFAP-Cre)	AA/ HG	100% by 5–8 months	Kwon et al. (2008)
$Nf1$; $p53$	Nestin	RCAS/tv-a; (RCAS:sh-Nf1, RCAS:shp53)	LG/HG	100% by 8 months	Ozawa et al. (2014)
$Nf1$; $p53$	GFAP	RCAS/tv-a; (RCAS:sh-Nf1, RCAS:shp53)	HG	100% by 5 months	Ozawa et al. (2014)
$Nf1^{-/lox}$	GFAP	Conditional and classical KO; Transgenic (GFAP:cre)	Optic HG	100% by 3 months	Bajenaru et al. (2003, 2005)
$Nf1$; $p53$; $Pten$; $Cas9$		CRISPR/Cas9. in utero electroporation	HG	100% by 6–10 weeks	Chen et al. (2015), Zuckermann et al. (2015)
FIG-ROS; $Ink4a/Arf^{-/-}$		Conditional transgenic (Adeno:Cre) and classical KO	A/variable	100% by 3 months	Charest et al. (2006)
SV40-Tag	GFAP	Transgenic.	A	100% by 1 month	Danks et al. (1995)
v-src	GFAP	Transgenic	A/AA/Schwannoma	15% by 1 year	Weissenberger et al. (1997)
GFAP-T121	GFAP	Transgenic. T121 (a truncated SV40 T antigen)	A/LG	100% by 10–12 months	Xiao et al. (2002)
GFAP-T121; $Pten^{loxlox}$	MSCV	Transgenic; Conditional KO (MSCV-Cre)	AA/HG	100% by 6 months	Xiao et al. (2005)
GFAP-H-RAS^{G12V}	GFAP	Transgenic	A/HG	100% by 0.5–3 months	Ding et al. (2001)
GFAP-H-RAS^{G12V}, EGFRvIII	GFAP	Transgenic; EGFRvIII delivered by adenovirus	O/OA/HG	100% by 3 months	Hao Ding et al. (2003)
GFAP-H-RAS^{G12V},$Pten^{-/-}$	GFAP	Transgenic; Classical KO	A/HG	100% by 6 weeks	Wei et al. (2006)
$S100\beta$-v-erbB	$S100\beta$	Transgenic	O/LG	60% by 1 year	Weiss et al. (2003)
$S100\beta$-v-erbB;$Ink4a/Arf^{-/-}$	$S100\beta$	Transgenic; Classical KO	O/HG	100% by 1 year	Weiss et al. (2003)
$S100\beta$-v-erbB; $p53^{+/-}$	$S100\beta$	Transgenic; Classical KO	O/OA	100% by 1 year	Weiss et al. (2003)
PDGF-B	MoMuLV	MoMuLV injected in C57Bl6 mice	O/HG/PNET	40% by 10 months	Uhrbom et al. (1998)
$KRAS^{G12D}$, $AKT^{Myr\Delta11-60}$	Nestin	RCAS/tv-a (RCAS-$KRAS^{G12D}$, RCAS- $AKT^{Myr\Delta11-60}$)	A/HG	25% by 3 months	Holland et al. (2000)
$KRAS^{G12D}$, $Pten^{-/-}$	Nestin	RCAS/tv-a; Conditional KO (RCAS-$KRAS^{G12D}$, RCAS-Cre)	A/HG	60% by 3 months	Hu et al. (2005)

Genotype	Nestin / GFAP	Method	Tumor type	Penetrance	Reference
$KRAS^{G12D}$; $AKT^{Myr11-60}$; $Ink4aArf^{-/-}$	Nestin / GFAP	RCAS/tv-a; ClassicalKO ($RCAS$-$KRAS_{G12D}$, $RCAS$- $AKT_{Myr11-60}$)	A/ spindle cell GBM, giant cell GBM	30% (GFAP)-50% (Nestin) in 3 months	Uhrbom et al. (2002)
GFAP: PDGF-B;	GFAP	Transgenic	OA/HG	65% by 6 months	Hitoshi et al. (2008)
PDGF-B-IRESβGeo; $p53^{-/-}$;	GFAP	Transgenic	O/HG	68% by 6 months	Hede et al. (2009)
GFAP:tTA:TRE: PDGF-B;	GFAP	Tetracycline regulated expression; Transgenic	OA/HG	50% by 3 months	Hitoshi, Harris, Liu, Popko, & Israel (2008)
PDGF-B	Nestin/GFAP	RCAS/tv-a; (RCAS-PDGF-B)	O/variable	60–100% by 3 months	Dai et al. (2001), Shih et al. (2004)
PDGF-B	CNP	Transgenic	A, AO, OA	33% by 3 months	Lindberg et al. (2014)
PDGF-B-IRESβGeo; $p53^{-/-}$;	GFAP	Transgenic	O/HG	68% by 6 months	Hede et al. (2009)
PDGF-B; $Ink4aArf^{-/-}$;	Nestin	RCAS/tv-a; Classical KO; (RCAS-PDGF-B)	O/HG	100% by 1.5 month	Dai et al. (2001), Fomchenko et al. (2011), Hambardzumyan et al. (2009)
PDGF-B; $Ink4aArf^{-/-}$; $Pten^{loxflox}$	Nestin	RCAS/tv-a; Classical KO; Conditional KO (RCAS-PDGF-B, RCAS-Cre)	O/HG	100% by 1 month	Dai et al. (2001), Fomchenko et al. (2011)
PDGF-B; $p53^{-/-}$	Nestin	RCAS/tv-a; Classical KO; (RCAS-PDGF-B)	HG	100% by 1 month	Squatrito et al. (2010)
PDGF-A; p53	Nestin/GFAP	RCAS/tv-a; (RCAS:PDGF-A, RCAS:shp53)	HG	100% by 3–4 months	Ozawa et al. (2014)
PDGF-A; Nf1; p53	Nestin/GFAP	RCAS/tv-a; (RCAS:PDGF-A, RCAS:shp53, RCAS:shNf1)	HG	100% by 2 months	Ozawa et al. (2014)

KO Knock-out, A astrocytoma, O oligodendroglioma, AA Aanaplastic astrocytoma, AO Anaplastic oligodendroglioma, OA Oligo astrocytoma, HG High grade, LG Low Grade. HG Glioblastoma Multiforme, PNET primitive neuroectodermal tumor, L lymphomas, S Sarcomas. GFAP Glial Fibrillary Acidic Protein, CNP 2′-3′-cyclic nucleotide 3′-phosphodiesterase, TRE tetracycline-responsive element, CRISPR Clustered Regularly Interspaced Short Palindromic Repeats. IRES Internal Ribosome Entry Site, β-Geo fusion gene formed from the β-galactosidase gene and the neomycin-resistance gene

In germ line models gene alteration occurs in all cells and not in a restricted population mimicking human hereditable cancer and predisposition syndromes. Moreover, embryonic lethality precludes study of genes critical for development in knockout models (Chen et al. 2012). To overcome this limitation conditional strategies have been designed to control in a spatial and time specific-manner such as the use of site-specific recombinases like Cre (Lakso et al. 1992; Talmadge et al. 2007; Macleod and Jacks 1999). The most popular Cre transgenic strains in GBM models express Cre recombinase under the glial fibrillary acidic protein (GFAP) to target astrocytes and glial precursors or nestin promoters to target neural stem cells and intermediate neural progenitor cells. Several strains have been generated and can be found at virtual "Cre Zoo" repositories (Chandras et al. 2012; Smedley et al. 2011; Birling et al. 2009). In addition several somatic gene transfer methods have been generated using retroviral, lentiviral and adenoviral vectors to deliver Cre recombinase for gene expression or inactivation of conditional alleles (Gierut et al. 2014; Ahmed et al. 2004). A temporal control of modified alleles can be achieved using ligand-inducible site-specific recombinases such as CreERT (Feil et al. 1996) which requires exposure to 4-hydroxytamoxifen.

Many of the GEMMs described in this chapter achieve their effects largely through the expression of an oncogenic mutation or tumor suppressor loss in an extensive area. The presence of a tumor initiating mutation in a large number of cells might reduce heterogeneity (Weiss and Shannon 2003). While these strategies generate molecularly and histologically relevant gliomas, these models frequently develop multifocal lesions or even fulminant widespread pathology (Ding et al. 2001; Xiao et al. 2005). Recent work demonstrated that histologically and molecularly distinct GBMs can arise from a set of progressively more restricted neural progenitors using identical genetic drivers (Alcantara Llaguno et al. 2015). Understanding the requirements and vulnerabilities of different progenitor cell types in the brain that are susceptible to malignant transformation might offer therapeutic opportunities.

The use of viruses for more localized gene delivery has emerged as an alternative mechanism for the production of brain tumors in GEMMs. Viral systems allow for the simultaneous delivery of multiple genes, in a variety of combinations and in a rapid way in opposing to germ line mutagenesis that requires the generation and breeding of multiple and different transgenic or gene targeted lines. The weaknesses of viral systems reside in the procedure to deliver the viruses (typically by intracranial injection), the limited DNA length that can be effectively packaged that impede the study of some genes and a reduced tumor incidence in some models (Huse and Holland 2009).

One of the first feasible somatic gene transfer models consisted in a murine retrovirus (MoMuLV) to deliver the PDGF-B into the forebrains of newborn mouse pups (Uhrbom et al. 1998). More evolved viral systems induce GBM in adult immunocompetent mice by injecting Cre-controlled lentiviral vectors expressing oncogenes in a region and cell type-specific manner in adult mice (Marumoto et al. 2009). These models show variable histology and incidence when transduced in different areas highlighting the importance and the need of selection of the cell type to be infected.

A series of GEMMs have been generated based on the somatic introduction of multiple genes into genetically engineering mouse strains that express a receptor (tv-a) for subgroup-A avian sarcoma leukosis viruses (ASLVs) (Federspiel et al. 1994). These mice strains express *tv-a* under the GFAP or nestin promoters (*Gtv-a* and *Ntv-a*, respectively) (Holland and Varmus 1998; Holland et al. 1998). Replication-Competent Avian leukosis virus Splice acceptor (RCAS) vectors are derived from ASLVs. RCAS vectors have been genetically engineered to accept insertion of DNA fragments of interest (Greenhouse et al. 1988). This system represents an advantage over other viral systems as it allows control not only the geographic area and timing of delivery but also allows the selection of the cell type to be infected, limiting it to astrocytes (*Gtv-a*) and glioneural progenitors (*Ntv-a*). This model allows the somatic gene transfer of oncogenes, shRNAs to knock down tumor suppressor genes as well as Cre recombinase and other genetic tools.

Ntv-a or *Gtv-a* mice injected with RCAS-*PDGF-B* form oligodendroglial or mixed oligoastrocytic gliomas at high incidence at 3 months depending on gene dosage (Shih et al. 2004). The combination of constitutive active variants of K-*RAS* and *AKT* yields to astrocytic tumors in the *Ntv-a* background in 3 months with 25% incidence (Holland et al. 2000). As in other models, loss of tumor suppressors such as *Pten* or *Ink4a/Arf* increase the appearance of high-grade glioma features and reduce latency (Dai et al. 2001; Uhrbom et al. 2002).

The RCAS/tv-a model is efficient, feasible, quick, flexible and safe. It has been informative to test new therapies such as mTOR inhibitors (Hu et al. 2005), to optimize of radiation dosing schedules for proneural glioblastoma (Leder et al. 2014) or to assess metabolic nutrient uptake in gliomas in vivo that may serve as a valuable tool in the clinical management of patients suffering from gliomas (Venneti et al. 2015). This model has been very useful to address the role of several components of the TME and to uncover new therapeutic strategies for targeting cells in the glioma microenvironment such as the tumor associated macrophages and microglia (Pyonteck et al. 2013; Quail et al. 2016).

In the past years, an important role for *IDH1* and *IDH2* mutant genes in low-grade gliomas and a small subset of GBM with a better prognosis has been reported (Noushmehr et al. 2010; Yan et al. 2009; Ceccarelli et al. 2016; Eckel-Passow et al. 2015; Network 2015; TCGA Network 2015). A GEMM for conditional activation of a heterozygous floxed *Idh1^{R132H}* mutant allele using *Nestin-Cre* or *Gfap-Cre* failed to elicit gliomagenesis in the developing mouse brain (Sasaki et al. 2012) despite the production of D-2-hydroxyglutarate. This oncometabolite led to brain hemorrhage and embryonic lethality by blocking collagen maturation and altered vascular basementmembranes. Activation of the *Idh1^{R132H}* floxed allele in the adult brain has not been reported so far.

While none of the GEMMs described above completely phenocopies their respective human conditions, their combined value in the preclinical testing of new drugs and novel regimens remains obvious. In the past years, rational drug design has led to numerous small molecule inhibitors targeting many of the pathways involved in gliomagenesis. GEMMs offer a great opportunity to study their effects on their molecular targets and the consequences for tumorigenesis, to evaluate their toxicity and to formulate strategies to follow clinical course.

9.2.3   CRISPR/Cas9 Models

It has been progressively established that the vast majority of human cancers are extremely heterogeneous at a genetic level. To properly recapitulate this complexity, it is now clear that in vivo animal models will require to recreate not just a handful of genetic alterations, but possibly dozens. The growing level of sophistication in making gene knockouts using novel genome editing system has made it possible to target almost any candidate cancer gene in the in vivo setting. The CRISPR (Clustered Regularly Interspaced Short Palindromic repeats) – Cas (CRISPR-associated), is probably the most powerful genome editing technology that ever existed. Such a methodology has revolutionized research in many fields, including cancer animal modelling, by allowing specific manipulation of the genome of individual cells. Its applications span from the inactivation of tumor suppressor gene, to the generation of somatic point mutations and more complex genomic rearrangements. Although there are some concerns related to possible off-target effects, it is generally believed that the CIRSPR/Cas9 is sufficiently specific and is less likely prone to off-targets as compared to RNAi or shRNA techniques.

A possibly relevant caveat of CRISPR-based in vivo somatic genome editing is the requirement to concurrently deliver the guide RNA and the Cas9 enzyme to the specific tissue of interest. To deal with this issue, various groups recently generated transgenic mice expressing Cas9 in a Cre- or tetracycline- dependent manner (Platt et al. 2014; Chiou et al. 2015; Dow et al. 2015). Moving forward with the use of CRISPR/Cas9 in tumor modelling, the combination of somatic genome editing with the huge collection of currently available genetically engineered mouse models, previously discussed in this chapter, will provide the chance to introduce precise genetic lesions into specific cell types, leading to the development of novel and more accurate tumor models.

Since various recent reviews have described the basic concept and applications of CRISPR/Cas9 (for example see Heidenreich and Zhang 2015; Kannan and Ventura 2015; Sánchez-Rivera and Jacks 2015), here we will be focusing only on its relevance to glioma mouse models.

Due to the very recent advancement in the CRISPR/Cas9 technology, only two mouse models using this methodology brain tumorigenesis (Zuckermann et al. 2015; Chen et al. 2015) have been reported at the time of writing of this book.

To induce GBM tumors with the CRISPR/Cas9 system Zuckerman and collaborators applied *in utero* electroporation (IUE) of the forebrain of E13.5 mouse embryos. By transducing simultaneously three independent plasmids, encoding Cas9 in combination with gRNAs targeting *Nf1*, *Trp53* and *Pten*, they were able to induce highly aggressive tumours, resembling human GBMs. Using a very similar approach and the same combination of gRNAs targeting *Nf1*, *Trp53* and *Pten*, Chen and colleagues were also able to induce very aggressive tumors that had histopathological characteristic typical of human GBMs.

In our opinion there are at least two main issues with the use of IUE for glioma CRISPR/Cas9 modelling: timing of the gRNA delivery and lack of specificity of the targeted cells. Electroporation is normally performed at E14.5 or E15.5, and genetic alterations at this gestational stage might not be necessarily reflecting the biology of gliomas in the adult. The second issue is that the expression of the Cas9 enzyme from a constitutive promoter, as it has been used in both studies, does not allow genome editing in a cell-type-specific manner thus not restricting the genetic alteration to the putative cells of origin of gliomas.

To overcome such limitations, our laboratory is currently working in combining the extensively used RCAS/tv-a glioma model with the incredibly powerful CRISPR/Cas9 genome editing technology (unpublished).

9.3 Other Animal Models

9.3.1 *Drosophila*

During decades, lower-model organisms like *Drosophila melanogaster* have provided critical information regarding the role of numerous human cancer-related proteins and their spatiotemporal organization in molecular signalling pathway that are relevant for the human disease (Brumby and Richardson 2005). Drosophila strains that are engineered to recapitulate important features of certain forms of human cancer have been very useful to elucidate the tumorigenesis process and served as platforms for therapeutic drug discovery (Gonzalez 2013).

Most human genes, including major signal transduction pathways, have functional *Drosophila melanogaster* orthologue (Reiter and Bier 2002). Lately, drosophila arose as a model system for human neurological diseases because the CNS shows significant evolutionary conservation in cellular structure and neurodevelopmental pathways (Bilen and Bonini 2005).

Flies present various advantages as compared to more complex organisms, as the mouse: small size, simple husbandry, short generation time and highly prolific nature; thousands of mutants, and stock collections of approximately genome-wide double-stranded RNAs for RNA interference; high-resolution microscopy of living cells and organs. On the other hands they also have numerous limitations: fly strains cannot be kept frozen; lack of some tissue types and organs that are present in mammals (e.g. pancreas, liver, adipose tissue and blood); absence of adaptive immune response and open circulatory system (Gonzalez 2013). GEMMs and xenograft mouse models have not been extensively used to systematically screen for novel genes that contribute to GBM, mainly because forward functional genetic assays are very lengthy and expensive to perform in these systems. On the contrary, drosophila might represent a very resourceful genetic model system in which cell-type specific gene function can be controlled with single-cell precision in vivo in an intact complex nervous system (Read 2011).

Drosophila models of glioblastoma, have been recently developed in which glial progenitor cells give rise to proliferative and invasive neoplastic cells that create transplantable tumors in response to constitutive co-activation of the EGFR-Ras and PI3K signalling pathways and inactivation of the E2F/Rb pathway (Read 2011; Read et al. 2009; Witte et al. 2009). While only a handful of tumor drivers were used in drosophila models of GBM (e.g. *dEGFRλ* and *dp110^{CAAX}*), various key rate-limiting genes have been identified, such as *dCyclinE*, *Stg*, *dMyc*, and also genes only needed for abnormal neoplastic glial proliferation, such as *dSin1*, *dRictor*, *dCdk4*, *dRIOK1* and *dRIOK2* (Read et al. 2009; Read et al. 2013). Moreover, consistent with a high frequency of RB pathway mutations in human GBM, the loss of *Rbf1*, one of the two *RB* genes in flies, boosts tumor development in Drosophila.

An important potential application of a Drosophila cancer model is the identification and design of novel therapeutic molecules that target GBM signalling pathways. The fly model has numerous advantages for testing novel compounds: drugs can be directly fed to animals, tumors develop quickly, inhibition of neoplastic proliferation can be detected in live animals using fluorescence microscopy. Moreover, screening in live flies readily identify those compounds that are toxic to the animal or that cannot reach their targets due to lack of stability or because they cannot reach the organ of interest, a very important aspect at the preclinical stage (Gonzalez 2013).

Although fly-based models hold great potential for further depicting pathways involved in gliomagenesis, there might be an important biological difference to be taken into consideration. While the exact cell of origins of human GBM has not been clearly identified, through the use of mouse models, it has been shown that both neural stem cells and committed progenitor cells can be readily transformed. Possibly differently to the human pathology, in fly-based models, using lineage tracing and cell-type specific markers, tumorigenic glial cells were established to derive from committed glial progenitor cells, rather than from multipotent neuroblasts, which are fly neural stem cells (Read et al. 2009).

9.3.2   Zebrafish

While well established as a system for the study of developmental processes, the zebrafish (*Danio rerio*) is progressively becoming an accepted system for modelling human diseases including cancer. At the genomic level, orthologues of approximately 70% of human genes can be found in the zebrafish genome (Howe et al. 2013). At the molecular levels signalling pathways controlling embryonic development and anatomy are extensively conserved between zebrafish and humans (Santoriello and Zon 2012).

The unique research advantages that zebrafish offers for genetic studies includes high fecundity, the rapid generation of transparent embryos, the conservation of vertebrate organs, which allows comparison with humans, presence of blood circulation, lack of an adaptive immune system for the first 4–6 weeks, quite inexpensive maintenance costs and most significantly the flexibility to genome editing techniques and high throughput forward genetic screens (White et al. 2013; Shive 2013). Another important practicality of zebrafish models is that the aqueous environment facilitates drug as well as studies using ionizing radiation (immersion in water provides radiation dose homogeneity) (Geiger et al. 2008). Particularly, by combining drug discovery and animal testing, in vivo screening of small molecules in zebrafish has allowed fast translation of anti-cancer compounds to the clinic, mostly through the repurposing of FDA-approved drugs (Dang et al. 2016).

Zebrafish develop cancer spontaneously, after exposure to mutagenic compounds and also through genetic manipulations. Such tumors resemble human tumors at multiple levels: histological, gene expression and genomic (White et al. 2013). Zebrafish cancer models have been generated by multiple approaches: chemical carcinogenesis, forward and reverse genetics screens, transgenic models and xeno-transplantation in embryos (Shive 2013).

The first zebrafish brain cancer model was established through the combined deletion of the *nf1a/nf1b* (orthologs of human *NF1*) and *p53* tumor suppressor genes: heterozygous inactivation of *nf1a* and homozygous inactivation of *nf1b* in a *p53*-deficient background resulted in an accelerated onset and increased penetrance of high-grade gliomas and malignant peripheral nerve sheath tumors (MPNSTs) in adult zebrafish (Shin et al. 2012). Immunohistochemical analysis showed hyperac-tivation of MAPK and mTOR pathways in some of the brain tumors in *nf1* and *p53* null animals, consistent with mouse and human *NF1*-derived MPNSTs and gliomas.

Newer brain tumor models utilized the expression of oncogenes to disrupt the PI3K-AKT-mTOR and RAF-MEK-ERK signalling pathways, which leads to the development of glioma. Transgenic zebrafish overexpressing a dominant-active form of Akt (DAAkt1) in the hindbrain developed at a high frequency glioma of varying histological grades within the cerebellum (Jung et al. 2013). While expres-sion of *darac1*, a dominant active mutant of RAC1, was not sufficient to induce tumor by itself, it did greatly accelerate DAAkt1-induced tumorigenesis. The co-expression of *darac1* not only boosted tumor incidence but also increased histologic grade and invasiveness (Jung et al. 2013), underlying the cooperativity between the two signalling pathways.

Most recently, transient transgenic expression of oncogenic *kras*(G12V) in neu-ral within the head region (Ju et al. 2015). Histological analyses revealed that only 20% of the tumors presented histopathological features consistent with glioma and were located in the ventricular zone, while the majority were MPNSTs in the cranial cavity. However, expressing *kras*(G12V) by the *gfap* promoter led to an increased frequency of high-grade gliomas in both VZs and brain parenchyma.

Until recently the inadequate reverse genetic techniques available for use in zebrafish have limited its use to generate genetic models for brain and CNS cancer. However, the highly powerful targeted nuclease methods including transcription activator-like effector nucleases (TALENs) and the CRISPR/Cas9 system have also been recently established in zebrafish and will be extremely useful to develop the next generation zebrafish cancer models (Yen et al. 2014).

Taking advantage of the lack of an adaptive immune system in the early zebrafish developmental phases, in parallel to the genetic models, zebrafish embryos xenografted with human glioblastoma cell lines have been recently used in a variety of studies (Geiger et al. 2008; Yang et al. 2013; Wehmas et al. 2016; Welker et al. 2015). These reports provide a noteworthy technique that goes past what is nor-mally feasible in mouse xenografts since they let for comprehensive, three-dimensional analysis of single cells within an engrafted tumor (White et al. 2013). Moreover, due to the microscopic size of the embryo recipients, thousands of recipi-ents can be used at a time, allowing high-throughput drug screening approaches.

9.3.3 Canine

Dogs are important spontaneous models of human complex disorders including cancers. Besides the benefits of working with large animal models, dogs and human cancers share both genetic and environmental factors. Although, avian sarcoma virus (ASV)-induced and allogeneic transplanted canine brain tumor models were developed in the past (Britt et al. 1985; Warnke et al. 1995; Berens et al. 1999), the ethics of these procedures were brought into question and lately researchers have been focusing mostly on naturally occurring tumor models.

Spontaneous gliomas in dogs exhibit similar pathological subtypes, molecular alterations and neuroimaging characteristics to their human counterparts and are usually classified and graded using the human WHO criteria. While the frequency of certain glioma subtypes varies between humans and dogs, with dogs having more high-grade oligodendrogliomas and humans having more GBMs (Dickinson 2014), some recent studies showed that similar signalling pathway alterations are also present in dogs (Boudreau et al. 2015).

The size and structure of the dog's brain, histopathology and molecular appearances of canine brain tumours, together with an intact immune system, are encouraging characteristics for the potential success of a canine model (Hicks et al. 2015). Moreover, some brachycephalic dog breeds, such as Boxer, Bulldog and Boston Terrier have a substantially increased risk of glioma (Song et al. 2013), making the dog an appropriate model also for identifying genes possibly important for the development of human glioma. Indeed, a recent genome wide association study (GWAS), in dogs of a variety of breeds, identified three candidate genes (*DENR, CAMKK2* and *P2RX7),* possibly representing potential glioma susceptibility genes in humans (Truvé et al. 2016).

Numerous small-scale pre-clinical treatment trials (e.g. immunotherapy, gene therapy, convection-enhanced delivery (CED) and cell-encapsulated anti-angiogenic therapy) have employed the dog as a spontaneous model providing significant information for both human and veterinary medicine (Hicks et al. 2015). However, progression of naturally occurring cancer in dogs, though faster than in humans, is much slower than most small animal models, limiting its application in the translational settings.

9.4   Future Perspective

The use of animal models is absolutely indispensable to better understand the biology of any complex disease like cancer. Animal research has played a fundamental role in virtually every medical breakthrough over the last few decades. However, there is not such thing as a "perfect animal model", all of them present caveats and pitfalls. In particular for what concerns the development of novel therapeutic approaches, as said by Thomas Hartung, director of the Center for Alternatives to Animal Testing at the Johns Hopkins Bloomberg School of Public Health in Baltimore, the ideal model simply doesn't exist: "*If there was an animal model good enough to substitute for people, we would not have a 92% failure rate in clinical trials*" (Dolgin 2013).

Despite decades of research, the approved drugs armamentarium against GBM remains limited. The scientific community will have to work together in order to better refine the current available models to integrate the comprehensive genomic characterization and novel GBM classification. We firmly believe that the novel genome editing technologies, such as the CRISPR/Cas9, will play an essential role in the development of the next-generation models of human cancer.

Acknowledgement We are very grateful to the Seve Ballesteros Foundation for the generous support of our laboratory.

Bibliography

Ahmed, B.Y., et al. 2004. Efficient delivery of Cre-recombinase to neurons in vivo and stable transduction of neurons using adeno-associated and lentiviral vectors. *BMC Neuroscience* 5: 4.

Alcantara Llaguno, S.R., et al. 2015. Adult lineage-restricted CNS progenitors specify distinct glioblastoma subtypes. *Cancer Cell* 28 (4): 429–440.

Antunes, L., et al. 2000. Analysis of tissue chimerism in nude mouse brain and abdominal xenograft models of human glioblastoma multiforme: What does it tell us about the models and about glioblastoma biology and therapy? *Journal of Histochemistry & Cytochemistry* 48 (6): 847–858.

Aparicio, S., M. Hidalgo, and A.L. Kung. 2015. Examining the utility of patient-derived xenograft mouse models. *Nature Reviews Cancer* 15 (5): 311–316.

Bajenaru, M.L., et al. 2003. Optic nerve glioma in mice requires astrocyte Nf1 gene inactivation and Nf1 brain heterozygosity. *Cancer Research* 63 (24): 8573–8577.

Bajenaru, M.L., et al. 2005. Natural history of neurofibromatosis 1-associated optic nerve glioma in mice. *Annals of Neurology* 57 (1): 119–127.

van den Bent, M.J. 2010. Interobserver variation of the histopathological diagnosis in clinical trials on glioma: A clinician's perspective. *Acta Neuropathologica* 120 (3): 297–304.

Berens, M.E., et al. 1999. Allogeneic astrocytoma in immune competent dogs. *Neoplasia (New York, N.Y.)* 1 (2): 107–112.

Biedermann, K.A., et al. 1991. scid mutation in mice confers hypersensitivity to ionizing radiation and a deficiency in DNA double-strand break repair. *Proceedings of the National Academy of Sciences of the United States of America* 88 (4): 1394–1397.

Bilen, J., and N.M. Bonini. 2005. Drosophila as a model for human neurodegenerative disease. *Annual Review of Genetics* 39: 153–171.

Birling, M.C., F. Gofflot, and X. Warot. 2009. Site-specific recombinases for manipulation of the mouse genome. *Methods in Molecular Biology* 561: 245–263.

Bjerkvig, R., et al. 1990. Multicellular tumor spheroids from human gliomas maintained in organ culture. *Journal of Neurosurgery* 72 (Table 1): 463–475.

Boudreau, C.E., et al. 2015. Molecular signalling pathways in canine gliomas. *Veterinary and Comparative Oncology* 15: 133–150.

Brennan, C.W., et al. 2013. The somatic genomic landscape of glioblastoma. *Cell* 155 (2): 462–477.

Brinster, R.L., et al. 1984. Transgenic mice harboring SV40 t-antigen genes develop characteristic brain tumors. *Cell* 37 (2): 367–379.

Britt, R.H., et al. 1985. Immunohistochemical study of glial fibrillary acidic protein in avian sarcoma virus-induced gliomas in dogs. *Journal of Neuro-Oncology* 3 (1): 53–59.

Brumby, A.M., and H.E. Richardson. 2005. Using Drosophila melanogaster to map human cancer pathways. *Nature Reviews Cancer* 5 (8): 626–639.

Camphausen, K., B. Purow, M. Sproull, T. Scott, T. Ozawa, D.F. Deen, et al. 2005a. Influence of in vivo growth on human glioma cell line gene expression: Convergent profiles under orthotopic conditions. *Proceedings of the National Academy of Sciences of the United States of America* 102 (23): 8287–8292.

————. 2005b. Orthotopic growth of human glioma cells quantitatively and qualitatively influ- ences radiation-induced changes in gene expression. *Cancer Research* 65 (22): 10389–10393.

Candolfi, M., et al. 2007. Intracranial glioblastoma models in preclinical neuro-oncology: Neuropathological characterization and tumor progression. *Journal of Neuro-Oncology* 85 (2): 133–148.

Ceccarelli, M., et al. 2016. Molecular profiling reveals biologically discrete subsets and pathways of progression in diffuse glioma. *Cell* 164 (3): 550–563.

Chandras, C., et al. 2012. CreZOO-The European virtual repository of Cre and other targeted conditional driver strains. *Database* 2012: 1–5.

Charest, A., et al. 2006. ROS fusion tyrosine kinase activates a SH2 domain-containing phospha- tase-2/phosphatidylinositol 3-kinase/mammalian target of rapamycin signaling axis to form glioblastoma in mice. *Cancer Research* 66 (15): 7473–7481.

Chen, J., R.M. McKay, and L.F. Parada. 2012. Malignant glioma: Lessons from genomics, mouse models, and stem cells. *Cell* 149 (1): 36–47.

Chen, F., et al. 2015. Tracking and transforming neocortical progenitors by CRISPR/Cas9 gene targeting and PiggyBac transposase lineage labeling. *Development* 142: 3601–3611.

Chiou, S.-H., et al. 2015. Pancreatic cancer modeling using retrograde viral vector delivery and in vivo CRISPR/Cas9-mediated somatic genome editing. *Genes & Development* 29 (14): 1576–1585.

Cook, N., D.I. Jodrell, and D.A. Tuveson. 2012. Predictive in vivo animal models and translation to clinical trials. *Drug Discovery Today* 17 (5–6): 253–260.

Dai, C., et al. 2001. PDGF autocrine stimulation dedifferentiates cultured astrocytes and induces oligodendrogliomas from and oligoastrocytomas neural progenitors and astrocytes in vivo. *Genes and Development* 15 (15): 1913–1925.

Dang, M., R. Fogley, and L.I. Zon. 2016. Identifying novel cancer therapies using chemical genet- ics and zebrafish. *Advances in Experimental Medicine and Biology* 916: 103–124.

Danks, R.A., et al. 1995. Transformation of astrocytes in transgenic mice expressing SV40 T anti- gen under the transcriptional control of the glial fibrillary acidic protein promoter. *Cancer Research* 55 (19): 4302–4310.

Dickinson, P.J. 2014. Advances in diagnostic and treatment modalities for intracranial tumors. *Journal of Veterinary Internal Medicine* 28 (4): 1165–1185.

Ding, H., et al. 2001. Astrocyte-specific expression of activated p21-ras results in malignant astro- cytoma formation in a transgenic mouse model of human gliomas. *Cancer Research* 61 (9): 3826–3836.

Ding, H., et al. 2003. Oligodendrogliomas result from the expression of an activated mutant epi- dermal growth factor receptor in a RAS transgenic mouse astrocytoma model. *Cancer Research* 63 (5): 1106–1113.

Dolgin, E. 2013. Animal rule for drug approval creates a jungle of confusion. *Nature Medicine* 19 (2): 118–119.

Dow, L.E., et al. 2015. Inducible in vivo genome editing with CRISPR-Cas9. *Nature Biotechnology* 33 (4): 390–394.

Eckel-Passow, J.E., et al. 2015. Glioma groups based on 1p/19q, IDH, and TERT promoter muta- tions in tumors. *The New England Journal of Medicine* 372 (26): 2499–2508.

Federspiel, M.J., et al. 1994. A system for tissue-specific gene targeting: Transgenic mice suscep- tible to subgroup A avian leukosis virus-based retroviral vectors. *Proceedings of the National Academy of Sciences of the United States of America* 91 (23): 11241–11245.

Fei, X.F., et al. 2010. Development of clinically relevant orthotopic xenograft mouse model of metastatic lung cancer and glioblastoma through surgical tumor tissues injection with trocar. *Journal of Experimental & Clinical Cancer Research : CR* 29 (1): 84.

Feil, R., et al. 1996. Ligand-activated site-specific recombination in mice. *Proceedings of the National Academy of Sciences of the United States of America* 93 (20): 10887–10890.

Fomchenko, E.I., and E.C. Holland. 2006. Mouse models of brain tumors and their applications in preclinical trials. *Clinical Cancer Research* 12 (18): 5288–5297.

Fomchenko, E.I., et al. 2011. Recruited cells can become transformed and overtake PDGF-induced murine gliomas in vivo during tumor progression. *PLoS One* 6 (7): e20605.

Frese, K.K., and D.A. Tuveson. 2007. Maximizing mouse cancer models. *Nature Reviews Cancer* 7 (9): 654–658.

Geiger, G.A., W. Fu, and G.D. Kao. 2008. Temozolomide-mediated radiosensitization of human glioma cells in a zebrafish embryonic system. *Cancer Research* 68 (9): 3396–3404.

Gierut, J.J., T.E. Jacks, and K.M. Haigis. 2014. Producing and concentrating lenti-cre for mouse infections. *Cold Spring Harbor Protocols* 2014 (3): 304–306.

Gonzalez, C. 2013. Drosophila melanogaster: A model and a tool to investigate malignancy and identify new therapeutics. *Nature Reviews Cancer* 13 (3): 172–183.

Greenhouse, J.J., et al. 1988. Helper-independent retrovirus vectors with Rous-associated virus type O long terminal repeats. *Journal of Virology* 62 (12): 4809–4812.

Guha, A. 1998. Ras activation in astrocytomas and neurofibromas. *The Canadian Journal of Neurological Sciences* 25 (4): 267–281.

Günther, H.S., et al. 2008. Glioblastoma-derived stem cell-enriched cultures form distinct subgroups according to molecular and phenotypic criteria. *Oncogene* 27: 2897–2909.

Hambardzumyan, D., et al. 2009. Modeling adult gliomas using RCAS/t-va technology. *Translational Oncology* 2 (2): 89–95.

———. 2011. Genetic modeling of gliomas in mice: New tools to tackle old problems. *Glia* 59 (8): 1155–1168.

Hede, S.M., et al. 2009. GFAP promoter driven transgenic expression of PDGFB in the mouse brain leads to glioblastoma in a Trp53 null background. *Glia* 57 (11): 1143–1153.

Heidenreich, M., and F. Zhang. 2015. Applications of CRISPR–Cas systems in neuroscience. *Nature Reviews Neuroscience* 17 (1): 36–44.

Henson, J.W., et al. 1994. The retinoblastoma gene is involved in malignant progression of astrocytomas. *Annals of Neurology* 36 (5): 714–721.

Hicks, J., et al. 2015. Canine brain tumours: A model for the human disease? *Veterinary and comparative oncology* 15: 252–272.

Hitoshi, Y., et al. 2008. Spinal glioma: Platelet-derived growth factor B-mediated oncogenesis in the spinal cord. *Cancer Research* 68 (20): 8507–8515.

Holland, E.C., and H.E. Varmus. 1998. Basic fibroblast growth factor induces cell migration and proliferation after glia-specific gene transfer in mice. *Proceedings of the National Academy of Sciences of the United States of America* 95 (3): 1218–1223.

Holland, E.C., et al. 1998. A constitutively active epidermal growth factor receptor cooperates with disruption of G1 cell-cycle arrest pathways to induce glioma-like lesions in mice. *Genes and Development* 12 (23): 3675–3685.

———. 2000. Combined activation of Ras and Akt in neural progenitors induces glioblastoma formation in mice. *Nature Genetics* 25 (1): 55–57.

Howe, K., et al. 2013. The zebrafish reference genome sequence and its relationship to the human genome. *Nature* 496 (7446): 498–503.

Hu, X., et al. 2005. mTOR promotes survival and astrocytic characteristics induced by Pten/AKT signaling in glioblastoma. *Neoplasia (New York, N.Y.)* 7 (4): 356–368.

Huse, J.T., and E.C. Holland. 2009. Genetically engineered mouse models of brain cancer and the promise of preclinical testing. *Brain Pathology* 19 (1): 132–143.

Huszthy, P.C., et al. 2012. In vivo models of primary brain tumors: Pitfalls and perspectives. *Neuro-Oncology* 14 (8): 979–993.

Joo, K.M., et al. 2013. Patient-specific orthotopic glioblastoma xenograft models recapitulate the histopathology and biology of human glioblastomas in situ. *Cell Reports* 3 (1): 260–273.

Ju, B., et al. 2015. Oncogenic KRAS promotes malignant brain tumors in zebrafish. *Molecular Cancer* 14 (1): 1–11.

Jue, T.R., and K.L. McDonald. 2016. The challenges associated with molecular targeted therapies for glioblastoma. *Journal of Neuro-Oncology* 127 (3): 427–434.

Jung, I.H., et al. 2013. Glioma is formed by active Akt1 alone and promoted by active Rac1 in transgenic zebrafish. *Neuro-Oncology* 15 (3): 290–304.

Kannan, R., and A. Ventura. 2015. The CRISPR revolution and its impact on cancer research. *Swiss Medical Weekly* 145: w14230.

Kühn, R., et al. 1995. Inducible gene targeting in mice. *Science (New York, N.Y.)* 269 (5229): 1427–1429.

Kwon, C.H., et al. 2008. Pten haploinsufficiency accelerates formation of high-grade astrocytomas. *Cancer Research* 68 (9): 3286–3294.

Laks, D.R., et al. 2009. Neurosphere formation is an independent predictor of clinical outcome in malignant glioma. *Stem Cells* 27 (4): 980–987.

Lakso, M., et al. 1992. Targeted oncogene activation by site-specific recombination in transgenic mice. *Proceedings of the National Academy of Sciences of the United States of America* 89 (14): 6232–6236.

Leder, K., et al. 2014. Mathematical modeling of pdgf-driven glioblastoma reveals optimized radiation dosing schedules. *Cell* 156 (3): 603–616.

Lee, J., et al. 2006. Tumor stem cells derived from glioblastomas cultured in bFGF and EGF more closely mirror the phenotype and genotype of primary tumors than do serum-cultured cell lines. *Cancer Cell* 9 (5): 391–403.

Lindberg, N., et al. 2014. Oncogenic signaling is dominant to cell of origin and dictates astrocytic or oligodendroglial tumor development from oligodendrocyte precursor cells. *The Journal of Neuroscience : The Official Journal of the Society for Neuroscience* 34 (44): 14644–14651.

Louis, D.N., et al. 2016a. The 2016 World Health Organization classification of tumors of the central nervous system: A summary. *Acta Neuropathologica* 131 (6): 803–820.

Louis, D.N., H. Ohgaki, O.D. Wiestler, and W.K. Cavenee. 2016b. *WHO classification of tumours of the central nervous system*. 4th ed. Lyon: International Agency For Research On Cancer.

Macleod, K.F., and T. Jacks. 1999. Insights into cancer from transgenic mouse models. *Journal of Pathology* 187 (1): 43–60.

Marumoto, T., et al. 2009. Development of a novel mouse glioma model using lentiviral vectors. *Nature Medicine* 15 (1): 110–116.

McNeill, R.S., et al. 2015. Contemporary murine models in preclinical astrocytoma drug development. *Neuro-Oncology* 17 (1): 12–28.

Morgan, R.A. 2012. Human tumor xenografts: The good, the bad, and the ugly. *Molecular Therapy* 20 (5): 882–884.

Noushmehr, H., et al. 2010. Identification of a CpG island methylator phenotype that defines a distinct subgroup of glioma. *Cancer Cell* 17 (5): 510–522.

Ohgaki, H., and P. Kleihues. 2013. The definition of primary and secondary glioblastoma. *Clinical Cancer Research : An Official Journal of the American Association for Cancer Research* 19 (4): 764–772.

Ozawa, T., et al. 2014. Article most human non-GCIMP glioblastoma subtypes evolve from a common proneural-like precursor glioma. *Cancer Cell* 26 (2): 288–300.

Parsons, D.W., et al. 2008. An integrated genomic analysis of human glioblastoma multiforme. *Science* 321 (5897): 1807–1812.

Platt, R.J., et al. 2014. CRISPR-Cas9 knockin mice for genome editing and cancer modeling. *Cell* 159 (2): 440–455.

Pyonteck, S.M., et al. 2013. CSF-1R inhibition alters macrophage polarization and blocks glioma progression. *Nature Medicine* 19: 1–12.

Quail, D.F., et al. 2016. The tumor microenvironment underlies acquired resistance to CSF-1R inhibition in gliomas. *Science* 352 (6288): aad3018.

Ramaswamy, V., and M.D. Taylor. 2016. Fall of the optical wall: Freedom from the tyranny of the microscope improves glioma risk stratification. *Cancer cell* 29 (2): 137–138.

Read, R.D. 2011. Drosophila melanogaster as a model system for human brain cancers. *Glia* 59 (9): 1364–1376.

Read, R.D., et al. 2009. A drosophila model for EGFR-Ras and PI3K-dependent human glioma. *PLoS Genetics* 5 (2): e1000374.

———. 2013. A kinome-wide RNAi screen in Drosophila Glia reveals that the RIO kinases mediate cell proliferation and survival through TORC2-Akt signaling in glioblastoma. *PLoS Genetics* 9 (2): e1003253.

Reilly, K.M., et al. 2000. Nf1;Trp53 mutant mice develop glioblastoma with evidence of strain-specific effects. *Nature Genetics* 26 (1): 109–113.

Reiter, L.T., and E. Bier. 2002. Using Drosophila melanogaster to uncover human disease gene function and potential drug target proteins. *Expert Opinion on Therapeutic Targets* 6 (3): 387–399.

Robertson, G., et al. 1995. Position-dependent variegation of globin transgene expression in mice. *Proceedings of the National Academy of Sciences of the United States of America* 92 (12): 5371–5375.

Sakariassen, P.Ø., et al. 2006. Angiogenesis-independent tumor growth mediated by stem-like cancer cells. *PNAS* 103 (44): 16466–16471.

Sánchez-Rivera, F.J., and T. Jacks. 2015. Applications of the CRISPR–Cas9 system in cancer biology. *Nature Reviews Cancer* 15 (7): 387–395.

Santoriello, C., and L.I. Zon. 2012. Hooked! Modeling human disease in zebrafish. *The Journal of Clinical Investigation* 122 (7): 2337–2343.

Sasaki, M., et al. 2012. D-2-hydroxyglutarate produced by mutant Idh1 perturbs collagen maturation and basement membrane function. *Genes and Development* 26 (18): 2038–2049.

Schmid, R.S., M. Vitucci, and C.R. Miller. 2012. Genetically engineered mouse models of diffuse gliomas. *Brain Research Bulletin* 88 (1): 72–79.

Schönig, K., et al. 2002. Stringent doxycycline dependent control of CRE recombinase in vivo. *Nucleic Acids Research* 30 (23): e134.

Shih, A.H., et al. 2004. Dose-dependent effects of platelet-derived growth factor-B on glial tumorigenesis. *Cancer Research* 64 (14): 4783–4789.

Shin, J., et al. 2012. Zebrafish neurofibromatosis type 1 genes have redundant functions in tumorigenesis and embryonic development. *Disease Models & Mechanisms* 5 (6): 881–894.

Shive, H.R. 2013. Zebrafish models for human cancer. *Veterinary Pathology* 50 (3): 468–482.

Shultz, L.D., F. Ishikawa, and D.L. Greiner. 2007. Humanized mice in translational biomedical research. *Nature reviews Immunology* 7 (2): 118–130.

Smedley, D., E. Salimova, and N. Rosenthal. 2011. Cre recombinase resources for conditional mouse mutagenesis. *Methods* 53 (4): 411–416.

Song, R.B., et al. 2013. Postmortem evaluation of 435 cases of intracranial neoplasia in dogs and relationship of neoplasm with breed, age, and body weight. *Journal of Veterinary Internal Medicine / American College of Veterinary Internal Medicine* 27 (5): 1143–1152.

Squatrito, M., et al. 2010. Loss of ATM/Chk2/p53 pathway components accelerates tumor development and contributes to radiation resistance in gliomas. *Cancer Cell* 18 (6): 619–629.

Squatrito, M., and E.C. Holland. 2011. DNA damage response and growth factor signaling pathways in gliomagenesis and therapeutic resistance. *Cancer Research* 71 (18): 5945–5949.

Stupp, R., et al. 2005. Radiotherapy plus concomitant and adjuvant temozolomide for glioblastoma. *The New England Journal of Medicine* 352 (10): 987–996.

———. 2009. Effects of radiotherapy with concomitant and adjuvant temozolomide versus radiotherapy alone on survival in glioblastoma in a randomised phase III study: 5-year analysis of the EORTC-NCIC trial. *The Lancet Oncology* 10 (5): 459–466.

Taillandier, L., L. Antunes, and K.S. Angioi-Duprez. 2003. Models for neuro-oncological preclinical studies: Solid orthotopic and heterotopic grafts of human gliomas into nude mice. *Journal of Neuroscience Methods* 125 (1–2): 147–157.

Talmadge, J.E., et al. 2007. Murine models to evaluate novel and conventional therapeutic strategies for cancer. *The American Journal of Pathology* 170 (3): 793–804.

Network, T.C.G.A. 2008. Comprehensive genomic characterization defines human glioblastoma genes and core pathways. *Nature* 455 (7216): 1061–1068.

———. 2015. Comprehensive, integrative genomic analysis of diffuse lower-grade gliomas. *The New England Journal of Medicine* 372 (26): 2481–2498.

Theeler, B.J., and M.R. Gilbert. 2015. Advances in the treatment of newly diagnosed glioblastoma. *BMC Medicine* 13: 293.

Truvé, K., et al. 2016. Utilizing the dog genome in the search for novel candidate genes involved in glioma development-genome wide association mapping followed by targeted massive parallel sequencing identifies a strongly associated locus. *PLoS Genetics* 12 (5): e1006000.

Ueki, K., et al. 1996. CDKN2/p16 or RB alterations occur in the majority of glioblastomas and are inversely correlated. *Cancer Research* 56 (1): 150–153.

Uhrbom, L., et al. 1998. Induction of brain tumors in mice using a recombinant platelet-derived growth factor B-chain retrovirus. *Cancer Research* 58 (23): 5275–5279.

———. 2002. Ink4a-Arf loss cooperates with KRas activation in astrocytes and neural progenitors to generate glioblastomas of various morphologies depending on activated Akt. *Cancer Research* 62 (19): 5551–5558.

Venneti, S., et al. 2015. Glutamine-based PET imaging facilitates enhanced metabolic evaluation of gliomas in vivo. *Science Translational Medicine* 7 (274): 274ra17.

Verhaak, R.G.W., et al. 2010. Integrated genomic analysis identifies clinically relevant subtypes of glioblastoma characterized by abnormalities in PDGFRA, IDH1, EGFR, and NF1. *Cancer Cell* 17 (1): 98–110.

Voskoglou-Nomikos, T., J.L. Pater, and L. Seymour. 2003. Clinical predictive value of the in vitro cell line, human xenograft, and mouse allograft preclinical cancer models. *Clinical Cancer Research : An Official Journal of the American Association for Cancer Research* 9 (11): 4227–4239.

de Vries, N.A., J.H. Beijnen, and O. van Tellingen. 2009. High-grade glioma mouse models and their applicability for preclinical testing. *Cancer Treatment Reviews* 35 (8): 714–723.

Wang, J., et al. 2009. A reproducible brain tumour model established from human glioblastoma biopsics. *BMC Cancer* 9: 465.

Warnke, P.C., et al. 1995. The effects of dexamethasone on transcapillary transport in experimental brain tumors: II. Canine brain tumors. *Journal of Neuro-Oncology* 25 (1): 29–38.

Wehmas, L.C., et al. 2016. Developing a novel embryo-larval zebrafish xenograft assay to prioritize human glioblastoma therapeutics. *Zebrafish* 13: 317–329.

Wei, Q., et al. 2006. High-grade glioma formation results from postnatal Pten loss or mutant epidermal growth factor receptor expression in a transgenic mouse glioma model. *Cancer Research* 66 (15): 7429–7437.

Weiss, B., and K. Shannon. 2003. Mouse cancer models as a platform for performing preclinical therapeutic trials. *Current Opinion in Genetics and Development* 13 (1): 84–89.

Weiss, W.A., et al. 2003. Genetic determinants of malignancy in a mouse model for oligodendroglioma. *Cancer Research* 63 (7): 1589–1595.

Weissenberger, J., et al. 1997. Development and malignant progression of astrocytomas in GFAP-v- src transgenic mice. *Oncogene* 14 (17): 2005–2013.

Welker, A.M., et al. 2015. Standardized orthotopic xenografts in zebrafish reveal glioma cell line specific characteristics and tumor cell heterogeneity. *Disease Models & Mechanisms* 9: 199–210.

White, R., K. Rose, and L. Zon. 2013. Zebrafish cancer: The state of the art and the path forward. *Nature reviews Cancer* 13 (9): 624–636.

Witte, H.T., et al. 2009. Modeling glioma growth and invasion in Drosophila melanogaster. *Neoplasia (New York, N.Y.)* 11 (9): 882–888.

Xiao, A., et al. 2002. Astrocyte inactivation of the pRb pathway predisposes mice to malignant astrocytoma development that is accelerated by PTEN mutation. *Cancer Cell* 1 (2): 157–168.

———. 2005. Somatic induction of Pten loss in a preclinical astrocytoma model reveals major roles in disease progression and avenues for target discovery and validation. *Cancer Research* 65 (12): 5172–5180.

Xie, Y., et al. 2015. The human glioblastoma cell culture resource: Validated cell models representing all molecular subtypes. *eBioMedicine* 2 (10): 1351–1363.

Yan, H., et al. 2009. IDH1 and IDH2 mutations in gliomas. *The New England Journal of Medicine* 360 (8): 765–773.

Yang, X.J., et al. 2013. A novel zebrafish xenotransplantation model for study of glioma stem cell invasion. *PLoS One* 8 (4): 1–9.

Yen, J., R.M. White, and D.L. Stemple. 2014. Zebrafish models of cancer: Progress and future challenges. *Current Opinion in Genetics & Development* 24: 38–45.

Zhang, X., et al. 2013. A renewable tissue resource of phenotypically stable, biologically and ethnically diverse, patient-derived human breast cancer xenograft models. *Cancer Research* 73 (15): 4885–4897.

Zhu, Y., et al. 2005. Early inactivation of p53 tumor suppressor gene cooperating with NF1 loss induces malignant astrocytoma. *Cancer Cell* 8 (2): 119–130.

Zuckermann, M., et al. 2015. Somatic CRISPR/Cas9-mediated tumour suppressor disruption enables versatile brain tumour modelling. *Nature Communications* 6: 7391.

Chapter 10
Pediatric High Grade Glioma

Chitra Sarkar, Suvendu Purkait, Pankaj Pathak, and Prerana Jha

Abstract Pediatric high grade gliomas (phGGs) constitute about 20% of childhood gliomas and show poor survival. The underlying molecular pathogenesis of phGGs is significantly distinct from histologically similar adult GBMs. Frequent driver mutations within chromatin remodeling genes histone H3.1-H3.3 (K27M-G34R/V)-ATRX-DAXX, in addition to alterations in ACVR1, SETD2, FGFR1, BRAF, PDGFRA, NTRK, MYCN, MYC and TP53 genes play a central role in the phGG pathogenesis. Genome-wide methylation data of pediatric GBM (pGBM) has shown four biologically distinct subgroups, associated with enrichment for mutations (K27 and G34), PDGFRA-amplification, and/or mesenchymal gene expression signatures. pGBMs show rare IDH1-mutation/G-CIMP (Glioma-CpG-Island Methylator Phenotype) and are associated with reactive oxygen species production. Genome-wide miRNA profile of phGGs has shown a set of uniquely expressed miRNAs distinct from adult GBMs which target PDGFR-b pathway. Functional consequences of histone H3.3 mutation in phGGs show reprogramming of H3K27 methylation in conjunction with EZH2 over a set of biologically significant genes leading to tumorigenesis. A major loss of expression of global histone trimethylation (H3K-27/−9/−4) code has also been shown in pGBMs.

C. Sarkar, MD, FRC (Path) (✉)
Department of Pathology, All India Institute of Medical Sciences, New Delhi, India, 110029
e-mail: sarkar.chitra@gmail.com

S. Purkait, MD
Department of Pathology and Laboratory Medicine, All India Institute of Medical Sciences, Bhubaneswar, India, 751019
e-mail: dr.suvendu.mch@gmail.com

P. Pathak, PhD
Department of Pathology, All India Institute of Medical Sciences, New Delhi, India, 110029
e-mail: pankgem@gmail.com

P. Jha, PhD
Division of Neuro-oncology, The Ohio State University Comprehensive Cancer Center, Columbus, OH, USA, 43210
e-mail: praiims25@gmail.com

© Springer International Publishing AG 2017
K. Somasundaram (ed.), *Advances in Biology and Treatment of Glioblastoma,*
Current Cancer Research, DOI 10.1007/978-3-319-56820-1_10

Patients with H3F3A-G34R/V shown better overall survival compared with H3F3A-wild type and -K27M. However H3F3A-K27M show poorest prognosis in pHGGs. Clinical trial designs should now focus on distinct molecular subgrouping in pHGGs and stratify patients applying markers associated with specific subgroup. Targeting chromatin modifiers, central to pHGG pathogenesis offers a rational way to develop highly selective treatment strategies.

Keywords Pediatric glioblastoma • Diffuse intrinsic pontine glioma • Diffuse midline glioma H3K27M–mutant • H3F3A • HIST1H3B • ATRX • Histone methylation • Glioma • CNS tumor

10.1   Introduction

Central nervous system (CNS) tumors are the most prevalent solid tumor of childhood, of which gliomas are the commonest. Low grade gliomas comprise the largest fraction of pediatric glial tumors and are associated with better prognosis; however, about 15%–20% of pediatric gliomas are high grade with poor outcome (Baker et al. 2016). High grade gliomas (HGGs) in pediatric age group are infrequent as compared to adults, and comprise a heterogeneous group of WHO grade III and IV tumors, similar to their adult counterpart. Thus among pediatric high grade gliomas (pHGGs), most common are glioblastoma which mainly occur in supratentorial locations and diffuse intrinsic pontine gliomas (DIPG) which are exclusively located in the brainstem and constitute approximately 10% of all pediatric CNS tumors (Donaldson et al. 2006). Both these tumors are very invasive in nature, therefore respond poorly to even most aggressive treatments and show dismal prognosis and generally poor clinical outcome. In general, these tumors show a two-year survival outcome of less than 20% and are one of the most aggressive human cancers with limited therapeutic options (Gottardo and Gajjar 2008). Recently, in 2016 update of the WHO classification of CNS tumors, a new entity viz. diffuse midline glioma, H3 K27M–mutant has been defined- characterised by midline location (thalamus, brain stem, and spinal cord), K27M mutation in the histone H3.1/3.3 (H3F3A and HIST1H3B gene) and a diffuse growth pattern (Louis et al. 2016; Castel et al. 2015).

Majority of adult GBMs (~95%) develop *de novo* (Primary GBM), but approximately 5% also arise from lower-grade diffuse astrocytoma (WHO grade II) and anaplastic astrocytoma (WHO grade III) (Secondary GBM). Unlike adults, progression from a lower-grade glioma is rarely seen in pediatric GBMs (pGBMs), as these arise almost exclusively *de novo* (Sturm et al. 2012).

Histologically, pHGGs are indistinguishable from adult GBMs. Recent advancement in high throughput genomic analyses has unfolded the different layers of genetic and epigenetic alterations that distinguish pediatric and adult gliomagenesis. Various studies using next generation sequencing have shown that pGBMs have unique pattern of genetic alterations, gene expression, DNA methylation profile and miRNA expression, distinct from their adult counterparts (Sturm et al. 2012; Schwartzentruber et al. 2012; Wu et al. 2012; Jha et al. 2015). These findings have brought about a tectonic shift in understanding of pHGG biology and integration of this information has contributed to reclassification of these tumors beyond histological characterisation to different molecular subgroups. These subgroups differ distinctly in terms of cell of origin, clinical features viz. age at presentation, anatomical location of tumor and prognostic outcome as well as response to therapeutic targets (Northcott et al. 2015; Jones and Baker 2014; Northcott et al. 2012; Pajtler et al. 2015; Sturm et al. 2014a; Taylor et al. 2012). Prior studies have also suggested that fundamental biological differences exist between pediatric and adult HGGs, with each responding in different manner to similar therapies (Jones et al. 2012a; Paugh et al. 2010). Hence, pGBMs should be considered as a distinct clinicopathological entity separate from adults as they have fundamental genetic and epigenetic differences. Therefore, it is now imperative to think about clinical management of pHGGs beyond therapeutic strategies developed primarily based on studies on adult GBMs. The discovery of aberrant chromatin level regulations in pHGGs suggest a need to design novel therapeutic approaches targeting epigenetic regulators for improved patient outcome in these diseases.

10.2 Epidemiology

The incidence of GBMs increases with age and they are much rarer in pediatric population. Importantly, even within the pediatric age group, the disease incidence peaks during adolescence (Perkins et al. 2011). Owing to the lower incidence in children, most of the studies on pediatric gliomas have traditionally combined GBMs, anaplastic astrocytomas and diffuse intrinsic pontine gliomas (DIPGs) together and termed as pediatric HGG. The estimated incidence of pHGG is approximately 0.85 per 100,000 children (<19 years) per year which makes them the most common group of malignant CNS neoplasms in pediatric age group alongside the embryonal tumors (Dolecek et al. 2012). Based on tumor site, infratentorial malignant brainstem gliomas represent 10% of pHGGs and 80% of these constitute DIPGs (Hargrave et al. 2006a). DIPGs are most commonly diagnosed in pediatric patients between ages of 5–10 years and are located within brainstem (midbrain, pons, or medulla). Frequency of supratentorial HGG is more in young children than in juveniles or adults. Thalamic pHGG represents 12% of cases and occurs more frequently in childhood than adults (Kramm et al. 2011; Wolff et al. 2008). Malignant gliomas in the spine are less common, with 3% occurrence rate in both children and adults (Wolff et al. 2012). Although, the exact frequency of diffuse midline glioma-H3K27M tumor has yet not been systematically estimated, they constitute about 70%–80% of previously referred DIPGs (Solomon et al. 2015). These tumors are predominantly present in children with peak age at diagnosis between 5 and 11 years and tend to be in midline locations. The pontine tumors arise on an average earlier (~7 years) than their thalamic counterparts (~11 years). There is no specific sex predilection reported in pHGGs. Presently, the only established risk factor associated with developing pHGG is prior radiation therapy (Pettorini et al. 2008). Genetic disorders associated with increased risk to develop brain tumor include Neurofibromatosis type 1 and 2, Li-Fraumeni syndrome (characterized by germline TP53 mutations), Gorlin syndrome (PTCH1 and SUFU) and Turcot syndrome (APC) (Cage et al. 2012).

10.3 Histopathology

Histologically, pGBMs are not distinguishable from their adult counterparts. They typically show high cellularity and are usually composed of poorly differentiated, pleomorphic tumor cells with nuclear atypia and brisk mitotic activity. Prominent endothelial proliferation and/or necrosis are essential diagnostic features. The distribution of these key elements within the tumor is variable, but large necrotic areas usually occupy the tumor centre, while microvascular proliferation is usually most marked around necrotic foci and in the peripheral zone of infiltration. DIPGs show poorly differentiated cells, with scant cytoplasm and round nuclei. Intra-tumoral histopathological heterogeneity and intracranial leptomeningeal dissemination are also common in DIPGs. Diffuse midline glioma-H3K27M shows predominantly small and monomorphic cells infiltrating the grey and white matter structures. However, cells can also be large and pleomorphic. Although, they typically show an astrocytic morphology, an oligodendroglial morphology is also a consistent pattern. Mitotic activity is present in majority of cases, but is not mainstay for diagnosis. Approximately 10% cases lack mitotic figures, microvascular proliferation and necrosis and thus morphologically mimic grade II. The remaining cases are high-grade, with one fourth of cases containing mitotic figures and the remainder containing, in addition, foci of necrosis and microvascular proliferation.

10.4 Molecular-Genetic Alterations in Pediatric HGGs

Gene expression profiling studies have identified three molecular subgroups of pHGG viz. Proliferative, Proneural and Mesenchymal, which overlap with the subgroups earlier classified in adult HGGs (Phillips et al. 2006). High frequency of mutations within the H3.3/ATRX/DAXX chromatin remodeling pathway occur in pGBMs (Schwartzentruber et al. 2012). Similarly, frequent H3.3 mutation along with mutation within the gene HIST1H3A (coding for the canonical histone H3.1) has been reported in DIPGs (Wu et al. 2012). These tumors also show significantly higher frequency of TP53 and PDGFRA alterations (Wu et al. 2012). Conversely, prototypic alterations of adult primary GBM (e.g., *EGFR* amplification, *CDKN2A/B* homozygous deletions *PTEN* mutations) are rarely present in pHGGs. Diffuse midline glioma-H3K27M harbours characteristic mutations in H3F3A, HIST1H3B, and HIST1H3C genes. Frequent mutation in TP53, ACVR1 and amplification of - PDGFRA gene are also common in this newly classified pHGG tumor entity.

10.4.1 Copy Number Alterations

The most prevalent genomic aberration identified in pGBMs and DIPGs is PDGFRA amplification (4q12) (Paugh et al. 2010; Bax et al. 2010). Gain of Chromosome 7 (74%–83%) and loss of 10q (80%–86%), the most frequent genetic aberration in adult GBMs are uncommon in pHGGs (13–19% and 16%–38%, respectively) (Network 2013; Brennan et al. 2013). Similarly, deletion of CDKN2A/B (9p21) is observed in about 53% adult HGGs but very infrequently seen in pHGGs (Brennan et al. 2013). Integration of TCGA copy number and sequencing data in adult GBMs identified somatic alterations in core components of the RB, TP53 and RTK pathways in 79%, 86% and 90% of patients (Brennan et al. 2013; Cancer Genome Atlas Research Network 2008). Focal chromosomal gains and/or losses in pHGGs are primarily associated with aberrant gene function within the p53, PI3K/RTK, and RB pathways (Verhaak et al. 2010; Frezza et al. 2010), however; at significantly lower frequency (RTK/PI3K:25%, p53:19% and RB:22% (Bax et al. 2010) compared to adults. pHGGs typically display chromosome 1q gain (19–20%) and small proportion of tumors are also associated with losses of chromosome 16q (7%–18%) and 4q (2%–15%) (Jones et al. 2012b). Diffuse midline glioma-H3K27M shows amplification of PDGFRA (30%), MYC/PVT1 (15%), and CDK4/6 or CCND1–3 (20%) in addition to infrequent homozygous deletion of CDKN2A/B in <5% cases (Castel et al. 2015). Overall, as compared to adults, pHGGs harbour significantly fewer DNA copy number alterations, and about 15% of these tumors are devoid of any evident copy number alterations (Sturm et al. 2012; Paugh et al. 2010; Bax et al. 2010; Jones et al. 2012b).

10.4.1.1 PDGFRA Amplification

Activation of the *PDGFRA* gene is present in approximately one third of pHGGs which include three principal forms of alterations – (i) Focal amplification, (ii) mutation and (iii) Intragenic deletion (Sturm et al. 2014b). Various studies show that recurrent focal amplification of *PDGFRA* is a key oncogenic event in DIPG (Paugh et al. 2011; Zarghooni et al. 2010). However, with increasing amounts of molecular data on treatment-naive DIPG, the occurrence of this alteration appears to be slightly lower than previously documented (<40%) and predominantly enriched in DIPGs that harbors histone H3.3/3.1 mutations (Sturm et al. 2012). Similar to EGFR, a fraction of *PDGFRA*-amplified GBMs from both pediatric as well as adults harbor age-specific intragenic deletion rearrangements of this kinase that result in constitutively increased activity (Ozawa et al. 2010; Paugh et al. 2013). Recent studies have also identified novel oncogenic mutations in *PDGFRA* in a group of pHGGs, and this often occurs in combination with amplification of the *PDGFRA* locus (Paugh et al. 2013; Puget et al. 2012). PDGFR signaling has also been shown to be activated upon up-regulation of PDGF ligands (A–D) in approximately 30% of gliomas and also in cell lines (Fleming et al. 1992; Hermanson et al. 1992; Lokker et al. 2002; Smith et al. 2000). Amplification of PDGF and *PDGFR* appear to promote aggressive glioma growth. Expression of genes associated with PDGFR signaling and genes involved in oligodendrocyte development (*OLIG2, NKX2–2*, and *PDGF*) have been documented in a large proportion of pHGGs (Paugh et al. 2010; Puget et al. 2012) which correlate with the higher frequency of *PDGFRA* amplification (Sturm et al. 2012; Paugh et al. 2010; Bax et al. 2010; Paugh et al. 2011; Qu et al. 2010).

10.4.2   Gene Mutation Profile

Studies have reported TP53 mutations to be present in 40%–54% of pHGGs (Appin and Brat 2014) as compared to 34%–37% of adults (Sturm et al. 2014b). HGG in infants show a lower frequency of TP53 mutation (9%) whereas DIPGs are associated with more frequent TP53 alteration (42%–64%) (Zarghooni et al. 2010; Wu et al. 2014; Pollack et al. 2001; Taylor et al. 2014). Lower frequency of somatic mutations in NF1 (25%), PDGFRA (8%) and EGFR (4%) have been reported in pHGGs when compared to adults (Wu et al. 2014). IDH1 and IDH2 mutations are rare and reported in <10% of pHGGs. Further, these are confined only to patients with age >13 years (Jones et al. 2012a). However, most frequent genetic alteration in pHGGs includes mutations in chromatin remodelling genes histone H3.3/3.1 and ATRX/DAXX.

10.4.2.1   Histone H3.3/H3.1 Mutation

The most significant mutation in pHGGs which invariably distinguishes these tumors from their adult counterparts is the newly discovered histone H-3.3/3.1 (H3F3A or HIST1H3B/ HIST1H3C gene) mutations (Schwartzentruber et al. 2012; Wu et al. 2012). These recurrent mutations, result in a p. Lys27Met (K27M) substitution in H3F3A or HIST1H3B/C gene and p.Gly34Arg/Val (G34R/V) substitution confined only to H3F3A (Schwartzentruber et al. 2012; Wu et al. 2012; Fontebasso et al. 2014). These mutations arise on the histone tail, at or near important post translational modification sites. H3F3A mutations are restricted to pediatric and young adult (<30 years) HGGs (Sturm et al. 2014b), but rarely reported in older adults and are mutually exclusive with IDH1 mutation (Schwartzentruber et al. 2012; Pathak et al. 2015). H3F3A mutations identify distinct subgroups of pGBMs and have been reported in 30%–52% of cases. The K27M tends to occur predominantly in midline pediatric GBMs (thalamus, pons, and spinal cord) while the G34R/V occur in cerebellar hemispheres. DIPGs frequently show K27M mutation in H3.3 gene (70%–88%) and less frequently (11%–31%) in *HIST1H3A* gene (K27M-H3.1), coding for the canonical histone H3.1 (Frattini et al. 2013). K27M-H3.1 mutations are mutually exclusive with K27M-H3.3 mutations. Further *TP53* mutations often co-occur with *H3F3A* and/or *ATRX* mutation in pGBMs and are identified in approximately 86% of cases that harbour *H3F3A-ATRX* alterations (reported in all G34R and about 67% of K27M mutants) (Schwartzentruber et al. 2012; Wu et al. 2012). Diffuse midline glioma-H3K27M presents recurrent characteristic mutations of H3F3A, HIST1H3B, and HIST1H3C genes in approximately 80%, 50% and 60% of tumors located in pons, thalamus and spinal cord respectively. Differences have also been reported in the gene expression, DNA methylation and prognostic outcome of H3.3 mutant versus wild types as well as K27M versus G34R/V mutant types (Sturm et al. 2012; Schwartzentruber et al. 2012).

10.4.2.2 ATRX/DAXX Mutation

ATRX mutations are less common in DIPGs (9%) as compared to supratentorial pHGGs (29%). ATRX-DAXX encodes a subunit of chromatin remodelling complex required for H3.3 incorporation at pericentric heterochromatin and telomeres (Schwartzentruber et al. 2012). Mutation in ATRX (alpha-thalassemia/mental-retardation syndrome X-linked) and DAXX (Death-Domain Associated Protein) leads to ALT (alternative lengthening telomeres) phenotype, frequently seen in pGBM, which maintains or increases telomere length (Schwartzentruber et al. 2012) in the absence of telomerase reverse transcriptase (TERT) promoter mutations. Mutations in ATRX along with DAXX gene have been identified in 31%–48% of pGBMs. DAXX mutations occur mostly in pGBMs and reported in about 6% of these tumors. ATRX-DAXX mutations are significantly associated with H3F3A mutations and particularly with 100% of H3F3A-G34R/V mutant cases (Schwartzentruber et al. 2012). Pathak P et al. identified association of ATRX mutation with 75% of G34R mutation as compared to only 60% in K27M mutant cases (Pathak et al. 2015). In another study, the mutations in H3.3/ARTX/ DAXX/TP53 were also found to associate with alterations in the telomere lengthening and specific gene expression profiles (Paugh et al. 2010; Paugh et al. 2011; Faury et al. 2007a; Haque et al. 2007). Unlike pHGGs, *ATRX* alterations are frequently seen together with *IDH1/2* and *TP53* mutations in adult diffuse astrocytic tumors across WHO grade 2 and 3 and in secondary adult GBMs (Jiao et al. 2012).

10.4.2.3 Other Recurrent Genetic Alterations

DIPGs exclusively harbour recurrent mutations in the ACVR1 (activin A receptor, type I) gene (20%–32%) which is a member of the bone morphogenic protein (BMP) signaling pathway (Buczkowicz et al. 2014a; Fontebasso et al. 2014).

ACVR1 mutation is the third most common genetic alteration in DIPGs, significantly overlaps with K27M mutations in histone H3.1 and is tightly associated with wild-type TP53 as well as younger age and longer survival (Wu et al. 2012; Taylor et al. 2014). Diffuse midline glioma-H3K27M also shows mutation in ACVR1 gene in 20% of these tumors (Fontebasso et al. 2014). Frequent somatic mutations in several histone writers, erasers and chromatin remodelling related genes namely MLL, KDM5C, KDM3A, JMJD1C etc. have also been identified in pHGGs recently (Wu et al. 2012) and these mutations often co-occur with mutations in H3.3/3.1 genes. Approximately 91% of DIPGs and 48% of hemispheric HGG harbour these mutations in histone genes and/or this group of epigenetic regulators (Wu et al. 2012). Mutations have been also identified in SETD2 gene, associated with global decrease in H3K36me3 levels, indicating another loss-of-function phenomenon in pHGGs (Fontebasso et al. 2013). In nonbrainstem tumors and/or DIPGs, MYCN and to a lesser extent, MYC amplifications have been also reported. Nevertheless, it is yet unidentified to what extent they mark a distinct subgroup (Wu et al. 2012; Taylor et al. 2014; Buczkowicz et al. 2014a; Fontebasso et al. 2014). Among pHGGs, notably tumors of juvenile and/or young adults situated in the cerebral hemispheres demonstrate defects in H3K36-methylation in about 50% of cases, acquired by mutations either in *H3F3A* (G34R/V), *IDH1* or *SETD2* (Sturm et al. 2012; Fontebasso et al. 2013). *TERT* gene promoter (pTERT) mutations are present at a much lower frequency (3%–11%) in pGBMs (Killela et al. 2013; Koelsche et al. 2013) which instead frequently display a loss of ATRX/DAXX and an alternative lengthening of telomeres (ALT) phenotype, associated with maintenance or increase in telomere length (Wu et al. 2012; Heaphy et al. 2011). Although BRAF-V600E mutation is strongly associated with pediatric pleomorphic xanthoastrocytomas (PXA), gangliogliomas, and pilocytic astrocytomas, a subset of pHGGs (5%–10%), predominantly cortical have been identified with this alteration (Korshunov et al. 2015). These pHGGs also display a histological and genome wide methylation signature similar to PXA and have a better clinical outcome (Korshunov et al. 2015). However, unlike lower-grade gliomas with characteristic MAP-K pathway activation, these tumors frequently co-occur with CDKN2A/CDKN2B (p16) deletions (Sturm et al. 2012; Korshunov et al. 2015). Nevertheless, BRAF-V600E mutation is extremely rare in adult GBMs.

In recent times, sequencing drive in pHGGs has led to the identification of the first fusion gene in these tumors (Wu et al. 2012). Importantly, gene fusion involving the kinase domain of each of the three *NTRK* (neurotrophin receptor) genes with five different N-terminal fusion partners has been reported in nearly 4% of DIPGs and 10% of non-brainstem HGGs. Interestingly, about 40% of nonbrainstem HGGs occur in infants (<3 years of age). NTRK fusions are linked with gliomagenesis *in vivo* and direct activation of PI3K/MAPK signalling (Wu et al. 2012). Recently, in a high throughput genome and transcriptome study on three pHGG cell lines, 17 novel fusion genes were identified and all associated with amplified chromosomal regions (Carvalho et al. 2014) Table 10.1.

Table 10.1 Frequency of different genetic alterations in pediatric and adult GBMs

Gene	Type of genetic alteration	Frequency (%)		Reference
		Pediatric HGG	Adult GBM	
H3F3A	G34R/V mutation	12–14	0–3	Castel et al. (2015), Sturm et al. (2012), Schwartzentruber et al. (2012), Wu et al. (2012), Brennan et al. (2013)
	K27M mutation	23–60	0–1	
HIST1H3B or HIST1H3C	K27M mutation	12–31	0	
	K27I mutation	2	0	
HIST2H3C	K27M mutation	2	0	
ATRX	Mutation/IHC	14–29	6–7	Schwartzentruber et al. (2012), Brennan et al. (2013), Heaphy et al. (2011)
PDGFRA	Focal amplification	8–39	11–26	Sturm et al. (2012), Paugh et al. (2010, 2012), Bax et al. (2010), Brennan et al. (2013), Verhaak et al. (2010), Ozawa et al. (2010), Paugh et al. (2013), Phillips et al. (2013), Barrow et al. (2011)
	Intragenic deletion/ Point mutation	4–9	3–18	
ACVR1	Mutation	20–32	0	Buczkowicz et al. (2014a), Fontebasso et al. (2014)
TP53	Mutation	34–37	20–29	Schwartzentruber et al. (2012), Brennan et al. (2013), Verhaak et al. (2010), Pollack et al. (2001), Noushmehr et al. (2010)
BRAF V600E	Mutation	10–25	2–8	Schwartzentruber et al. (2012), Brennan et al. (2013), Korshunov et al. (2015), Dahiya et al. (2014), Takahashi et al. (2015), Schiffman et al. (2010)
IDH1	Mutation	0–16	5–12	Sturm et al. (2012), Schwartzentruber et al. (2012), Paugh et al. (2010), Brennan et al. (2013), Verhaak et al. (2010), Suri et al. (2009), Noushmehr et al. (2010), Parsons et al. (2008), Yan et al. (2009)
EGFR	Focal amplification	1–11	40–43	Sturm et al. (2012), Schwartzentruber et al. (2012), Paugh et al. (2010), Bax et al. (2010), Brennan et al. (2013), Noushmehr et al. (2010), Bax et al. (2009)
	Intragenic deletion	17	10–64	
	Point mutation	4	18–26	
PTEN	Focal deletion	0–1	8–10	Schwartzentruber et al. (2012), Paugh et al. (2010), Bax et al. (2010), Brennan et al. (2013), Pollack et al. (2006), Raffel et al. (1999)
TERT	Promoter mutation	3–11	55–83	Brennan et al. (2013), Killela et al. (2013), Arita et al. (2013), Nonoguchi et al. (2013), Vinagre et al. (2013)
CDKN2A and 2B	Focal deletion	10–19	53–62	Paugh et al. (2010), Bax et al. (2010), Brennan et al. (2013), Verhaak et al. (2010), Barrow et al. (2011), Purkait et al. (2013)

10.5 Epigenetic Alterations in Pediatric GBM

10.5.1 MGMT Gene Promoter Methylation

Hypermethylation of O^6-methylguanine-DNA methyltransferase (MGMT) promoter region, which encodes a DNA repair enzyme associated with resistance in adult glioblastoma to alkylating agents, particularly temozolomide (TMZ) holds significant clinical relevance (Hegi et al. 2005). A variable frequency of MGMT promoter methylation has been noted in pGBMs owing to the various methodologies used for its assessment. Donson et al. (2007) and Srivastava et al. (2010) identified 40–50% of pGBMs with MGMT promoter methylation using MS-PCR (methylation-specific polymerase chain reaction). In another study (Lee et al. 2011), applying both MS-PCR and MS-MLPA (methylation-specific multiplex ligation-dependent probe amplification), it was identified in only 6% and 16% of cases respectively. There has been scant data on pHGGs regarding the role of MGMT promoter methylation either as an independent predictive and/or prognostic marker. Few studies, including phase 1 and 2 trials, evaluating the activity of TMZ in childhood CNS tumors have shown some promising results (Nicholson et al. 2007; Broniscer et al. 2005, 2006; Verschuur et al. 2004; Barone et al. 2006; Jakacki et al. 2008; Lashford et al. 2002; Estlin et al. 1998; Loh et al. 2005). Donson et al. (2007) reported the average survival time of 13.7 months for TMZ-treated children with methylated MGMT compared to 2.5 months for patients with an unmethylated MGMT. A correlation with overall survival, regardless of treatment in patients with methylated MGMT promoter (median survival of methylated patients: 13.6 months and unmethylated patients: 2.5 months) was also shown by Donson et al. (2007). In another study by Schlosser et al. (2010), slightly improved median event-free survival (EFS) and overall survival (OS) in children with MGMT promoter methylation (5.5 months versus 0.9 months) was noted. Even though both H3.3-K27M and G34R/V genetic alteration result in a reduction in DNA methylation throughout the epigenome (K27M globally and G34R/V mostly at subtelomeric regions) (Sturm et al. 2012), there exist few notable exceptions. Thus, MGMT promoter methylation is primarily associated with H3.3-G34R/V subgroup and rarely occurs in tumors with H3.3-K27M mutations (Korshunov et al. 2015). Hence, it has been suggested that this likely contributes to the lack of clinical response to TMZ in majority of pHGGs including DIPG. This has also been noted across various clinical trials (Cohen et al. 2011; Rizzo et al. 2015; Chassot et al. 2012; Hargrave et al. 2006b).

10.5.2 G-CIMP Status and DNA Methylation Profile in pHGGs

Analysis of epigenetic changes in 272 adult GBMs from TCGA revealed a distinct subset of GBMs with highly concordant DNA methylation of a subset of loci, indicative of a glioma CpG island methylator phenotype (G-CIMP). Distinctly, the

G-CIMP cases associated with younger age, proneural subtype, frequent IDH1 mutation and significantly improved survival, thus representing a distinct subset of human gliomas. However, pHGGs are largely G-CIMP negative (Sturm et al. 2012; Jha et al. 2014), correlating with absence of IDH mutation. Nevertheless, a small proportion of pGBMs have been reported with mutations in the IDH1/2 genes (5%), which associate with global hypermethylation (G-CIMP) (Sturm et al. 2014b). The major clinical impact of these findings is that IDH1 and G-CIMP are important prognostic markers in adult GBMs but are rarely seen in pGBMs.

Recently, Jha P et al. (2014) showed distinct differences between methylomes of pediatric and adult GBM. pGBMs showed 94 hypermethylated and 1206 hypomethylated cytosine–phosphate–guanine (CpG) islands, with three distinct clusters, with discrete differences in methylation levels and a trend to prognostic correlation. Further, pGBM methylome was shown to associate with reactive oxygen species (ROS) production, suggesting a possible role of ROS in pGBM pathogenesis. Patients with H3F3A mutation presented a unique methylome as compared to H3F3A-wild type and this exemplifies the presence of epigenetic subgroups within pGBMs. Functional annotation analysis using differentially methylated genes between H3F3A mutant and wild-type H3F3A identified pGBMs to be enriched in processes related to neuronal development, differentiation, cell proliferation, and cell-fate commitment. These results suggest that pGBM with H3F3A mutation is likely to be different from H3F3A-wild-type with respect to biological functions/pathways.

10.6   Molecular Subclasses of Pediatric GBMs

Integration of genomewide CpG island methylation with whole genome and transcriptome, and copy number profiling has identified H3F3A-K27M, −G34R/V and H3F3A-wild type as three distinct molecular subgroups in pGBMs (Sturm et al. 2012). A similar approach has shown three molecularly distinct subgroups; MYCN, Silent, and H3-K27M in DIPGs (Buczkowicz et al. 2014a). The detailed molecular sub-grouping of pHGGs is discussed below.

10.6.1   Gene Expression Profile Based Subclassification

The first gene expression profiling study on pHGG by Paugh et al. (2010) identified three major groups designated as HC1, HC2 and HC3 which overlapped with the subgroups previously identified in adult HGGs (Proliferative, Proneural and Mesenchymal) (Phillips et al. 2006). Notably, about 90% of PDGFR driven tumors cluster within Proliferative/HC1 subgroup, indicating this pathway as a fundamental driver of proliferation in pHGG, and distinct from the strong PDGFRA/IDH1/ Proneural association present in adult HGGs (Paugh et al. 2010). Proliferative/HC1 and Proneural/HC2 subgroups frequently associate with 1q gain (Paugh et al. 2010). The PDGFRA driven gene expression profile in pHGGs associate with cell cycle regulators and proliferation, but are different when compared to adults, as pHGGs are preferentially and differentially driven by *PDGFRA* amplification, in contrast to *EGFR* amplification in adult GBMs (Paugh et al. 2010).

10.6.2   DNA Methylation Profile Based Molecular Subtypes

The discovery of H3F3A mutation as a driver event led to enhanced understanding of epigenetic regulation and GBMs across all age continuums were classified together based on their methylation profile, gene expression, mutational status and copy number (Sturm et al. 2012). These efforts identified that the hotspot H3F3A mutation (K27 and G34) and IDH1 mutant tumors segregate into distinct epigenetic subgroups of GBMs. The adult GBMs have been classified into Classical, Mesenchymal, Neural and Proneural subtypes based on their gene-expression patterns, somatic mutations and DNA copy number variations (Network 2013). Similar to adult tumors, genetic heterogeneity and DNA methylation patterns in pGBMs resulted in their separation into different molecular subclasses. Sturm et al. (2012) investigated a cohort of pediatric and adult GBMs by genomic DNA methylation array and identified six distinct epigenetic subgroups within pGBMs, closely associated with specific genetic alterations. The different molecular subgroups termed as IDH, K27, G34, RTK-I (PDGFRA), mesenchymal, and RTK-II (classic). H3F3A mutations are exclusively associated with the K27 and G34 subgroups. Patients of K27 tend to be youngest with a median age of 10.5 years while the G34 subtype encompasses mostly adolescent and young adult patients (median age, 18 years). The IDH subclass shows enriched IDH1/2 mutations and association with young to middle-aged adults (median age, 40 years). IDH subclass is mutually exclusive compared to G34 and K27 and show a direct association with global hypermethylation (G-CIMP positive), while the *H3F3A*–G34 is linked to a hypomethylated signature of the genome (G-CIMP negative). The RTK-I subclass shows a patient age nearly similar to that of the IDH subclass (median age, 36 years). The RTK-II or classic subclass demonstrates an older adult patient age (median age, 58 years) and are enriched within tumors that encompass chromosome 7 gains, EGFR amplification, chromosome 10 losses and CDKN2A deletion, all the alterations typically present in adult primary GBMs. Interestingly, the RTK-II (EGFR) subclass shows significant overlap with Verhaak's classic subclass and the RTK-I (PDGFRA), IDH, and K27 subclasses show significant overlap with Verhaak's Proneural subclass (Sturm et al. 2012; Verhaak et al. 2010; Appin and Brat 2015). Also, recent multidimensional studies of DIPGs show a global landscape of DNA hypomethylation in K27 M-DIPGs, and distinct subgroups of tumors with activated Hedgehog (Hh) or N-Myc (MYCN) (Saratsis et al. 2014). MYCN alterations occur independently of H3-K27M and ACVR1 mutations and these three form individual epigenetic subgroups with distinct DNA methylation signatures. Moreover, recent DNA methylation profile study has identified a unique methylome of pGBM and showed substantial epigenetic differences from adult GBM, especially in terms of lack of G-CIMP methylation profile and involvement of ROS in the pathogenesis of pGBMs

(Jha et al. 2014). Thus, overall a more precise recapitulation of the DNA methylation signatures are robustly now known in pHGGs and this indicate a bright future for progress in understanding the biology of subgroups of HGGs.

An integrated analysis of DNA methylation and gene expression data have identified specifically hypermethylated promoter of FOXG1 (forkhead box protein 1) and associated loss of FOXG1 gene expression in K27M mutant pGBMs. It is now clear that concerted hypermethylation of promoter of OLIG1 and OLIG2 genes (two oligodendrocyte lineage marker genes) along with low level of their expression exclusively associated with G34R mutant pGBMs. These observations also suggest a surrogate marker to categorize H3.3 mutated pGBMs using OLIG1/2 and FOXG1 immunohistochemical analysis (Sturm et al. 2012).

10.7   miRNA Profile in Pediatric GBMs

Pediatric GBMs have remained uncharacterized for miRNA profile till recent times, whereas the role of miRNA has been widely studied in adult GBMs. In a small scale miRNA profile study, Miele E et al. (2014) reported a specific microRNA pattern in pHGGs with an overexpression and a proliferative role of the miR-17-92 cluster. Very recently, Jha P et al. (2015) examined genome wide miRNA profile of pGBM and showed that 21 upregulated and 24 downregulated miRNAs were uniquely expressed in pHGGs as compared to adult GBMs. The pHGGs also showed a significant upregulation of miR-17/92 and its paralog clusters miR-106b/25 and miR-106a/363 (Jha et al. 2015; Miele et al. 2014). These miRNA clusters are potentially oncogenic in nature and regulate tumor development and maintenance. Downregulation of miRNAs located on 14q32 locus (members of miR-379/656 and miR493/136 clusters) which is associated with neuronal developmental pathway was common to both pediatric and adult GBMs (Jha et al. 2015). Some novel miR-NAs such as miR-3613, 23,651, 24,429, 24,521 and 24,668-5p were identified exclusively in pHGGs (Jha et al. 2015), though their role still remains to be elucidated. The pathway enrichment analyses of the miRNAs identified PDGFR-b signaling as most affected pathway in pHGGs as compared to adult GBMs. This is exciting as the distinctions between EGFR- and PDGFR mediated receptor tyrosine kinase signaling pathways have been shown in adult vs pHGGs. Other pathways actively regulated by the unique miRNAs in pGBMs are SMAD2/3, ErBB1, cdc42 and calcineurin signaling pathways (Jha et al. 2015). H3F3A-K27M mutation specific pHGG patients identified with a specific set of up- and down-regulated miR-NAs which target a number of genes implicated in apoptosis, cell cycle regulation and proliferation. Notably, pHGGs with K27M mutation show aberrant expression of several known epigenetically regulated miRNAs such as miR-101, −224, −130b, −374c and −301b etc. Recently, first description of snoRNAs in pGBM was reported with global downregulation of snoRNA HBII-52 cluster (SNORD115) that potentially regulates the editing and/or alternative splicing of the serotonin receptor, 5-HT2CR. The pathological implication of this cluster has also been described in a neuro-developmental disorder viz. Prader-Willi syndrome. The major features of miRNA expression in pHGGs are summarized in Table 10.2.

Table 10.2 Top deregulated miRNAs in pediatric and adult GBMs

S.No.	Patient group	miRNAs
1	Pediatric and Adult HGGs	Top most commonly upregulated: miR-10b, miR-182, miR-21, miR-155, miR-130b, miR-106b, miR-542, miR-503, miR-201, miR-25 and miR-320d
2	Pediatric and Adult HGG	Top most common highly downregulated: miR-7, miR-124, miR-129, miR-137 and miR-203
3	Pediatric HGGs	Novel: miR-3613, −3651, −4429, −4521 and −4668-5p.
4	H3F3A-mutant pHGGs	upregulation of 62 miRNAs
5	H3F3A-wt pHGGs	downregulation of 35 miRNAs
6	Pediatric HGGs with K27M mutation	Epigenetically regulated: miR-101, −130b, −224, −301b and -374c.

Based on data from Jha et al. (2015)

10.8 Biological Implication of Chromatin Remodeling Alterations in pHGG: Histone Code Alterations

Frequent histone H3.3 mutation in pHGGs has gained considerable attention regarding its role in tumorigenesis. Genome-wide studies applying ChIP-seq on H3.3-K27M mutant tumors showed a global reduction in levels of H3K27 di- and trimethylation (H3K27me2 and H3K27me3) (Lewis et al. 2013; Chan et al. 2013). Moreover, significant enrichment of H3K27me3 and EZH2 (the catalytic subunit H3K27 methyltransferase) at numerous gene loci associated with various cancer pathways was noted in H3.3K27M patient derived cell line. These changes reprogram the epigenetic landscape and gene expression that may drive tumorigenesis. In contrast, the G34R substitution was shown to diminish K36 trimethylation in vitro (Lewis et al. 2013) as well as impair differentiation of mesenchymal progenitor cells. It was shown that H3K36M mutant inhibits the enzymatic activities of several H3K36 methyltransferases which leads to the loss of H3K36 methylation and a genome-wide gain in H3K27 methylation (Lu et al. 2016). This reprogrammed H3K27 pattern directs redistribution of PRC1 and de-repression of their target genes and ultimately obstructs mesenchymal differentiation and result in tumorigenesis (Lu et al. 2016). Additionally, Venneti et al. (2013) reported absent and/or lowered expression of H3K27me3 in K27M mutants. Bjerke et al. (2013) discovered MYCN gene as most strongly enriched for H3K36me3 marks in a G34V mutant pGBM cell line (KNS42) and this was also associated with transcriptional upregulation of this locus.

Mutations in H3.3, a regulatory histone, triggered interest in understanding how this affects different histone post translational modifications (PTMs) that regulate gene expression. The most widely understood histone modification is histone lysine (H3K) methylation. These can be an activator or repressor of transcription, primarily depending on the particular histone residue being methylated. Conventionally, methylation of H3K9 and H3K27 is associated with silencing of transcription, whereas H3K4 and H3K36 methylation associates with activation of transcription (Martin and Zhang 2005). Importantly, Pathak et al. (2015) reported status of all four global histone trimethylation marks (H3K-4/9/27/36me3) in pGBMs and noted association of H3F3A mutation with loss of histone trimethylation at H3K27 (H3K27me3, 60% cases), H3K4me3 (45.5%) and H3K9me3 (18.2%) (Pathak et al. 2015). Thus, in majority of pGBMs, H3F3A mutation was found to be invariably associated with combinatorial loss of one or more histone-trimethylation marks (Pathak et al. 2015). The H3K27me3 loss in non H3F3A-K27M was also reported, although; the underlying pathology that leads to alteration in global H3K4, H3K27 and H3K9 trimethylation levels in these cases was not explainable in pGBMs and evaluation of histone lysine methylases and demethylases were suggested as probable mechanism. To further support this hypothesis, recently, a mutation in SETD2, a H3K36 trimethyltransferase was identified in 15% of pHGGs with substantial decrease in H3K36me3 (Fontebasso et al. 2013). Hence, it is likely that histone methylases and demethylases are deregulated and lead to aberrant histone code in pGBMs.

10.9   Prognostic and Predictive Biomarkers of Pediatric HGGs

The overall clinical outcome of pHGGs is dismal as updated trial results show 3 years event-free survival (EFS) and OS rates of 10% and 20%, respectively (Cohen et al. 2011). In general, extent of surgical resection, histological grade, age at diagnosis, and ability to tolerate adjuvant therapies determine individual survival rate. Patients who undergo gross total resection (GTR) show improved 5-year PFS as compared to those who receive only stereotactic tumor resection (STR) or biopsy (Vanan and Eisenstat 2014). Infants show improved clinical outcome as compared to older children and adults (Fangusaro et al. 2012).

Among various genetic alterations and molecular subgroups of pHGGs, IDH1 mutations (tightly coupled with G-CIMP), TP53 wild-type (wt), H3F3A-wt and MGMT promoter methylation show favorable prognosis (Sturm et al. 2012). The IDH1 mutant group (mainly present in young adults and rarely in pHGGs) shows a significantly longer overall survival than patients with H3F3A and IDH1-wt tumors. pGBMs with G34 mutation also show a trend toward a better OS than G34-wt patients. K27 mutated patients show a trend toward an even shorter OS than patients with K27-wt tumors as these are associated with (1) deep midline locations and, as a result have limited options for tumor resection; (2) frequent craniospinal tumor dissemination after treatment and (3) absence of MGMT promoter methylation in almost all cases, implying a low efficacy of TMZ-based adjuvant therapy. G34 and IDH1 mutant tumors carry a more favorable prognosis, as these tumors usually have a hemispheric location, hence surgically accessible. Additionally, they show frequent MGMT promoter methylation which correlates with enhanced responsiveness to TMZ and thus better outcomes (Sturm et al. 2012; Korshunov et al. 2015). Korshunov et al. (2015) identified a subset of pGBMs with DNA methylation pattern nearly similar to LGGs or PXAs along with higher frequency of BRAFV-600E mutation and CDKN2A deletion. This subgroup was associated with significantly better OS as compared to molecularly confirmed GBM, with best prognosis in LGG like subgroup. Other molecular alterations which have an association with clinical outcome in pHGGs include genomic amplification involving PDGFRA, EGFR or MYC (associated with poor prognosis) and 9p21 homozygous deletion (associated with poor prognosis) (Korshunov et al. 2015; Schlosser et al. 2010). Moreover, reports have highlighted that diffuse midline gliomas with histone H3-K27M mutation are associated with aggressive clinical course and poor prognosis (Sturm et al. 2012; Korshunov et al. 2015; Fangusaro et al. 2012) irrespective of tumors with only low grade histological morphology (Buczkowicz et al. 2014b) with 2-year survival rate of <10%.

10.10   Novel Strategies in Pediatric Glioblastoma Therapy

The treatments that are the standard of care for pHGG include radiation therapy and alkylating agents such as temozolomide (Stupp et al. 2005). The continuing unmet medical need for new therapeutic strategies against HGGs has promoted research on a range of new drugs and therapeutic modalities. Most of these drugs specifically target key signaling pathways of gliomagenesis, such as RTK signalling (anti PDGFRA, Anti EGFR) or angiogenesis (Anti VEGF) and have been used in various clinical trials. Unfortunately, majority of the drugs have not provided a significant survival benefit when tested singly, or in combination with other therapies in unselected GBM patient cohorts despite the fact that activation of both of the above mentioned pathways are seen in pHGGs (Sturm et al. 2014b; Tanaka et al. 2013). A phase II trial of the ErbB inhibitor (lapatinib) in refractory pediatric glial tumors reported low intratumoral drug concentrations of target agents, hence a poor drug delivery that resulted in failed treatment benefit (Holdhoff et al. 2010; Razis et al. 2009; Vivanco et al. 2012; Fouladi et al. 2013). The histone deacetylase (HDAC) inhibitor valproic acid has the potential to sensitize cells to other chemotherapeutic agents and is often used as a part of highly intensified chemotherapy regimens. DIPGs have shown the potential therapeutic value of epigenetic modifying drugs targeting HDACs and histone demethylases (KDMs) (Grasso et al. 2015; Hashizume et al. 2014). Each of these epigenetic agents program restoration of trimethylation of H3K27 via distinct mechanisms, and show synergy when used in a combination (Grasso et al. 2015). A phase I clinical trial of the HDAC inhibitor (panobinostat) in DIPGs is also in progress in the Pediatric Brain Tumor Consortium (PBTC 047). Other histone deacetylase inhibitors, such as vorinostat are now under investigation (MacDonald et al. 2011; Children's Oncology Group, National Cancer Institute). PLX4032, a specific inhibitor of BRAF-V600E, is being considered for clinical trial for cases carrying these alterations in pGBMs (Cage et al. 2012).

The identification of histone mutations in a significant proportion of pHGGs (Schwartzentruber et al. 2012; Wu et al. 2012) has raised expectations for targeted treatment approaches (Sturm et al. 2012, 2014b; Bjerke et al. 2013). Although the exact mechanism of K27M-mediated PRC2 inhibition is not well-understood, pharmacological intervention that targets K27M-mutant H3.3 or downstream effectors of this change might represent an important therapeutic target. A number of small molecular inhibitors against EZH2 and DNA methyl transferases (DNMTs) are now available and currently under investigation for their possible utility in treating a variety of tumors including pGBMs (Nakagawa et al. 2014; Qi et al. 2012; Kim et al. 2012). Recently, it has been reported that EZH2 inhibition did not induce significant cytotoxicity in pHGG cells independently of H3.3 mutations but its inhibition might not present an effective single agent treatment choice for pHGGs (Wiese et al. 2016). H3K27me3 loss in K27M mutant group also affects other histone marks (methylation of H3-K4/9/36) or chromatin machinery and therefore presents a pharmacologically actionable target. Evidential support has shown that inhibition of menin (trithorax group member and antagoniser of K27me3 that deposits polycomb repressive complex) decreased the proliferation of DIPGs (Funato et al. 2014). This implies that mechanistic understanding of H3.1/3.3 mutation driven information of genome-wide transcriptome, DNA methylome and post translational histone modification may provide a new insight for identification of novel prognostic and targeted therapeutic approaches in pHGGs. The targeted therapies against the miRNAs are also potential area of current interest (Costa et al. 2015) and some pHGG specific novel miRNAs with possible therapeutic benefit could be targeted in these tumors Table 10.3.

Table 10.3 Investigational therapeutic agents used in pHGGs

Mechanism of action	Therapeutic agent
VEGF/EGFR inhibitor	Bevacizumab, Vandetanib
EGF receptor tyrosine kinase inhibitor	Erlotinib, Gefitinib, Nimotuzumab, Cediranib (AZD2171), Cetuximab
Anti-angiogenic; protein kinase C inhibitor	Enzastaurin (LY317615)
PDGFRA inhibitor	Imatinib
avb3 and avb5 integrin inhibitor	Cilengitide
Inhibitor of BRAF V600E	Vemurafenib (PLX4032)
Histone deacetylase inhibitor	Valproic acid
Gamma secretase inhibitor	MK-0752
Poly(ADP-ribose) polymerase inhibitor	Veliparib (ABT-888)
mTOR inhibitor	Temsirolimus
Farnesyltransferase inhibitor	Tipifarnib

Based on data from Stupp et al. (2005), MacDonald et al. (2011), Morton et al. (2012), Kilburn et al. (2015), MacDonald et al. (2013), Bautista et al. (2014), Felix et al. (2014), Hoffman et al. (2015), Chornenkyy et al. (2015)

10.11   Future Direction

It has been now clear that the molecular pathogenesis of pHGG is distinct and there is limited overlap in mutational/methylation/copy number profile between pediatric and adult GBM subtypes (Sturm et al. 2012; Paugh et al. 2010; Buczkowicz et al. 2014a). The growing body of evidence now suggest that pHGG is a biologically diverse group of tumor rather than a homogenous tumor entity. The recent studies have highlighted the tumor heterogeneity (each tumor comprising a mixture of cells) within adult and pGBMs (Patel et al. 2014; Meyer et al. 2015), representing different subtypes. Increasing evidence show that clinical manifestation of a tumor is more closely associated with its underlying genome and epigenome profile rather than cellular morphology or histopathological grading or other radiological/neurosurgical parameters. None of the GBMs are homogenous; they are actually diverse cells with possibly different genetic/epigenetic characteristics and are in continuous status of evolutionary selection pressure to evade the tumor microenvironment and escape the current mode of therapy. Owing to the relatively small cohort sizes and/or heterogeneity of the applied treatment modalities, various studies investigating the prognostic implications of mutations, gene expression patterns and copy number aberrations in pGBM remained inconsistent or contradictory (Bax et al. 2010; Puget et al. 2012; Haque et al. 2007; Korshunov et al. 2015; Donson et al. 2007; Srivastava et al. 2010; Lee et al. 2011; Buttarelli et al. 2010; Faury et al. 2007b; Korshunov et al. 2005; Phillips et al. 2013; Suri et al. 2009). Therefore, cohort size is of particular importance to address the extensive biological heterogeneity of these tumors. Tumor heterogeneity has a crucial role in disease development, progression and treatment resistance. Moreover, novel and emerging drugs for the treatment of HGG will likely target only a subset of pHGG, resulting in relatively small eligible populations for targeted clinical trials. Thus tumor heterogeneity and molecular subgrouping has profound implications for the design and planning of future clinical trials. Emergence of defective chromatin remodelling as key pathogenic player in pHGGs, it appears imminent that candidate histone mutation or post translational histone modification will be considered for treatment in near future. The ongoing clinical trials exploring histone modifier inhibitors in conjunction with presently practiced chemo-radiological therapies to examine antitumor activity may possibly improve outcomes in pHGGs. The emergence of the miRNA as the mediator of gene expression renders them as promising potential diagnostic marker for malignancy. With current emphasis on miRNA based therapeutics, the chracterization of miRNA expression pattern in cancers may have noticeable value for prognostic decision as well as for ultimate therapeutic intervention in pHGGs. It would be interesting to know the roles of novel and specific miRNAs recently identified in pHGGs and thereafter their therapeutic implications towards patient management.

References

Appin, C.L., and D.J. Brat. 2014. Molecular genetics of gliomas. *Cancer Journal* 20 (1): 66–72.

Appin, C.L., and D.J. Brat. 2015. Molecular pathways in gliomagenesis and their relevance to neuropathologic diagnosis. *Advances in Anatomic Pathology* 22 (1): 50–58.

Arita, H., Y. Narita, S. Fukushima, K. Tateishi, Y. Matsushita, A. Yoshida, et al. 2013. Upregulating mutations in the TERT promoter commonly occur in adult malignant gliomas and are strongly associated with total 1p19q loss. *Acta Neuropathologica* 126 (2): 267–276.

Baker, S.J., D.W. Ellison, and D.H. Gutmann. 2016. Pediatric gliomas as neurodevelopmental disorders. *Glia* 64 (6): 879–895.

Barone, G., P. Maurizi, G. Tamburrini, and R. Riccardi. 2006. Role of temozolomide in pediatric brain tumors. *Child's Nervous System* 22: 652–661.

Barrow, J., M. Adamowicz-Brice, M. Cartmill, D. MacArthur, J. Lowe, K. Robson, et al. 2011. Homozygous loss of ADAM3A revealed by genome-wide analysis of pediatric high-grade glioma and diffuse intrinsic pontine gliomas. *Neuro-Oncology* 13 (2): 212–222.

Bautista, F., A. Paci, V. Minard-Colin, C. Dufour, J. Grill, L. Lacroix, et al. 2014. Vemurafenib in pediatric patients with BRAFV600E mutated high-grade gliomas. *Pediatric Blood & Cancer* 61 (6): 1101–1103.

Bax, D.A., N. Gaspar, S.E. Little, L. Marshall, L. Perryman, M. Regairaz, et al. 2009. EGFRvIII deletion mutations in pediatric high-grade glioma and response to targeted therapy in pediatric glioma cell lines. *Clinical Cancer Research* 15 (18): 5753–5761.

Bax, D.A., A. Mackay, S.E. Little, D. Carvalho, M. Viana-Pereira, N. Tamber, et al. 2010. A distinct spectrum of copy number aberrations in pediatric highgrade gliomas. *Clinical Cancer Research* 16 (13): 3368–3377.

Bjerke, L., A. Mackay, M. Nandhabalan, A. Burford, A. Jury, S. Popov, et al. 2013. Histone H3.3. mutations drive pediatric glioblastoma through upregulation of MYCN. *Cancer Discovery* 3 (5): 512–519.

Brennan, C.W., R.G. Verhaak, A. McKenna, B. Campos, H. Noushmehr, S.R. Salama, et al. 2013. The somatic genomic landscape of glioblastoma. *Cell* 155 (2): 462–477.

Broniscer, A., L. Iacono, M. Chintagumpala, M. Fouladi, D. Wallace, et al. 2005. Role of temozolomide after radiotherapy for newly diagnosed diffuse brainstem glioma in children: Results of a multiinstitutional study (SJHG-98). *Cancer* 103: 133–139.

Broniscer, A., M. Chintagumpala, M. Fouladi, M.J. Krasin, M. Kocak, D.C. Bowers, et al. 2006. Temozolomide after radiotherapy for newly diagnosed high-grade glioma and unfavorable low-grade glioma in children. *Journal of Neuro-Oncology* 76: 313–319.

Buczkowicz, P., C. Hoeman, P. Rakopoulos, S. Pajovic, L. Letourneau, M. Dzamba, et al. 2014a. Genomic analysis of diffuse intrinsic pontine gliomas identifies three molecular subgroups and recurrent activating ACVR1 mutations. *Nature Genetics* 46 (5): 451–456.

Buczkowicz, P., U. Bartels, E. Bouffet, O. Becher, and C. Hawkins. 2014b. Histopathologic spectrum of paediatric diffuse intrinsic pontine glioma: Diagnostic and therapeutic implications. *Acta Neuropathologica* 128: 573–581.

Buttarelli, F.R., M. Massimino, M. Antonelli, L. Lauriola, P. Nozza, V. Donofrio, et al. 2010. Evaluation status and prognostic significance of O6-methylguanine-DNA methyltransferase (MGMT) promoter methylation in pediatric high grade gliomas. *Child's Nervous System* 26 (8): 1051–1056.

Cage, T.A., S. Mueller, D. Haas-Kogan, and N. Gupta. 2012. High-grade gliomas in children. *Neurosurgery Clinics of North America* 23 (3): 515–523.

Cancer Genome Atlas Research Network. 2008. Comprehensive genomic characterization defines human glioblastoma genes and core pathways. *Nature* 455 (7216): 1061–1068.

Carvalho, D., A. Mackay, L. Bjerke, R.G. Grundy, C. Lopes, R.M. Reis, et al. 2014. The prognostic role of intragenic copy number breakpoints and identification of novel fusion genes in paediatric high grade glioma. *Acta Neuropathologica Communications* 2: 23.

Castel, D., C. Philippe, R. Calmon, L. Le Dret, N. Truffaux, N. Boddaert, et al. 2015. Histone H3F3A and HIST1H3B K27M mutations define two subgroups of diffuse intrinsic pontine gliomas with different prognosis and phenotypes. *Acta Neuropathologica* 130 (6): 815–827.

Chan, K.M., D. Fang, H. Gan, R. Hashizume, C. Yu, M. Schroeder, et al. 2013. The histone H3.3K27M mutation in pediatric glioma reprograms H3K27 methylation and gene expression. *Genes & Development* 27 (9): 985–990.

Chassot, A., S. Canale, P. Varlet, S. Puget, T. Roujeau, L. Negretti, et al. 2012. Radiotherapy with concurrent and adjuvant temozolomide in children with newly diagnosed diffuse intrinsic pontine glioma. *Journal of Neuro-Oncology* 106 (2): 399–407.

Children's Oncology Group, National Cancer Institute. Vorinostat and radiation therapy followed by maintenance therapy with vorinostat in treating younger patients with newly diagnosed pontine glioma. Available at: http://www.clinicaltrials.gov/ct2/show/NCT01189266?

Chornenkyy, Y., S. Agnihotri, M. Yu, P. Buczkowicz, P. Rakopoulos, B. Golbourn, et al. 2015. Poly-ADP-Ribose polymerase as a therapeutic target in pediatric diffuse intrinsic pontine glioma and pediatric high-grade astrocytoma. *Molecular Cancer Therapeutics* 14 (11): 2560–2568.

Cohen, K.J., R.L. Heideman, T. Zhou, E.J. Holmes, R.S. Lavey, E. Bouffet, et al. 2011. Temozolomide in the treatment of children with newly diagnosed diffuse intrinsic pontine gliomas: A report from the Children's Oncology Group. *Neuro-Oncology* 13 (4): 410–416.

Costa, P.M., A.L. Cardoso, M. Mano, and M.C. de Lima. 2015. MicroRNAs in glioblastoma: Role in pathogenesis and opportunities for targeted therapies. *CNS & Neurological Disorders Drug Targets* 14 (2): 222–238.

Dahiya, S., R.J. Emnett, D.H. Haydon, J.R. Leonard, J.J. Phillips, A. Perry, et al. 2014. BRAF-V600E mutation in pediatric and adult glioblastoma. *Neuro-Oncology* 16 (2): 318–319.

Dolecek, T., J. Propp, N. Stroup, and C. Kruchko. 2012. CBTRUS statistical report: Primary brain and central nervous system tumors diagnosed in the United States in 2005–2009. *Neuro-Oncology* 14 (Suppl. 5): 49.

Donaldson, S.S., F. Laningham, and P.G. Fisher. 2006. Advances toward an understanding of brainstem gliomas. *Journal of Clinical Oncology* 24 (8): 1266–1272. Review.

Donson, A.M., S.O. Addo-Yobo, M.H. Handler, L. Gore, and N.K. Foreman. 2007. MGMT promoter methylation correlates with survival benefit and sensitivity to temozolomide in pediatric glioblastoma. *Pediatric Blood & Cancer* 48 (4): 403–407.

Estlin, E.J., L. Lashford, S. Ablett, L. Price, R. Gowing, A. Gholkar, et al. 1998. Phase I study of temozolomide in paediatric patients with advanced cancer. United Kingdom Children's Cancer Study Group. *British Journal of Cancer* 78 (5): 652–661.

Fangusaro, J. 2012. Pediatric high grade glioma: A review and update on tumor clinical characteristics and biology. *Frontiers in Oncology* 2: 105; 92. Khuong-Quang, D.A., P. Buczkowicz, P. Rakopoulos, X.Y. Liu, A.M. Fontebasso, E. Bouffet, et al. 2012. K27M mutation in histone H3.3 defines clinically and biologically distinct subgroups of pediatric diffuse intrinsic pontine gliomas. *Acta Neuropathologica* 124: 439–447.

Faury, D., A. Nantel, S.E. Dunn, M.C. Guiot, T. Haque, P. Hauser, et al. 2007a. Molecular profiling identifies prognostic subgroups of pediatric glioblastoma and shows increased YB-1 expression in tumors. *Journal of Clinical Oncology* 25 (10): 1196–1208.

Faury, D., A. Nantel, S.E. Dunn, M.C. Guiot, T. Haque, P. Hauser, et al. 2007b. Molecular profiling identifies prognostic subgroups of pediatric glioblastoma and shows increased YB-1 expression in tumors. *Journal of Clinical Oncology: Official Journal of the American Society of Clinical Oncology* 25 (10): 1196–1208.

Felix, F.H., O.L. de Araujo, K.M. da Trindade, N.M. Trompieri, and J.B. Fontenele. 2014. Retrospective evaluation of the outcomes of children with diffuse intrinsic pontine glioma treated with radiochemotherapy and valproic acid in a single center. *Journal of Neuro-Oncology* 116 (2): 261–266.

Fleming, T.P., A. Saxena, W.C. Clark, J.T. Robertson, E.H. Oldfield, S.A. Aaronson, et al. 1992. Amplification and/or overexpression of platelet-derived growth factor receptors and epidermal growth factor receptor in human glial tumors. *Cancer Research* 52 (16): 4550–4553.

Fontebasso, A.M., J. Schwartzentruber, D.A. Khuong-Quang, X.Y. Liu, D. Sturm, A. Korshunov, et al. 2013. Mutations in SETD2 and genes affecting histone H3K36 methylation target hemispheric high-grade gliomas. *Acta Neuropathologica* 125 (5): 659–669.

Fontebasso, A.M., S. Papillon-Cavanagh, J. Schwartzentruber, H. Nikbakht, N. Gerges, P.O. Fiset, et al. 2014. Recurrent somatic mutations in ACVR1 in pediatric midline high-grade astrocytoma. *Nature Genetics* 46 (5): 462–466.

Fouladi, M., C.F. Stewart, S.M. Blaney, A. Onar-Thomas, P. Schaiquevich, R.J. Packer, et al. 2013. A molecular biology and phase II trial of lapatinib in children with refractory CNS malignancies: A pediatric brain tumor consortium study. *Journal of Neuro-Oncology* 114 (2): 173–179.

Frattini, V., V. Trifonov, J.M. Chan, A. Castano, M. Lia, F. Abate, et al. 2013. The integrated landscape of driver genomic alterations in glioblastoma. *Nature Genetics* 45 (10): 1141–1149.

Frezza, C., D.A. Tennant, and E. Gottlieb. 2010. IDH1 mutations in gliomas: When an enzyme loses its grip. *Cancer Cell* 17 (1): 7–9.

Funato, K., T. Major, P.W. Lewis, C.D. Allis, and V. Tabar. 2014. Use of human embryonic stem cells to model pediatric gliomas with H3.3K27 M histone mutation. *Science* 346 (6216): 1529–1533.

Gottardo, N.G., and A. Gajjar. 2008. Chemotherapy for malignant brain tumors of childhood. *Journal of Child Neurology* 23: 1149–1159.

Grasso, C.S., Y. Tang, N. Truffaux, N.E. Berlow, L. Liu, M.A. Debily, et al. 2015. Functionally defined therapeutic targets in diffuse intrinsic pontine glioma. *Nature Medicine* 21 (6): 555–559.

Haque, T., D. Faury, S. Albrecht, E. Lopez-Aguilar, P. Hauser, M. Garami, et al. 2007. Gene expressionprofiling from formalin-fixed paraffin-embedded tumors of pediatric glioblastoma. *Clinical Cancer Research* 13 (21): 6284–6292.

Hargrave, D., U. Bartels, and E. Bouffet. 2006a. Diffuse brainstem glioma in children: Critical review of clinical trials. *The Lancet Oncology* 7 (3): 241–248.

Hashizume, R., N. Andor, Y. Ihara, R. Lerner, H. Gan, X. Chen, et al. 2014. Pharmacologic inhibition of histone demethylation as a therapy for pediatric brainstem glioma. *Nature Medicine* 20 (12): 1394–1396.

Heaphy, C.M., R.F. de Wilde, Y. Jiao, A.P. Klein, B.H. Edil, C. Shi, et al. 2011. Altered telomeres in tumors with ATRX and DAXX mutations. *Science* 333 (6041): 425.

Hegi, M.E., A.C. Diserens, T. Gorlia, M.F. Hamou, N. de Tribolet, M. Weller, et al. 2005. MGMT gene silencing and benefit from temozolomide in glioblastoma. *The New England Journal of Medicine* 352 (10): 997–1003.

Hermanson, M., K. Funa, M. Hartman, L. Claesson-Welsh, C.H. Heldin, B. Westermark, et al. 1992. Platelet-derived growth factor and its receptors in human glioma tissue: Expression of messenger RNA and protein suggests the presence of autocrine and paracrine loops. *Cancer Research* 52 (11): 3213–3219.

Hoffman, L.M., M. Fouladi, J. Olson, V.M. Daryani, C.F. Stewart, C. Wetmore, et al. 2015. Phase I trial of weekly MK-0752 in children with refractory central nervous system malignancies: A pediatric brain tumor consortium study. *Child's Nervous System* 31 (8): 1283–1289.

Holdhoff, M., J.G. Supko, G.L. Gallia, C.L. Hann, D. Bonekamp, et al. 2010. Intratumoral concentrations of imatinib after oral administration in patients with glioblastoma multiforme. *Journal of Neuro-Oncology* 97 (2): 241–245.

Jakacki, R.I., A. Yates, S.M. Blaney, T. Zhou, R. Timmerman, A.M. Ingle, et al. 2008. A phase I trial of temozolomide and lomustine in newly diagnosed high-grade gliomas of childhood. *Neuro-Oncology* 10 (4): 569–576.

Jha, P., I.R. Pia Patric, S. Shukla, P. Pathak, J. Pal, V. Sharma, et al. 2014. Genome-wide methylation profiling identifies an essential role of reactive oxygen species in pediatric glioblastoma multiforme and validates a methylome specific for H3 histone family 3A with absence of G-CIMP/isocitrate dehydrogenase 1 mutation. *Neuro-Oncology* 16 (12): 1607–1617.

Jha, P., R. Agrawal, P. Pathak, A. Kumar, S. Purkait, S. Mallik, et al. 2015. Genome-wide small noncoding RNA profiling of pediatric high-grade gliomas reveals deregulation of several miRNAs, identifies downregulation of snoRNA cluster HBII-52 and delineates H3F3A and TP53 mutant-specific miRNAs and snoRNAs. *International Journal of Cancer* 137 (10): 2343–2353.

Jiao, Y., P.J. Killela, Z.J. Reitman, A.B. Rasheed, C.M. Heaphy, R.F. de Wilde, et al. 2012. Frequent ATRX, CIC, FUBP1 and IDH1 mutations refine the classification of malignant gliomas. *Oncotarget* 3 (7): 709–722.

Jones, C., and S.J. Baker. 2014. Unique genetic and epigenetic mechanisms driving paediatric diffuse high-grade glioma. *Nature Reviews. Cancer* 14 (10): 651–661.

Jones, C., L. Perryman, and D. Hargrave. 2012a. Paediatric and adult malignant glioma: Close relatives or distant cousins? *Nature Reviews. Clinical Oncology* 9 (7): 400–413.

Kilburn, L.B., M. Kocak, R.L. Decker, C. Wetmore, M. Chintagumpala, J. Su, et al. 2015. A phase 1 and pharmacokinetic study of enzastaurin in pediatric patients with refractory primary central nervous system tumors: A pediatric brain tumor consortium study. *Neuro-Oncology* 17 (2): 303–311.

Killela, P.J., Z.J. Reitman, Y. Jiao, C. Bettegowda, N. Agrawal, L.A. Diaz Jr., et al. 2013. TERT promoter mutations occur frequently in gliomas and a subset of tumors derived from cells with low rates of self-renewal. *Proceedings of the National Academy of Sciences of the United States of America* 110 (15): 6021–6026.

Kim, H.J., J.H. Kim, E.K. Chie, P.D. Young, I.A. Kim, and I.H. Kim. 2012. DNMT (DNA methyltransferase) inhibitors radiosensitize human cancer cells by suppressing DNA repair activity. *Radiation Oncology* 7: 39.

Koelsche, C., F. Sahm, D. Capper, D. Reuss, D. Sturm, D.T. Jones, et al. 2013. Distribution of TERT promoter mutations in pediatric and adult tumors of the nervous system. *Acta Neuropathologica* 126 (6): 907–915.

Korshunov, A., R. Sycheva, S. Gorelyshev, and A. Golanov. 2005. Clinical utility of fluorescence in situ hybridization (FISH) in nonbrainstem glioblastomas of childhood. *Modern Pathology* 18 (9): 1258–1263.

Korshunov, A., M. Ryzhova, V. Hovestadt, S. Bender, D. Sturm, D. Capper, et al. 2015. Integrated analysis of pediatric glioblastoma reveals a subset of biologically favorable tumors with associated molecular prognostic markers. *Acta Neuropathologica* 129 (5): 669–678.

Kramm, C.M., S. Butenhoff, U. Rausche, M. Warmuth-Metz, R.D. Kortmann, T. Pietsch, et al. 2011. Thalamic high-grade gliomas in children: A distinct clinical subset? *Neuro-Oncology* 13 (6): 680–689.

Lashford, L.S., P. Thiesse, A. Jouvet, T. Jaspan, D. Couanet, et al. 2002. Temozolomide in malignant gliomas of childhood: A United Kingdom Children's Cancer Study Group and French Society for Pediatric Oncology Intergroup study. *Journal of Clinical Oncology* 20: 4684–4691.

Lee, J.Y., C.K. Park, S.H. Park, K.C. Wang, B.K. Cho, and S.K. Kim. 2011. MGMT promoter gene methylation in pediatric glioblastoma: Analysis using MS-MLPA. *Child's Nervous System* 27 (11): 1877–1883.

Lewis, P.W., M.M. Müller, M.S. Koletsky, F. Cordero, S. Lin, L.A. Banaszynski, et al. 2013. Inhibition of PRC2 activity by a gain-of-function H3 mutation found in pediatric glioblastoma. *Science* 340: 857–861.

Loh, K.C., J. Willert, H. Meltzer, W. Roberts, B. Kerlin, R. Kadota, et al. 2005. Temozolomide and radiation for aggressive pediatric central nervous system malignancies. *Journal of Pediatric Hematology/Oncology* 27 (5): 254–258.

Lokker, N.A., C.M. Sullivan, S.J. Hollenbach, M.A. Israel, and N.A. Giese. 2002. Platelet-derived growth factor (PDGF) autocrine signaling regulates survival and mitogenic pathways in glioblastoma cells: Evidence that the novel PDGF-C and PDGF-D ligands may play a role in the development of brain tumors. *Cancer Research* 62 (13): 3729–3735.

Louis, D.N., A. Perry, G. Reifenberger, A. von Deimling, D. Figarella-Branger, W.K. Cavenee, H. Ohgaki, O.D. Wiestler, P. Kleihues, and D.W. Ellison. 2016. The 2016 World Health Organization Classification of Tumors of the central nervous system: A summary. *Acta Neuropathologica* 131: 803–820.

Lu, C., S.U. Jain, D. Hoelper, D. Bechet, R.C. Molden, L. Ran, et al. 2016. Histone H3K36 mutations promote sarcomagenesis through altered histone methylation landscape. *Science* 352 (6287): 844–849.

MacDonald, T.J., D. Aguilera, and C.M. Kramm. 2011. Treatment of high-grade glioma in children and adolescents. *Neuro-Oncology* 13 (10): 1049–1058.

MacDonald, T.J., G. Vezina, C.F. Stewart, D. Turner, C.R. Pierson, L. Chen, et al. 2013. Phase II study of cilengitide in the treatment of refractory or relapsed high-grade gliomas in children: A report from the Children's Oncology Group. *Neuro-Oncology* 15 (10): 1438–1444.

Martin, C., and Y. Zhang. 2005. The diverse functions of histone lysine methylation. *Nature Reviews. Molecular Cell Biology* 6 (11): 838–849. Review.

Meyer, M., J. Reimand, X. Lan, R. Head, X. Zhu, M. Kushida, et al. 2015. Single cell-derived clonal analysis of human glioblastoma links functional and genomic heterogeneity. *Proceedings of the National Academy of Sciences of the United States of America* 112 (3): 851–856.

Miele, E., F.R. Buttarelli, A. Arcella, F. Begalli, N. Garg, M. Silvano, et al. 2014. High-throughput microRNA profiling of pediatric high-grade gliomas. *Neuro-Oncology* 16 (2): 228–240.

Morton, C.L., J.M. Maris, S.T. Keir, R. Gorlick, E.A. Kolb, C.A. Billups, et al. 2012. Combination testing of cediranib (AZD2171) against childhood cancer models by the pediatric preclinical testing program. *Pediatric Blood & Cancer* 58 (4): 566–571.

Nakagawa, S., Y. Sakamoto, H. Okabe, H. Hayashi, D. Hashimoto, N. Yokoyama, et al. 2014. Epigenetic therapy with the histone methyltransferase EZH2 inhibitor 3-deazaneplanocin A inhibits the growth of cholangiocarcinoma cells. *Oncology Reports* 31 (2): 983–988.

Network, T.C. 2013. Corrigendum: Comprehensive genomic characterization defines human glioblastoma genes and core pathways. *Nature* 494 (7438): 506.

Nicholson, H.S., C.S. Kretschmar, M. Krailo, M. Bernstein, R. Kadota, D. Fort, et al. 2007. Phase 2 study of temozolomide in children and adolescents with recurrent central nervous system tumors. *Cancer* 110: 1542–1549.

Nonoguchi, N., T. Ohta, J.E. Oh, Y.H. Kim, P. Kleihues, and H. Ohgaki. 2013. TERT promoter mutations in primary and secondary glioblastomas. *Acta Neuropathologica* 126 (6): 931–937.

Northcott, P.A., D.T. Jones, M. Kool, G.W. Robinson, R.J. Gilbertson, Y.J. Cho, et al. 2012. Medulloblastomics: The end of the beginning. *Nature Reviews. Cancer* 12 (12): 818–834.

Northcott, P.A., S.M. Pfister, and D.T. Jones. 2015. Next-generation (epi)genetic drivers of childhood brain tumors and the outlook for targeted therapies. *The Lancet Oncology* 16 (6): e293–e302.

Noushmehr, H., D.J. Weisenberger, K. Diefes, H.S. Phillips, K. Pujara, B.P. Berman, et al. 2010. Identification of a CpG island methylator phenotype that defines a distinct subgroup of glioma. *Cancer Cell* 17 (5): 510–522.

Ozawa, T., C.W. Brennan, L. Wang, M. Squatrito, T. Sasayama, M. Nakada, et al. 2010. PDGFRA gene rearrangements are frequent genetic events in PDGFRA-amplified glioblastomas. *Genes & Development* 24 (19): 2205–2218.

Pajtler, K.W., H. Witt, M. Sill, D.T. Jones, V. Hovestadt, F. Kratochwil, et al. 2015. Molecular classification of ependymal tumors across all CNS compartments, histopathological grades, and age groups. *Cancer Cell* 27 (5): 728–743.

Parsons, D.W., S. Jones, X. Zhang, J.C. Lin, R.J. Leary, P. Angenendt, et al. 2008. An integrated genomic analysis of human glioblastoma multiforme. *Science* 321 (5897): 1807–1812.

Patel, A.P., I. Tirosh, J.J. Trombetta, A.K. Shalek, S.M. Gillespie, H. Wakimoto, et al. 2014. Single-cell RNA-seq highlights intratumoral heterogeneity in primary glioblastoma. *Science* 344 (6190): 1396–1401.

Pathak, P., P. Jha, S. Purkait, V. Sharma, V. Suri, M.C. Sharma, et al. 2015. Altered global histone-trimethylation code and H3F3A-ATRX mutation in pediatric GBM. *Journal of Neuro-Oncology* 121 (3): 489–497.

Paugh, B.S., C. Qu, C. Jones, Z. Liu, M. Adamowicz-Brice, J. Zhang, et al. 2010. Integrated molecular genetic profiling of pediatric high-grade gliomas reveals key differences with the adult disease. *Journal of Clinical Oncology* 28: 3061–3068.

Paugh, B.S., A. Broniscer, C. Qu, C.P. Miller, J. Zhang, R.G. Tatevossian, et al. 2011. Genome-wide analyses identify recurrent amplifications of receptor tyrosine kinases and cell-cycle regulatory genes in diffuse intrinsic pontine glioma. *Journal of Clinical Oncology* 29 (30): 3999–4006.

Paugh, B.S., X. Zhu, C. Qu, R. Endersby, A.K. Diaz, J. Zhang, et al. 2013. Novel oncogenic PDGFRA mutations in pediatric high-grade gliomas. *Cancer Research* 73 (20): 6219–6229.

Perkins, S.M., J.B. Rubin, J.R. Leonard, M.D. Smyth, I. El Naqa, J.M. Michalski, et al. 2011. Glioblastoma in children: A single-institution experience. *International Journal of Radiation Oncology, Biology, Physics* 80 (4): 1117–1121.

Pettorini, B.L., Y.S. Park, M. Caldarelli, L. Massimi, G. Tamburrini, and C. Di Rocco. 2008. Radiation-induced brain tumors after central nervous system irradiation in childhood: A review. *Child's Nervous System* 24 (7): 793–805.

Phillips, H.S., S. Kharbanda, R. Chen, W.F. Forrest, R.H. Soriano, T.D. Wu, et al. 2006. Molecular subclasses of high-grade glioma predict prognosis, delineate a pattern of disease progression, and resemble stages in neurogenesis. *Cancer Cell* 9 (3): 157–173.

Phillips, J.J., D. Aranda, D.W. Ellison, A.R. Judkins, S.E. Croul, D.J. Brat, et al. 2013. PDGFRA amplification is common in pediatric and adult high-grade astrocytomas and identifies a poor prognostic group in IDH1 mutant glioblastoma. *Brain Pathology* 23 (5): 565–573.

Pollack, I.F., S.D. Finkelstein, J. Burnham, E.J. Holmes, R.L. Hamilton, A.J. Yates, et al. 2001. Age and TP53 mutation frequency in childhood malignant gliomas: Results in a multi-institutional cohort. *Cancer Research* 61 (20): 7404–7407.

Pollack, I.F., R.L. Hamilton, C.D. James, S.D. Finkelstein, J. Burnham, A.J. Yates, et al. 2006. Rarity of PTEN deletions and EGFR amplification in malignant gliomas of childhood: Results from the Children's Cancer Group 945 cohort. *Journal of Neurosurgery* 105 (5 Suppl): 418–424.

Puget, S., C. Philippe, D.A. Bax, B. Job, P. Varlet, M.P. Junier, et al. 2012. Mesenchymal transition and PDGFRA amplification/mutation are key distinct oncogenic events in pediatric diffuse intrinsic pontine gliomas. *PloS One* 7 (2): e30313.

Purkait, S., P. Jha, M.C. Sharma, V. Suri, M. Sharma, S.S. Kale, et al. 2013. CDKN2A deletion in pediatric versus adult glioblastomas and predictive value of p16 immunohistochemistry. *Neuropathology* 33 (4): 405–412.

Qi, W., H. Chan, L. Teng, L. Li, S. Chuai, R. Zhang, et al. 2012. Selective inhibition of Ezh2 by a small molecule inhibitor blocks tumor cells proliferation. *Proceedings of the National Academy of Sciences of the United States of America* 109 (52): 21360–21365.

Qu, H.Q., K. Jacob, S. Fatet, B. Ge, D. Barnett, O. Delattre, et al. 2010. Genome-wide profiling using single-nucleotide polymorphism arrays identifies novel chromosomal imbalances in pediatric glioblastomas. *Neuro-Oncology* 12 (2): 153–163.

Raffel, C., L. Frederick, J.R. O'Fallon, P. Atherton-Skaff, A. Perry, R.B. Jenkins, et al. 1999. Analysis of oncogene and tumor suppressor gene alterations in pediatric malignant astrocytomas reveals reduced survival for patients with PTEN mutations. *Clinical Cancer Research* 5 (12): 4085–4090.

Razis, E., P. Selviaridis, S. Labropoulos, J.L. Norris, M.J. Zhu, et al. 2009. Phase II study of neoadjuvant imatinib in glioblastoma: Evaluation of clinical and molecular effects of the treatment. *Clinical Cancer Research* 15 (19): 6258–6266.

Rizzo, D., M. Scalzone, A. Ruggiero, P. Maurizi, G. Attinà, S. Mastrangelo, et al. 2015. Temozolomide in the treatment of newly diagnosed diffuse brainstem glioma in children: A broken promise? *Journal of Chemotherapy* 27 (2): 106–110.

Saratsis, A.M., M. Kambhampati, K. Snyder, S. Yadavilli, J.M. Devaney, B. Harmon, et al. 2014. Comparative multidimensional molecular analyses of pediatric diffuse intrinsic pontine glioma reveals distinct molecular subtypes. *Acta Neuropathologica* 127 (6): 881–895.

Schiffman, J.D., J.G. Hodgson, S.R. VandenBerg, P. Flaherty, M.Y. Polley, M. Yu, et al. 2010. Oncogenic BRAF mutation with CDKN2A inactivation is characteristic of a subset of pediatric malignant astrocytomas. *Cancer Research* 70 (2): 512–519.

Schlosser, S., S. Wagner, J. Mühlisch, M. Hasselblatt, J. Gerss, J.E. Wolff, et al. 2010. MGMT as a potential stratification marker in relapsed high-grade glioma of children: The HIT-GBM experience. *Pediatric Blood & Cancer* 54 (2): 228–237.

Schwartzentruber, J., A. Korshunov, X.Y. Liu, D.T. Jones, E. Pfaff, K. Jacob, et al. 2012. Driver mutations in histone H3.3 and chromatin remodelling genes in paediatric glioblastoma. *Nature* 482 (7384): 226–231. doi:10.1038/nature10833.

Smith, J.S., X.Y. Wang, J. Qian, S.M. Hosek, B.W. Scheithauer, R.B. Jenkins, et al. 2000. Amplification of the platelet-derived growth factor receptor-A (PDGFRA) gene occurs in oligodendrogliomas with grade IV anaplastic features. *Journal of Neuropathology and Experimental Neurology* 59 (6): 495–503.

Solomon, D.A., M.D. Wood, T. Tihan, A.W. Bollen, N. Gupta, J.J. Phillips, et al. 2015. Diffuse midline gliomas with histone H3-K27M mutation: A series of 47 cases assessing the spectrum of morphologic variation and associated genetic alterations. *Brain Pathology* 30: 569–580.

Srivastava, A., A. Jain, P. Jha, V. Suri, M.C. Sharma, S. Mallick, et al. 2010. MGMT gene promoter methylation in pediatric glioblastomas. *Child's Nervous System* 26 (11): 1613–1618.

Stupp, R., W.P. Mason, M.J. van den Bent, M. Weller, B. Fisher, M.J. Taphoorn, et al. 2005. Radiotherapy plus concomitant and adjuvant temozolomide for glioblastoma. *The New England Journal of Medicine* 352 (10): 987–996.

Sturm, D., H. Witt, V. Hovestadt, D.A. Khuong-Quang, D.T. Jones, C. Konermann, et al. 2012. Hotspot mutations in H3F3A and IDH1 define distinct epigenetic and biological subgroups of glioblastoma. *Cancer Cell* 22 (4): 425–437. doi:10.1016/j.ccr.2012.08.024.

Sturm, D., S. Bender, D.T. Jones, P. Lichter, J. Grill, O. Becher, et al. 2014a. Paediatric and adult glioblastoma: Multiform (epi)genomic culprits emerge. *Nature Reviews. Cancer* 14 (2): 92–107.

Suri, V., P. Das, P. Pathak, A. Jain, M.C. Sharma, S.A. Borkar, et al. 2009. Pediatric glioblastomas: A histopathological and molecular genetic study. *Neuro-Oncology* 11 (3): 274–280.

Takahashi, Y., T. Akahane, T. Sawada, H. Ikeda, A. Tempaku, S. Yamauchi, et al. 2015. Adult classical glioblastoma with a BRAF V600E mutation. *World Journal of Surgical Oncology* 13: 100.

Tanaka, S., D.N. Louis, W.T. Curry, T.T. Batchelor, and J. Dietrich. 2013. Diagnostic and therapeutic avenues for glioblastoma: No longer a dead end? *Nature Reviews. Clinical Oncology* 10 (1): 14–26.

Taylor, M.D., P.A. Northcott, A. Korshunov, M. Remke, Y.J. Cho, S.C. Clifford, et al. 2012. Molecular subgroups of medulloblastoma: The current consensus. *Acta Neuropathologica* 123 (4): 465–472.

Taylor, K.R., A. Mackay, Nathalène Truffaux, Yaron Butterfield, Olena Morozova, Cathy Philippe, David Castel, et al. 2014. Recurrent activating ACVR1 mutations in diffuse intrinsic pontine glioma. *Nature Genetics* 46: 457–461.

Vanan, M.I., and D.D. Eisenstat. 2014. Management of high-grade gliomas in the pediatric patient: Past, present, and future. *Neurooncology Practices* 1 (4): 145–157.

Venneti, S., M.T. Garimella, L.M. Sullivan, D. Martinez, J.T. Huse, A. Heguy, et al. 2013. Evaluation of histone 3 lysine 27 trimethylation (H3K27me3) and enhancer of Zest 2 (EZH2) in pediatric glial and glioneuronal tumors shows decreased H3K27me3 in H3F3A K27M mutant glioblastomas. *Brain Pathology* 23: 558–564.

Verhaak, R.G., K.A. Hoadley, E. Purdom, V. Wang, Y. Qi, M.D. Wilkerson, et al. 2010. Integrated genomic analysis identifies clinically relevant subtypes of glioblastoma characterized by abnormalities in PDGFRA, IDH1, EGFR, and NF1. *Cancer Cell* 17 (1): 98–110. 42.

Verschuur, A.C., J. Grill, A. Lelouch-Tubiana, D. Couanet, C. Kalifa, and G. Vassal. 2004. Temozolomide in paediatric high-grade glioma: A key for combination therapy? *British Journal of Cancer* 91: 425–429.

Vinagre, J., A. Almeida, H. Pópulo, R. Batista, J. Lyra, V. Pinto, et al. 2013. Frequency of TERT promoter mutations in human cancers. *Nature Communications* 4: 2185.

Vivanco, I., H.I. Robins, D. Rohle, C. Campos, C. Grommes, P.L. Nghiemphu, et al. 2012. Differential sensitivity of glioma- versus lung cancer-specific EGFR mutations to EGFR kinase inhibitors. *Cancer Discovery* 2 (5): 458–471.

Wiese, M., F. Schill, D. Sturm, S. Pfister, E. Hulleman, S.A. Johnsen, et al. 2016. No significant cytotoxic effect of the EZH2 inhibitor Tazemetostat (EPZ-6438) on pediatric glioma cells with Wildtype histone 3 or mutated histone 3.3. *Klinische Pädiatrie* 228 (3): 113–117.

Wolff, J.E., C.F. Classen, S. Wagner, R.D. Kortmann, S.L. Palla, T. Pietsch, et al. 2008. Subpopulations of malignant gliomas in pediatric patients: Analysis of the HIT-GBM database. *Journal of Neuro-Oncology* 87 (2): 155–164.

Wolff, B., A. Ng, D. Roth, K. Parthey, M. Warmuth-Metz, M. Eyrich, et al. 2012. Pediatric high grade glioma of the spinal cord: Results of the HITGBM database. *Journal of Neuro-Oncology* 107 (1): 139–146.

Wu, G., A. Broniscer, T.A. McEachron, C. Lu, B.S. Paugh, J. Becksfort, et al. 2012. Somatic histone H3 alterations in pediatric diffuse intrinsic pontine gliomas and non-brainstem glioblastomas. *Nature Genetics* 44 (3): 251–253.

Wu, G., A.K. Diaz, B.S. Paugh, S.L. Rankin, B. Ju, Y. Li, et al. 2014. The genomic landscape of diffuse intrinsic pontine glioma and pediatric non-brainstem high-grade glioma. *Nature Genetics* 46 (5): 444–450.

Yan, H., D.W. Parsons, G. Jin, R. McLendon, B.A. Rasheed, W. Yuan, I. Kos, I. Batinic-Haberle, S. Jones, G.J. Riggins, H. Friedman, A. Friedman, D. Reardon, J. Herndon, K.W. Kinzler, V.E. Velculescu, B. Vogelstein, and D.D. Bigner. 2009. IDH1 and IDH2 mutations in gliomas. *The New England Journal of Medicine* 360 (8): 765–773.

Zarghooni, M., U. Bartels, E. Lee, P. Buczkowicz, A. Morrison, A. Huang, et al. 2010. Whole-genome profiling of pediatric diffuse intrinsic pontine gliomas highlights platelet-derived growth factor receptor alpha and poly (ADP-ribose)polymerase as potential therapeutic targets. *Journal of Clinical Oncology* 28 (8): 1337–1344.

Index

A

Activating protein- 1 (AP-1), 123
Adjuvant chemotherapy (chemoRT), 58
5-Aminolevulinic acid (5-ALA), 9
Amphiregulin (AR), 119
Animal models
    brain tumors, 220
    glioma cell, 222
    in vivo models, 221
    PDX, 223
    pseudopalisades, 220
    signaling cascades, 220
    solid cancers, 221
    spheroids/cell suspension, 223
    tumor implantation, 224
    xenograft models, 222
Antiangiogenic agents, 63
Astrocytes, 162
ATRX mutation, 38
ATRX/DAXX mutation, 247
Autologous vaccine, 78
Avatar models, 223

B

Bacterial artificial chromosome (BAC), 170
BCNU Wafers, 61
Betacellulin, 119
Bevacizumab, 64, 65, 72
Biological therapies, 78
    genetically engineered T-cells, 80
    high grade glioma trials, 75–7
    immune checkpoint Inhibitors, 80
    immunotherapies, 78–80
    vaccine therapy (*see* Vaccine therapy)
    virus-based therapies, 73–8

Blood-Brain-Barrier (BBB), 129
Bridge amplification, 171

C

Cancer stem cells (CSCs)
    de novo isolation, 198
    epigenetic/ transcriptomic phenotypes, 193
    hematopoietic system, 193
    hierarchical model, 193, 194
    histone modifiers, 195
    in vivo, 192
    neurospheres, 197
    and tumor heterogeneity, 195, 196
Canonical EGFR signaling
    MAP/ERK pathway, 122–123 (*see also*
        Non canonical EGFR signaling)
    PI3K pathway, 123
    PKC-NF-kB pathway, 123–124
    STATs, 124
    tyrosine residues, 121
Central nervous system (CNS), 162, 167, 242
Chemoradiation Therapy, 60
Chemotherapy, 68, 163
Chimeric antigen receptor T cells (CART), 133
c-jun N-terminal kinase (JNK), 121
Cluster, 171
Comparative genomic hybridization
    (CGH), 32
Computational pathology
    biological mechanisms, 152
    molecular analysis, 151
    MVP, 151
    nuclei, 151
    oligodendroglioma component, 152
    principal component analysis/clustering, 152

© Springer International Publishing AG 2017
K. Somasundaram (ed.), *Advances in Biology and Treatment of Glioblastoma*,
Current Cancer Research, DOI 10.1007/978-3-319-56820-1

Computed tomography (CT), 145
Concurrent chemoradiation therapy, 58
Conventional therapy, 163
Cortical stimulation, 12
CpG island methylator phenotype
  (C-CIMP), 104
CRISPR/Cas9 model
  in vivo, 230
  IUE, 230
  RCAS/t-va glioma model, 231
Custom amplicon method, 173, 175
Custom enrichment, 173, 175
Cyclin-dependent kinase inhibitor 2A
  (CDKN2A), 36–7, 93
Cysteine-rich (CR) domains, 119
Cytogenetic abnormalities, 40

D
DAT. *See* Deformable anatomic templates
  (DAT)
De novo isolation, 198
Deformable anatomic templates (DAT), 7
De-multiplexing, 171
Dendritic-cell vaccines, 78
Diagnosed GBM, 63–67
  alternating electric fields, 62
  antiangiogenic strategies, 63
  BCNU Wafers, 61
  chemoradiation therapy, 60
  dose intensification of chemotherapy, 61
  phase III trials, 58
  recurrent GBM (*see* Recurrent GBM)
  surgical resection, 59
Diffuse intrinsic pontine gliomas (DIPG), 242
Diffuse midline glioma H3 K27M–mutant, 242
Diffusion spectrum imaging (DSI), 7
Diffusion tensor imaging (DTI) protocols, 5, 6
Direct cortical stimulation (DCS), 4
Direct electrical stimulation (DES), 9
Driver genetic alterations, 166
  passenger genetic alterations/hitchhikers,
    166
  SNVs/point mutations, 166, 167
  targeted sequencing, 167
Drug penetrance, 105

E
EGFR. *See* Epidermal Growth Factor Receptor
  (EGFR)
EGFR amplification and mutation, 41, 42
Epidermal growth factor receptor (EGFR), 41,
  70, 93, 121–4

activation, 118
amplifications, 118
canonical signaling (*see* Canonical EGFR
  signaling)
clinical trials, 128–31
ligand binding, factors, 119
pathway, 119
proto-onocogenes, 118
signaling, 119
STAT3, 121
strategies targeting, 133
structure and mutations, 119–21
therapeutic strategies, 128, 129, 131
therapies targeting, 133
Epithelioid glioblastoma, 31
Extracellular signal-regulated kinase
  (ERK), 122

F
Fluid-attenuated inversion recovery (FLAIR),
  59, 147
Fluoro-deoxyglucose (FDG), 147
Fotemustine, 66
Fractionated stereotactic radiotherapy
  (FSRT), 61
Functional MRI (fMRI), 3

G
GA-binding protein (GABP) transcription
  factor, 40
GEINO11 clinical trial, 130
Gene-set enrichment analysis (GSEA), 149
Genetically engineered mouse models
  (GEMM)
  astrocytic glioma model, 225
  canine, 234
  cDNA, 225
  CRISPR/Cas9 models, 230–1
  drosophila, 231–2
  embryonic stem cells, 225
  germ line models, 228
  Ntv-a/Gtv-a, 229
  RCAS/tv-a, 229
  somatic gene transfer models, 228
  sophisticated models, 225
  TME, 224, 225
  zebrafish, 232–3
Giant cell glioblastoma, 29
Glioblastoma
  adult patients, 67–9
  EGFR activation, 118
  EORTC/NCIC trial, 67

granular cell, 27
gross pathology, 22–32
histomorphology, 22–32
isocitrate dehydrogenase 1 and 2 (*IDH1/2*)
    wild-type, 118
molecules, 32–45
multiforme, 25
oligodendroglial component, 27
primitive neuronal component, 27, 28
small cell glioblastoma, 25, 27
Glioblastoma- IDH mutant, 22
Glioma
    molecular analysis, 151
    MRI, 147
    nuclei, 151
Glioma CpG island methylator phenotype
    (G-CIMP), 36, 250, 251
Glioma stem-like cells (GSC), 192–3, 200–3
    characterization, 198–199
    chemo-radio therapy, 204
    CSCs (*see* Cancer stem cells (CSCs))
    drug resistance (*see* Therapy resistance)
    immunotherapy, 204
    in vitro, 206
    intra- and inter-tumoral heterogeneity, 203
    NSCs, 204
    oxide nanoparticles, 203
    radiation, 196
    signaling pathways, 204, 205
    stem cell markers, 206
    tumor heterogeneity, 195–6
Gliomas, 19
Gliomatosis cerebri (GC), 69, 70
Gliosarcoma, 30, 31
GlioSeq, 167
Granular cell glioblastoma, 27
Granulocyte-macrophage colony-stimulating
    factor (GM-CSF), 78

H
Health-related quality of life (HRQOL), 63
Heat shock protein peptide complexes
    (HSPPCs), 79
Heat-shock protein vaccines, 79
Heavily lipidized glioblastoma, 27
Heparin- binding EGF-like growth factor
    (HB-EGF), 119
Herpes simplex type I – thymidine kinase
    construct (HSV-TK), 74
High angular resolution diffusion imaging
    (HARDI), 7
Histomics. *See* Computational pathology
Histone de-acetylase enzymes (HDACs), 178

Histone H3.3/H3.1 mutation, 246–7
Human Glioblastoma Cell Culture
    (HGCC), 223
2-Hydroxyglutarate (2-HG), 104

I
IDH. *See* Isocitrate dehydrogenase (IDH)
IDH mutant, 31–2, 118
IDH mutations, 34–6
IDH1/IDH2 mutations, 34, 35, 103–4
IDH-wild type
    epithelioid Glioblastoma, 31
    giant cell glioblastoma, 29
    gliosarcoma, 30, 31
Imaging-genomics. *See* Radiogenomics
imaging-proteomics. *See* Radioproteomics
Immune checkpoint Inhibitors, 80
Immunohistochemistry (IHC), 166
Immunotherapies, 78
In utero electroporation (IUE), 230
Inhibitor of nuclear factor kappa B kinase
    subunit alpha (IKKα), 123
Insulin growth factor receptor, 132
Inter-tumoral heterogeneity, 164, 182
Intraoperative adjuncts, tumor resection
    5-aminolevulinic acid, 9
    cortical stimulation, 12
    DES, 5
    functional cortical and subcortical
        mapping, 9–10
    intraoperative image guidance techniques,
        7–9
    language mapping, 12–13
    motor evoked potentials, 11
    resection principles, 13
    somatosensory evoked potentials, 11
    subcortical stimulation, 12
Intra-tumoral heterogeneity, 144, 165
Involved field radiation therapy (IFRT), 60
ISN Haarlem guidelines, 21
Isocitrate dehydrogenase (IDH), 20
Isocitrate dehydrogenase 1(IDH 1)
    gene, 93

L
Laser induced thermal therapy (LITT), 67
Leucine rich repeats and immunoglobulin-like
    domains-1 (LRIG1), 125
Ligand-binding (LB), 119
Ligand-independent EGFR signalling, 127–8
LITT. *See* Laser-induced thermal therapy
    (LITT)

M
Magnetic resonance imaging (MRI), 2, 59, 145
Magnetoencephalography (MEG), 4
Mammalian target of rapamycin (mTOR)
    signaling pathway, 71
Methyl Guanine DNA Methyl Transferase
    (MGMT), 37, 38
Methyltransferase (MGMT), 250
MicroRNAs (miRs), 145
Microvascular proliferation (MVP), 24, 151
Mitochondrial EGFR, 126
Mitogen-activated protein kinase (MAPK), 122
Mitogen-inducible gene 6 (MIG-6), 125
Molecular pathology, 43–45
    ATRX mutation, 38–39
    cytogenetic abnormalitics, 40–41
    EGFR amplification and mutation, 41–2
    IDH mutations, 34–7
    MGMT, 37–8
    NF1inactivation, 43
    PDGFRA, 42–3
    PTEN mutation, 42
    recurrence, 45–8
    signaling pathways (*see* Signaling
        pathways)
    TERT promoter mutation, 40
    TP53 mutation, 39–40
Motor evoked potentials (MEPs), 4, 11
Multiplexing, 171

N
National Cancer Institute (NCI), 92
National Human Genome Research Institute
    (NHGRI), 92
Neurofibromatosis type 1 (*NF1*), 118
Neurofibromatosis type 1 gene (NF1)
    inactivation, 43
Neurospheres
    enzymatic/chemical/mechanical
        disruption, 197
    in vitro, 197
    limitations, 197
Next generation sequencing (NGS), 167
    BAC, 170
    bridge amplification, 171
    computational skills, 175
    de-multiplexing, 171
    GATK, 177
    Illumina's Solexa sequencing, 175, 176
    multiplexing, 171
    NGS data analysis, 175–7
    polymerase-dependent sequencing
        approach, 171, 172

SNVs, 177
    targeted sequencing, 173, 175
    targeted sequencing panels, 177–8
    WES, 173
    WGS, 173
Nimotuzumab, 71, 131
Nitric oxide pathway (iNOS), 127
Nitrosoureas, 65, 66
Non canonical EGFR signaling
    EGFR turnover, 124–6
    ligand-independent EGFR signalling, 127–8
    mitochondrial EGFR, 126
    nuclear functions, 126–7
Nuclear EGFR, 127
Nuclear factor kappa-light-chain-enhancer of
    activated B cells (NF κB), 121
Nuclear localization sequence (NLS), 126

O
O-6-methylguanine DNA methyltransferase
    (MGMT), 60, 164
    gene promoter methylation, 37–8
Oncolytic virotherapy, 179
Overall survival (OS), 79, 128

P
p53-upregulated modulator of apoptosis
    (PUMA), 126
Passenger genetic alterations/hitchhikers, 166
Patient derived xenograft (PDX), 223
Patient reported outcomes (PRO), 63
PDGFRA. *See* Platelet derived growth factor
    receptor alpha(PDGFRA)
PDGFRA amplification, 245, 246
Pediatric GBMs (pGBMs)
    DNA methylation, 252–3
    MGMT gene promoter methylation, 250
    miRNA, 253–4
    pHGGs, 250–1
    subclassification, 251–2
Pediatric high grade gliomas (pHGGs)
    ATRX/DAXX, 247
    CNS, 242
    copy number alterations, 245–6
    epidemiology, 243–4
    H3F3A/HIST1H3B/C, 246
    HIST1H3B, 242
    histone code alterations, 254–5
    histone H3.3/H3.1, 246–7
    histopathology, 244
    molecular-genetic alterations, 244–50
    PDGFRA amplification, 245–6

prognostic and predictive biomarkers,
      255–6
recurrent genetic alterations, 247–50
therapeutic agents, 257
TP53 mutations, 246
treatments, 256, 257
Peptide vaccines, 79
Peripheral blood mononuclear cells
      (PBMC), 78
Peroxisome-proliferator-activated receptor γ
      (PPARγ), 122–123
Personalized therapy
inter-tumoral heterogeneity, 164
intra-tumoral heterogeneity, 165
MGMT, 164
patient stratification, 164
targeted therapy, 165
treatment, 163
Phosphatase and tensin homolog (*PTEN*)
      genes, 93, 118
Phosphatidylinositol 3-kinase, regulatory
      subunit 1 (*PIK3R1*), 118
Phosphatidylinositol-3-kinases (PI3Ks), 169
Phosphoinositide 3-kinase (PI3K) pathway,
      71, 121, 123
Phosphoserin phosphatase (PSPH), 121
Platelet-derived growth factor receptors
      (PDGFR), 95, 101, 102
Platelet-derived growth factor receptor A
      (PDGFRA), 42, 43, 118
Polymerase-dependent sequencing
      approach, 171
Positron emission tomography (PET), 145
Preoperative adjuncts, tumor and cortical areas
      DAT, 7
diffusion tensor imaging, 6–7
DTI, 6
fMRI, 3
magnetic resonance imaging, 2–3
magnetoencephalography, 4
navigated transcranial magnetic
      stimulation, 4–6
Principal components analysis (PCA), 149
Progression-free survival (PFS), 60, 79,
      95, 128
Protein kinase C (PKC), 123
PTEN mutation, 42

R
Radiation, 196
Radiation therapy (RT), 58, 163
Radiation Therapy Oncology Group
      (RTOG), 63

Radiogenomics
de novo mutations, 149
future, 152–3
GSEA, 149
MGMT, 149
radiological data acquisition, 150
Radioimmunotherapy, 61
Radiomics
CT, 145, 146
data acquisition, 147
data analysis, 148–9
feature extraction, 147–8
image pre-processing, 147
MR, 146
MRI, 145
PET, 145, 146
Radioproteomics, 150
RB pathway, 170
Recentin in GBM alone and with lomustine'
      (REGAL), 72
Receptor endocytosis, 126
Receptor tyrosine kinases (RTKs) pathway,
      42, 93–5, 145
EGFR, 96–101
PDGFR, 101–2
PI3K/AKT/PTEN/mTOR, 102–3
RAS/RAF/MEK/MAP (ERK)
      Kinase, 103
VEGFR, 95–6
Recurrence in glioblastoma tumors,
      45–7
Recurrent GBM
bevacizumab, 64, 65
LITT, 67
nitrosoureas, 65, 66
progression, bevacizumab
      treatment, 65
re-irradiation, 66
surgical resection, 64
Regulatory domain (RD), 119
Re-irradiation, recurrent GBM, 66
Replication-competent oncolytic viruses
      (OVs), 76–77
Replication-Deficient Viral Vectors, 75
Retinoblastoma (Rb) pathway, 95
Retinoblastoma (RB) pathways, 93
RTK/Ras/PI3K pathway, 168, 169

S
Septin 14 (SEPT14), 121
Sequencing by synthesis (SBS), 171
Signal transducer and activator of transcription
      3 (STAT3) signaling, 121

Signaling pathways
    CDKN2A/CDK4/retinoblastoma protein
        pathway, 45
    P53/MDM2/p14ARF pathway, 44
    receptor tyrosine kinase/ PI3K/ PTEN/
        AKT/mTOR pathway, 43
Single nucleotide polymorphism (SNP)
    arrays, 32
Single strand conformation polymorphism
    (SSCP), 166
Small cell glioblastoma, 25, 27
SNVs/point mutations
    carcinogens, 166
    genetic alterations, 167
    in situ hybridization techniques, 167
    SSCP, 166
    types, 166
Sodium/glucose cotransporter 1 (SGLT1), 127
Somatosensory evoked potentials, 11
Son of sevenless (SOS), 103
Src family kinases (SFK), 121
Stereotactic radiosurgery (SRS), 61
Subcortical stimulation, 12
Surgical resection, 59

T
Targeted agents
    EGFR inhibitors, 70–1
    PI3K and mTOR inhibitors, 71–2
    VEGF and VEGFR inhibitors, 72–3
Targeted sequencing, 167
    panels, 177–8
Targeted therapy, 92, 98, 100–97
    angiogenesis inhibitor, 178
    Bevacizumab, 178
    driver genetic alteration (*see* Driver genetic
        alterations)
    EGFR, 178
    epigenetic modifiers, 178
    Gleevec/Imatinib, 165
    novel therapeutic approaches, 179
    oncolytic virotherapy, 179
    types of cancer, 165
    types of cancers, 179–181
    VEGF, 165
Telomerase reverse transcriptase (TERT),
    40, 118
Temozolomide (TMZ), 58, 69, 199
TERT promoter mutation, 40
The Cancer Genome Atlas (TCGA), 32, 92,
    93, 144

Therapeutic failure, 131–133
Theraphy resistance
    anti apoptotic pathway, 200, 201
    CD133+clonal cells, 199, 200
    DNA repair, 200
    efflux of drugs, 200
    heterogeneity, 203
    hypoxia and high redox potential, 201
    metabolic circuit, 202
    quiescence, 202
    TMZ, 199
    vascular nich, 201, 202
TP53 mutation, 39, 40
TP53 pathway, 169
Transcription factors (TFs), 122
Transforming growth factor α (TGF α), 119
Tumor heterogeneity and clonal evolution, 105
Tumor protein P53 signaling pathway,
    93–94
Tumor treatment fields (TTF), 62
Tyrosine kinase (TK), 119
Tyrosine kinase inhibitors (TKIs), 128

U
Urokinase-type plasminogen activator receptor
    (uPAR), 121

V
Vaccine therapy
    cell-based vaccines, 78
    non-cell based vaccines, 79
Vascular endothelial growth factor (VEGF),
    64, 70, 95, 165, 178
VEGF and VEGFR inhibitors, 72, 73
VEGFR, 178
Virus-based therapies, 73, 74
Visually Accessible REMBRANDT Images
    (VASARI), 147

W
WHO 2007 Classification vs 2016
    classification, 21–22
WHO 2016, 21
Whole exome sequencing (WES), 173
Whole genome sequencing (WGS), 173

X
Xenograft models, 222